T0259621

Toxicology

Editors

STEVE ENSLEY
TIMOTHY J. EVANS

VETERINARY CLINICS
OF NORTH AMERICA:
FOOD ANIMAL PRACTICE

www.vetfood.theclinics.com

Consulting Editor
ROBERT A. SMITH

November 2020 • Volume 36 • Number 3

ELSEVIER

1600 John F. Kennedy Boulevard • Suite 1800 • Philadelphia, Pennsylvania, 19103-2899

http://www.vetfood.theclinics.com

VETERINARY CLINICS OF NORTH AMERICA: FOOD ANIMAL PRACTICE Volume 36, Number 3
November 2020 ISSN 0749-0720, ISBN-13: 978-0-323-75462-0

Editor: Katerina Heidhausen
Developmental Editor: Nicole Congleton

Veterinary Clinics of North America: Food Animal Practice (ISSN 0749-0720) is published in March, July, and November by Elsevier Inc., 360 Park Avenue South, New York, NY 10010-1710. Subscription prices are $259.00 per year (domestic individuals), $456.00 per year (domestic institutions), $100.00 per year (domestic students/residents), $283.00 per year (Canadian individuals), $601.00 per year (Canadian institutions), $335.00 per year (international individuals), $601.00 per year (international institutions), $100.00 per year (Canadian students), and $165.00 (international students). To receive student/resident rate, orders must be accompanied by name of affiliated institution, date of term, and the signature of program/residency coordinator on institution letterhead. *Clinics* subscription prices. All prices are subject to change without notice. **POSTMASTER:** Send address changes to *Veterinary Clinics of North America: Food Animal Practice*, Elsevier Health Sciences Division, Subscription Customer Service, 3251 Riverport Lane, Maryland Heights, MO 63043. Customer Service (orders, claims, online, change of address): Elsevier Health Sciences Division, Subscription **Customer Service, 3251 Riverport Lane, Maryland Heights, MO 63043. Tel: 1-800-654-2452 (U.S. and Canada); 314-447-8871 (ouside U.S. and Canada). Fax: 314-447-8029. E-mail: journalscustomerservice-usa@elsevier.com (for print support); journalsonlinesupport-usa@elsevier.com (for online support).**

Reprints. For copies of 100 or more, of articles in this publication, please contact the Commercial Reprints Department, Elsevier Inc., 360 Park Avenue South, New York, NY 10010-1710. Tel.: 212-633-3874; Fax: 212-633-3820; E-mail: reprints@elsevier.com.

Veterinary Clinics of North America: Food Animal Practice is covered in *Current Contents/Agriculture, Biology and Environmental Sciences, MEDLINE/PubMed (Index Medicus), and Excerpta Medica.*

Contributors

CONSULTING EDITOR

ROBERT A. SMITH, DVM, MS
Diplomate, American Board of Veterinary Practitioners; Veterinary Research and Consulting Services, LLC, Greeley, Colorado, USA; Veterinary Research and Consulting Services, LLC, Stillwater, Oklahoma

EDITORS

STEVE ENSLEY, DVM, PhD
Clinical Professor, Anatomy & Physiology, Kansas State University, Manhattan, Kansas

TIM J. EVANS, DVM, MS, PhD
Diplomate, American College of Theriogenologists; Diplomate, American Board of Veterinary Toxicology; Associate Professor, Department of Veterinary Pathobiology, Veterinary Medical Diagnostic Laboratory, University of Missouri, Columbia, Missouri

AUTHORS

MICHAEL J. CLAYTON, DVM
Veterinary Pathologist, USDA/ARS Poisonous Plant Research Laboratory, Logan, Utah

T. ZANE DAVIS, PhD
Molecular Toxicologist, USDA/ARS Poisonous Plant Research Laboratory, Logan, Utah

STEVE ENSLEY, DVM, PhD
Clinical Professor, Anatomy & Physiology, Kansas State University, Manhattan, Kansas

TIM J. EVANS, DVM, MS, PhD
Diplomate, American College of Theriogenologists; Diplomate, American Board of Veterinary Toxicology; Associate Professor, Department of Veterinary Pathobiology, Veterinary Medical Diagnostic Laboratory, University of Missouri, Columbia, Missouri

DALE R. GARDNER, PhD
Research Natural Product Chemist, USDA/ARS Poisonous Plant Research Laboratory, Logan, Utah

STEPHEN B. HOOSER, DVM, PhD
Diplomate, American Board of Veterinary Toxicology; Professor of Comparative Pathobiology, Head, Toxicology Section, Animal Disease Diagnostic Laboratory, Purdue University, College of Veterinary Medicine, West Lafayette, Indiana

BARRY J. JACOBSEN, PhD
Professor Emeritus of Plant Pathology, Montana State University, Bozeman, Montana

EDWARD L. KNOPPEL, MS
Research Technician, USDA/ARS Poisonous Plant Research Laboratory, Logan, Utah

MICHELLE S. MOSTROM, DVM, PhD
Diplomate, American Board Veterinary Toxicology; Diplomate, American Board
Toxicology; Veterinary Toxicologist, North Dakota State University, Veterinary Diagnostic
Laboratory, Fargo, North Dakota

ROBERT H. POPPENGA, DVM, PhD
Diplomate, American Board of Veterinary Toxicology; Professor of Veterinary and
Diagnostic Toxicology, California Animal Health and Food Safety Laboratory, University of
California, School of Veterinary Medicine, Davis, California

MERL F. RAISBECK, DVM, MS, PhD
Diplomate, American Board of Veterinary Toxicology; Emeritus Professor of Veterinary
Toxicology, Department of Veterinary Sciences, College of Agriculture, University of
Wyoming, Laramie, Wyoming

BRYAN L. STEGELMEIER, DVM, PhD
Diplomate, American College of Veterinary Pathologists; USDA/ARS Poisonous Plant
Research Laboratory, Logan, Utah

Contents

This article addresses the diagnostic challenges associated with suspected intoxications, the causes of which are actually multifactorial in nature, possibly involving sublethal exposures to multiple toxicants and/or other etiologies which are not toxic in nature. Gold standard toxicologic diagnostic approaches were developed for and are still applicable to obvious intoxications. However, a more integrated diagnostic approach, focusing on the initial problem list, is consistent with how veterinarians diagnose most cases of ruminant production inefficiency, morbidity, and/or mortality and helps ensure that all of the factors contributing to the development of the observed clinical signs are taken into appropriate consideration.

Determining mineral status of production animals is important when developing an optimum health program. Nutrition is the largest expense in food animal production and has the greatest impact on health and productivity of the animals. Knowing the bioavailability of minerals in the diet is difficult. Evaluating fluid or tissues from animals is the optimum method to determine bioavailability. Evaluating the diet provides some information. Serum/blood or liver from the animal needs to be analyzed to determine bioavailability of vitamin and minerals in the diet. This article reviews how to sample and the function of these minerals in cattle.

Water is the most important nutrient for rangeland livestock. However, competition with municipalities, industry, and other water users often results in grazing livestock being forced to use water supplies that are less than perfect. Surface water in western rangleands are often contaminated by mineral extraction, irrigation runoff and other human activities. Mineral contaminants in drinking water are additive with similar contaminants in feedstuffs. The goal of this and the subsequent article is to provide producers and veterinarians with the basic background to make informed decisions about whether a given water supply is "safe" for livestock.

Water is the most important nutrient for rangeland livestock. However, competition with municipalities, industry, and other water users often results in grazing livestock being forced to use water supplies that are less than perfect. Surface water in western rangelands are often contaminated by mineral extraction, irrigation runoff and other human activities. Mineral contaminants in drinking water are additive with similar contaminants in feedstuffs. The goal of this article is to provide producers and veterinarians with the basic background to make informed decisions about whether a given water supply is "safe" for livestock.

containing dehydropyrrolizidine alkaloids is used to provide examples and suggestions for investigating and sampling. It is also used to show how to recruit expert collaborators, diagnostic resources, and information sources to amass required expertise, information, and laboratory results to produce the best diagnosis.

In the western United States, poisonous plants most often affect grazing livestock, and the related livestock losses are estimated to cost the grazing livestock industry more than $200 million annually. Many of these toxic plants contain neurotoxins that damage or alter the function of neurologic cells in the central and peripheral nervous systems. The objectives of this article are to present common North American neurotoxic plants, including conditions of poisoning, clinical disease, pathologic changes, and available diagnostics, to identify poisoned animals and the potential prognosis for poisoned animals.

Many toxic plants, ingested by livestock while grazing or eating contaminated processed feed, produce myoskeletal or myocardial lesions that sometimes have irreversible consequences. Some myotoxic plants are lethal after ingestion of very small amounts whereas others require consumption for many days to several weeks to produce disease. Incorporation of field studies, clinical signs, gross and microscopic pathology, and chemical identification of plants, toxins, and metabolites in animal samples is essential for an accurate diagnosis. This review introduces toxic plants that cause myotoxicity, reviews toxins and lesions, discusses analyses for making an accurate diagnosis, and summarizes treatments and recommendations to avoid future poisonings.

Whether exposed by grazing toxic range or pasture plants or by eating contaminated feed, there are plant toxins that produce urinary tract disease, gastroenteritis, and other miscellaneous or multisystemic diseases. Diagnosis can be challenging and requires incorporation of field studies, clinical signs, gross and microscopic pathology, and chemical identification of plants, toxins, and metabolites in animal samples. The objectives of this review are to introduce poisonous plants that commonly poison livestock in North America; describe clinical and pathologic lesions they produce in livestock; and present current technology available to identify poisoning, treat affected animals, and minimize or avoid poisoning additional animals.

The liver is one of the most commonly affected organs by ingested toxicants. This article familiarizes veterinarians with clinical signs, serum biochemistry changes, necropsy findings, and field information found in livestock poisonings with hepatotoxic plants. The focus is on the most common plant-derived hepatotoxins important to livestock in North America. Pyrrolizidine alkaloids are covered in greater detail than the other toxins, because they are likely the most important plant-derived toxins worldwide in livestock, wildlife, and even human exposure. Additionally, many of the principles discussed regarding clinical diagnosis of pyrrolizidine alkaloid intoxication can be applied to the other poisonous plants listed.

Whether poisoned by grazing certain toxic plants, by eating contaminated feed, or by topical contact with plant toxins, certain plants poison livestock causing photosensitivity and dermatitis. These dermal lesions are rarely fatal, and with appropriate therapy and protection from additional exposure most lesions heal with few permanent sequelae. However, these lesions often result in costly production losses and missed opportunities. The objectives of this review are to briefly introduce toxic plants that result in photosensitivity and dermatitis, review the toxins and pathogenesis of plant-induced skin disease, and summarize treatments and recommendations to avoid poisoning.

Whether poisoned by grazing toxic plants or by eating feeds that are contaminated by toxic plants, affected livestock often have compromised reproductive function including infertility, abortion, and fetal deformities. Certainly all diagnostic tools—field studies, clinical signs, gross and microscopic pathology as well as chemical identification of plant and plant toxins in animal samples—are essential to make an accurate diagnosis, to develop intervening management strategies and to improve the reproductive performance. The objectives of this review are to briefly introduce toxic plants that are reproductive toxins, abortifacients, or teratogens.

This review focuses on factors associated with mold production in feedstuffs and major mycotoxins affecting ruminants in North America. Ruminants are often considered less sensitive to mycotoxins owing to rumen microflora metabolism to less toxic compounds. However, ruminants occupy wide agricultural niches that expose animals to diverse toxins under widely different environmental and nutritional conditions. Often the moldy and potentially highly contaminated feeds end up at feedlots. Less than optimal feedstuffs creating suboptimal rumen microbial flora could result in decreased ruminal capacity to detoxify certain mycotoxins and adverse effects. Numerous mycotoxins and clinical effects in ruminants are discussed.

Merl F. Raisbeck

Selenium (Se) is a metalloid that exists as a red amorphous powder, reddish crystal, silver-gray crystal, or brown-black solid. Its potency as a nutrient and a toxicant is such that few people have seen the pure element. It is easy to lose sight of the narrow margin between too little and too much. The most common cause of selenosis is accidental or intentional overuse of supplements. Many target organs and effects of Se toxicity are similar to those of Se deficiency, so laboratory confirmation is necessary. Prevention consists of minimizing exposure to seleniferous feedstuffs and optimizing dietary factors that might aggravate selenosis.

Toxicology

VETERINARY CLINICS OF NORTH AMERICA: FOOD ANIMAL PRACTICE

SERIES OF RELATED INTEREST

Veterinary Clinics of North America: Equine Practice

THE CLINICS ARE NOW AVAILABLE ONLINE!
Access your subscription at:
www.theclinics.com

Preface

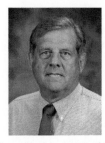 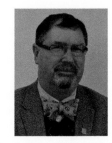

Steve Ensley, DVM, PhD   Tim J. Evans, DVM, MS, PhD
Editors

Food animal veterinary toxicology is an interesting part of veterinary medicine. I appreciate the time that Dr Gene Lloyd, Dr Gary Osweiler, and Dr Tom Carson spent mentoring me when I started my toxicology career.

Toxicology is an evolving science. With new analytical methods and increased sensitivities, new discoveries are possible. Food animal toxicology has changed its focus in the last 20 years because of agricultural production practices. Food animal agriculture in the United States has become an industry utilizing the latest science, becoming very capital intensive and charged with feeding the world. These changes have brought change and focus to veterinary food animal toxicology.

The topics in this updated *Veterinary Clinics: Food Animal Practice* include current topics in agriculture, such as drinking water for production animals, poisonous plants, mycotoxins, fescue/ergot toxicosis, biofuels used as co-products, and commercial and industrial hazards for ruminants.

Vet Clin Food Anim 36 (2020) xi–xii
https://doi.org/10.1016/j.cvfa.2020.09.001
0749-0720/20/© 2020 Published by Elsevier Inc.

vetfood.theclinics.com

As an aid to students and practitioners, there is a section on how to conduct a thorough diagnostic investigation into a potential toxicosis. There is a difference between suddenly finding an animal dead and finding an animal suddenly dying.

Steve Ensley, DVM, PhD
Department of Anatomy & Physiology
Kansas State University
1800 Denison Avenue, Mosier P217
Manhattan, KS 66506, USA

Tim J. Evans, DVM, MS, PhD
Department of Veterinary Pathobiology
Veterinary Medical Diagnostic Laboratory
University of Missouri
810 East Campus Loop
Columbia, MO 65211, USA

E-mail addresses:
sensley01@ksu.edu (S. Ensley)
evanst@missouri.edu (T.J. Evans)

Diagnostic Challenges and Guidelines Pertaining to Suspected Ruminant Intoxications

Tim J. Evans, DVM, MS, PhD

KEYWORDS

- Diagnostic challenges • Postmortem examination • Ruminant intoxications
- Toxicology

KEY POINTS

- The etiologies of an increasing number of cases of ruminant production inefficiency, morbidity, and/or mortality are actually multifactorial in nature.
- An integrated diagnostic approach, focusing on the initial problem list, is consistent with how veterinarians diagnose the causes of most ruminant health problems, other than those assumed to be intoxications, and helps ensure that all of the factors contributing to the development of clinical signs are taken into appropriate consideration.
- The basic steps in diagnosing suspected intoxications and/or cases of ruminant production inefficiency, morbidity, and/or mortality of initially unknown etiologies should include collection of historical information and a thorough physical examination, development of a problem list with a DAMNIT analysis, and an explanation of what about a given case suggests it represents an intoxication.
- Suspected intoxications or toxic exposures contributing to production inefficiency, morbidity, and/or mortality should be confirmed with plausible evidence of exposure to a specific toxicant and clinical signs which are consistent with the characteristic toxidrome of tat toxicant.

This article addresses some of the emerging toxicologic diagnostic challenges involving the increasing number of toxicology cases that actually are multifactorial in nature, often involving sublethal exposures to multiple toxicants and/or other etiologies that are not toxic in nature. The traditional, gold standard diagnostic approaches were developed under the assumption that the cases being investigated were undoubtedly intoxications, and they are still very applicable to those types of cases. A more integrated diagnostic approach, however, focusing on the initial problem list, is more consistent with how veterinarians generally diagnose most cases, other than those assumed to be intoxications. Likewise, livestock ownership attitudes

Department of Veterinary Pathobiology, Veterinary Medical Diagnostic Laboratory, University of Missouri, 901 East Campus Loop, Columbia, MO 65211, USA
E-mail address: evanst@missouri.edu

Vet Clin Food Anim 36 (2020) 509–524
https://doi.org/10.1016/j.cvfa.2020.08.007   vetfood.theclinics.com
0749-0720/20/© 2020 Elsevier Inc. All rights reserved.

need to continue to evolve into a more production-centered mindset, allowing for more efficient use of veterinary services. Finally, there needs to be continued concerns about how ongoing threats to the financial well-being of animal agriculture in the United States ultimately will have an impact on the ability of producers to maintain the health and performance of their livestock.

The intent of this article is 3-fold. Reviewing the aforementioned diagnostic challenges helps illustrate how the concept of multifactorial causality, as applied to sudden death (**Fig. 1**) and an example of suboptimal livestock performance (**Fig. 2**), has in an impact on how to look at the determinants of livestock health and production.[1] In addition, this article updates **Boxes 1–3** from the 2011 issue of *Ruminant Toxicology* (Veterinary Clinics of North America), which summarize traditional toxicology-focused diagnostics, and, while recognizing their utility for the types of cases for which they were formulated, integrates them with a problems list–based diagnostic approach, which hopefully ensures that the bare essentials of sample collection and analyses are performed for more cases.[2] The final intent of this article is to provides readily accessible, bulleted lists of (1) the basic steps in diagnosing suspected intoxications and cases of ruminant production inefficiency, morbidity, and/or mortality of initially unknown etiologies, including collection of historical information and physical examination, development of a problem list with DAMNIT analysis; (2) the basic characteristics of circumstances most likely to involve intoxications; (3) the attributes of an appropriate differential diagnosis for a given toxicant-induced clinical sign, with examples listed for sudden death without any premonitory signs in cattle as well as blindness in cattle; (4) a summary of critical historical information to collect and essential body systems to evaluate; and (5) confirmation of evidence of exposure to a toxicant (EET) and consistent clinical signs (CCSs) of that exposure as well as a list of standard diagnostic testing procedures that complement the diagnostic necropsy samples outlined in **Box 3**.[2]

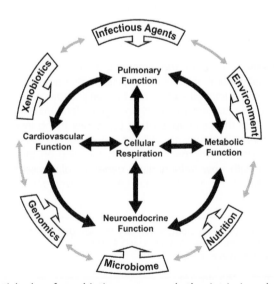

Fig. 1. The potential roles of xenobiotic exposure and other intrinsic and extrinsic factors in the etiology of sudden death in livestock.

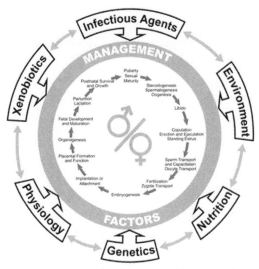

Fig. 2. Using reproduction as an example of a targeted function, the possible roles of multiple intrinsic and extrinsic factors, as well as interactions between these factors, in the pathogenesis of reproductive problems, is shown.

DIAGNOSTIC CHALLENGES
Emerging Diagnostic Challenges Associated with Multifactorial Ruminant Health Problems

As noted in the preface to this issue, the past 50 years generally have seen a decrease in poisoning cases related to exposure to solely 1 toxicant and without any other contributing factors, including those that are not toxic in nature.[2] **Fig. 1** shows some of the factors, including exposures to potentially toxic xenobiotics, which can potentially have an impact on occurrence of sudden death in ruminants. **Fig. 1** adds some more contemporary concepts, such as genomics and the microbiome, to the factors possibly affecting the major physiologic determinants of whether the body has sufficient oxygen to facilitate cellular respiration and the production of enough adenosine triphosphate (ATP) to survive. **Fig. 2** illustrates how impaired reproductive function in ruminant species, which is used as an example of a ruminant performance parameter, also be can impacted by many of these same factors. As shown in **Fig. 2**, a combination of management factors and livestock producer decisions forms a critical interface with external stressors, including xenobiotics infectious agents, environmental extremes, and nutritional quality, and also animal-based factors, such as physiology and genetics.[1] Whether talking about sudden death or suboptimal performance, the sum of all of the interactions occurring at a single point in time or over a more extended period of time ultimately determines ruminant health outcomes. Significant variations in these interactions, between individual animals within a population, help explain why different individual animals appear to respond to the same set of conditions. As viewed from this perspective, sudden death often represents a perfect storm, where it often is difficult to blame just 1 toxicant, disease, or stressor for the observed mortality. Anecdotally, the author has been involved in working-up many cases of livestock mortality, where 1 factor alone, such as mild to moderate pneumonia, was evident but did not fully explain the magnitude of the observed livestock mortality. It was discovered only later that poor nutrition and what normally would

---

Box 1
Checklist for pertinent information to be collected in a suspected ruminant poisoning or ruminant production inefficiency/illness/death of unknown etiology

Owner data

Owner/financially responsible individual:

Manager/caretaker:

Address:

Cell phone numbers:

E-mail addresses:

Home phone number:

Work phone number:

Fax number:

Web site:

Herd/flock health history

Illness past 6 months:

Exposure to other animals past 30 days (recent animal introduction):

Vaccination history past 12 months:

Herd/flock exposures to sprays, pour-on preparations, medicated ear tags, implants, dewormers past 6 months:

History of anaplasmosis/access to medications for anaplasmosis prevention:

History of abortions, stillbirths, subfertility past 12 months:

Unexplained deaths past 12 months:

Last examination by a veterinarian:

Environmental data

Location (pasture, woods, dry lot, near river or pond, confined indoors):

Buildings (ventilation; old or new construction; recent painting or renovation):

Weather conditions (tornados, hurricanes, precipitation; flooding, lightning, drought; extreme cold or heat):

Access to "routine" sources of potential toxicants (access to trash, burn piles, old construction materials, dipping tanks or vats, storage sheds, nonfunctional machinery or automobiles, automotive parts, recently burnt materials):

Unique exposure scenarios to potential toxicants (proximity to mining lands, seepage or tailings; access to oil drilling or petroleum storage; locations near Superfund sites, nuclear power plants, previous radioactive testing sites; nearby military installations):

Patient data

Species:

Breed:

Age:

Sex:

Reproductive status:

Recent health issues:

Body condition score:

Weight (loss, gain, stable):

Current clinical history

For herds/flocks, current size of group:

Other groups of same species on same premises:

Common feed or water amongst groups:

Morbidity:_____; mortality_____

Date first observed sick or dead

If found dead, last seen alive and healthy:

Onset and progression of signs (sudden death; acute onset moving to less severe; gradual onset becoming more severe):

Duration of problem in the herd:

Recent malicious threats:

Proximity to neighbors:

Changes in exposure

Escape of livestock from confinement:

Plant clippings discarded in livestock pastures:

Recent changes in location or environment (movement to new grazing areas or buildings on premises; transport to exhibitions or sales):

Recent changes in sources of water, feed, forage, or inclusion of feed additives:

Access to materials used for construction/renovation:

Specific recent use of parenteral medications (antibiotics; vitamin and/or mineral supplements; miscellaneous drugs) and specific types or names if available (ask for labels to identify):

Specific recent use of pesticides (insecticides, rodenticides, herbicides) and specific types or names if available (ask for tags or bags to identify):

Weed invasion into forage or grain crops; weed seeds in grain or feed:

Fungal contamination of grasses, grains, hays, or silage:

Outside services (eg, lawn care, pasture seeding, tree planting, fertilization, building renovation, fly control):

Diet and water sources

Type of diet:

Water source (flowing stream, pond, well, county, or city water):

Recent changes in total diet or a specific feed:

Changes in specific ingredient(s):

Feed type (whole grains; sweet feed; pelleted complete feed; total mixed ration):

Type of hay (eg, grass, alfalfa, mixed; weed contaminants):

Recent fertilization or pesticide application:

Pasture type (scant, abundant, weed contamination; trees or brush present):

Method of feeding (hand-feeding; full-feed, automated, or manual):

Presence of moldy or spoiled feed or hay:

Modified from Osweiler GD. Diagnostic guidelines for ruminant toxicosis. Vet Clin North Am Food Anim Pract. 2011;27(2):247-254; with permission.

Box 2
Checklist of clinical signs pertinent to suspected ruminant poisoning or ruminant production inefficiency/illness/death of unknown etiology

Sudden death without any premonitory clinical signs

Most often associated with acute abnormalities in neurologic/endocrine function, metabolic function, cardiovascular function, and pulmonary function (see **Fig. 1**), all of which can lead to systemic hypoxia and/or depletion of ATP

The absence of premonitory clinical signs is a function of the nature of causality and the level of animal supervision.

Neurologic signs

Blindness/visual impairment/frequent collision with structures and/or barriers

Seizures/convulsions

Ataxia

Salivation

Depression/recumbency

Weakness

Excitement

Head pressing

Cerebellar signs

Dysphonia

Dysphagia

Choke

Shifting leg lameness

Other (describe)

Cardiovascular/circulatory/hematologic signs

Exercise intolerance

Weakness

Edema

Anemia/pale mucous membranes

Hemorrhage

Hematuria

Hemolysis

Icterus

Hemoglobinuria

Methemoglobinemia

Arrhythmia

Bradycardia

Tachycardia

Leukopenia or leukocytosis

Dry gangrene

Hyperthermia or fever

Other (describe)

Respiratory signs

Exercise intolerance

Dyspnea

Persistent tachypnea

Nasal discharge/cough

Fever/hyperthermia

Other (describe)

Gastrointestinal signs (including problems involving the oropharynx)

Ruminal tympany or bloat

Rumen acidosis or rumen alkalosis

Salivation

Anorexia

Regurgitation

Constipation

Diarrhea

Melena

Polyphagia

Polydipsia

Dysphagia

Choke

Other (describe)

Hepatic/metabolic signs

Anorexia

Icterus

Weight loss

Photosensitization

Hypoglycemia

Hypoproteinemia

Other (describe)

Renal/urinary signs

Azotemia

Anuria

Polyuria

Hematuria

Hemoglobinuria

Dysuria

Other (describe)

Reproductive signs

Decreased pregnancy rates (decreased calving, lambing, kidding rates)

Anestrus or irregular estrous cycles

Hyperestrogenism

Abortion or stillbirth

Agalactia or dysgalactia

Teratogenesis

Prolonged gestation

Testicular and/or spermatozoal abnormalities

Other (describe)

Dermal signs

Achromotrichia

Alopecia

Photosensitization

Other (describe)

Modified from Osweiler GD. Diagnostic guidelines for ruminant toxicosis. Vet Clin North Am Food Anim Pract. 2011;27(2):247-254; with permission.

Box 3
Clinical and necropsy specimens for ruminant toxicology diagnosis

Blood: 5 mL to 10 mL in ethylenediaminetetraacetic acid anticoagulant. Chill and submit on ice.

Serum: centrifuge, remove from clot, store, and submit chilled or frozen.

Brain (half frozen, half formalin): leave midline in formalin for pathologist.

Cerebrospinal fluid (2–4 mL, chilled): submit in sterile container.

Ocular fluid or entire eye (frozen): useful for electrolytes, ammonia, nitrates, and nitrites

Injection site (100 g, frozen): for identifying drug injection residues

Rumen, abomasal, and intestinal contents (1 kg, frozen): samples of rumen should be taken from several locations; samples may be pooled from the same organ (eg, rumen) but not from different parts of gastrointestinal tract.

Colon contents (1 kg, frozen)

Liver (200 g, frozen): biopsy from live animals is useful for evaluating metals, especially copper, and selected organic compounds

Kidney (200 g, frozen)

Urine, if present (100 mL, half chilled, half frozen)

Data from Osweiler GD, Carson TL, Buck WB, et al. Diagnostic toxicology. In: Osweiler GD, Carson TL, Buck WB, et al., eds. Diagnostic and clinical veterinary toxicology, Dubuque, IA: Kendall Hunt; 1985: 44–51 and Galey FD. Diagnostic toxicology for the food animal practitioner. Vet Clin North Am Food Anim Pract 2000;16(3):409–21.

constitute sublethal exposures to potential toxicants likely pushed multiple animals over the edge. These examples, along with **Figs. 1** and **2**, show how discerning the role of a given xenobiotic exposure in the etiology of observed livestock production losses, including death, can be extremely challenging.[1]

Integrating the Gold Standard with a Problems-Based Approach

The first article in the 2011 *Ruminant Toxicology* issue reviewed the gold standards for diagnosing intoxications involving ruminants, with those standards summarized in **Boxes 1–3** in that article.[2] That information has been updated for this article in the current *Ruminant Toxicology* issue, with **Boxes 1–3** maintaining the same names and still representing an extremely detailed, standardized roadmap for diagnosing ruminant intoxications. This traditional, rigorous diagnostic approach is especially valuable when intoxications are most likely to be the sole cause of the observed clinical problems and when large populations of ruminants are involved. These types of crises inevitably initiate potential legal entanglements, possibly involving regulatory agencies, such as the Food and Drug Administration and the Environmental Protection Agency, and/or insurance companies, often taking years to resolve. Carefully detailed histories, clinical signs, and analytical results remain essential to diagnosing those types of intoxications. The occurrence of toxic catastrophes, however, involving exposures to a single toxicant, generally are becoming less common, and the types of toxic cases addressed today often are different from those observed 20 years ago.[2] Time and financial constraints, often in combination with owner attitudes and management factors, often limit the collection of essential samples and the performance of critical analyses. This article addresses the integration of key aspects of the gold standard, toxicant-focused, diagnostic approach with a problem list–based approach intended to help identify any potential causes of livestock production losses, including those possibly involving exposures to xenobiotics.

Developing a Production Mindset

Veterinarians providing services to livestock producers ultimately want to help their clients be financially successful. The general inclination of some livestock owners to use veterinary services primarily on an emergency basis, however, runs counter to this goal and the increasing need for producers to have a production mindset. A production mindset, where veterinarians and extension personnel are utilized to help make strategic, cost-effective management decisions, can address a variety of extrinsic and intrinsic factors having a negative impact on a given production system. The idea of livestock producers pursuing the standard diagnostic approach for suspected intoxications, only when they are trying to establish third-party financial responsibility for observed production losses, is not making full use of the wide range of services veterinarians can provide to their clients. Chalking up decreased livestock performance, morbidity, and mortality to simply bad luck or unproved presumptions of cause, usually involving a lightning strike, carbohydrate overload, or bad feed, ignores the likelihood that the root causality of an increasing number of negative health outcomes most likely is multifactorial in nature.[1]

An Unfortunate Reality Check

If the unprecedented events of 2020 have taught anything, other than that cows represent a social distance generally greater than 6 ft and 2 calves usually represent a similar distance, they have taught the potential financial impacts of extreme weather, international trade issues, and an ongoing human pandemic on animal agriculture. The challenges currently facing livestock production medicine require that veterinarians help lessen the financial losses and potentially facilitate a greater margin of profit for their livestock producer clientele, under difficult financial circumstances, while continuing to practice the quality of medicine that motivated them to become veterinarians in the first place. Suspected intoxications and decreased livestock production efficiency, illness, and death of unknown etiology can be particularly time-consuming and expensive.

DIAGNOSTIC GUIDELINES

As discussed previously, several articles have thoroughly reviewed traditional diagnostic approaches focused on intoxications, and there still are situations where all of this information can be essential for the optimal outcome.[2–4] The information that follows and the updated information in **Boxes 1–3** are intended to integrate toxicology with the other diagnostic ologies. It is hoped that, by facilitating the evaluation of multiple factors contributing to the clinical of the clinical signs being observed, appropriate management decisions can be made and suboptimal management practices can be altered, thereby addressing the root causes of decreased livestock performance and preventing illness and death in the future.[1]

How to Work-up a Suspected Intoxication or Ruminant Health Problems of Unknown Etiology

For the first few years the author worked as a clinical veterinary toxicologist, the most common emergency phone calls the author received pertained to the perceived unique nature of working-up a suspected intoxication and the special requirements of a toxicology necropsy. The first step in integrating the standard diagnostic approach for suspected intoxications with the diagnosis of other causes of morbidity and mortality requires some demystification of the diagnostic process when toxicant exposures are possible or the etiologies remain unknown. The process of working-up a suspected intoxication essentially is no different from working-up any other type of case. Because of the relative costs of working-up an intoxication, it often is just as important to rule out an intoxication as to confirm it.

Basic steps in the diagnostic work-up
- Collection of complete history and performance of a thorough physical examination
- Development of a problem list
- DAMNIT analysis
- Circumstances and clinical signs that are characteristic of an intoxication
- Formulation of a list of differential diagnoses
- Confirmation of EET and CCSs

Collection of Complete History and Performance of a Thorough Physical Examination

The initial steps in the diagnostic process require a complete history and a thorough physical examination. **Box 1** is a summary of the type of historical information that should be collected. Although this information is tailored for diagnosis of a suspected intoxication, it also applies to other causes of limited performance, illness, and death.[2] Although somewhat subjective, the author has asterisked the information, which in his experiences have yielded some of the most productive information, while not creating too many red herrings. **Box 2** summarizes a list of clinical signs that often are observed in cases of suspected intoxications; however, clinical signs that could be consistent with bovine respiratory disease complex also are included.[2] The clinical signs that the author has found to be most useful in developing a productive problem list or one that is likely to result in an accurate diagnosis have been asterisked. Although again this selection process is subjective, the clinical signs are ones that often are most obvious and more objective in nature. For this issue, sudden death without premonitory clinical signs has been added to **Box 2**. In many instances, death might be the only clinical sign observed. **Fig. 1** shows the potential for a variety of factors to have a negative impact on neuroendocrine function, cardiovascular function, pulmonary function, and metabolic function, ultimately resulting in systemic hypoxia and/or depletion of ATP, both of which can be responsible for sudden and rapid death. Whether premonitory clinical signs are observed or not observed in large part is a function of the causality of the observed mortality and the level to which the animals are monitored by owners and/or managers.

Development of a Problem List

The development of a problem list from certain aspects of the history (see **Box 1**) and the observed clinical signs (see **Box 2**) is the key element in a problem list–based approach to determining which types of disease processes might be involved as well as what further diagnostic and therapeutic steps might be indicated.

DAMNIT Analysis

There are a variety of permutations of this acronym, but the author has borrowed this acronym and has assigned the terms, *degenerative* and *developmental*; *anomaly*; *metabolic* and *mechanical*; *nutritional* and *neoplastic*; *infectious, inflammatory, immune-mediated*, and *idiopathic*; and *toxic and traumatic*, to describe the possible origins of the noted clinical problems represented by these six letters. The author often is left to NIT picking for the types of sudden death cases brought to his attention, most of which can be narrowed down to *nutritional, infectious, toxic*, and *traumatic* causes.

Circumstances characteristic of an intoxication
- Sudden death/similar clinical problems/signs in MULTIPLE animals
- Evidence of possible/confirmed exposure to common toxicants
- Evidence of confirmed exposure to toxic dosage of a known toxicant
- The exposure dosage does not have to be ≥median lethal dosage.
- Clinical problems/signs consistent with those of a common intoxication
- Remember that common intoxications happen commonly.
- Recent change in diet or environment
- Neighborhood feuds/love gone BAD
- Signs of unknown etiology/other causes ruled out
- Miscellaneous (just about anything)

Note: if toxic etiology appears unlikely, collect samples/change direction for now.

Formulation of list of differential diagnoses
An appropriate differential diagnosis for a given toxicant-induced clinical sign:
- Can be toxic or nontoxic in nature
- Has at least 1 target organ in common in the same species AND/OR
- Has at least 1 mechanism of action in common in the same species AND/OR
- Has at least 1 clinical problem/sign in common in the same species AND/OR
- Derived by DAMNIT for shared clinical problem(s)/sign(s) in the same species AND/OR
- Common things happen commonly in susceptible species

Common differential diagnoses for sudden death without premonitory signs in cattle

- Grain overload
- Lightning (requires a storm)
- Gunshot (yes, this really occurs)
- Neurotoxic/cardiotoxic plants
- Cyanide intoxication
- Nitrate/nitrite intoxication
- NPN/urea/ammonia toxicosis
- Inorganic arsenic from burnt CCA-treated lumber
- Lead from automotive batteries or lead-containing paint (only if blindness observed)
- Organophosphate/carbamate insecticides
- Organochlorine insecticides (potential residue issues/might need to contact state veterinarian)

Note: although some intoxications might NOT be associated with sudden death in a given species, such as copper toxicosis in sheep and acute bovine pulmonary edema and emphysema in cattle, the typical earlier signs of these common toxicoses might not always be observed when animal supervision is limited.

Common differential diagnoses for blindness in cattle

- Polioencephalomalacia from lead intoxication, sodium ion intoxication/water deprivation syndrome, thiaminase-containing plants, and excessive dietary sulfur
- Hypovitaminosis A
- Listeriosis

Confirmation of Evidence of Exposure to a Toxicant and Consistent Clinical Signs

Some might argue that the author has taken a circuitous route to get to this point in the discussion, and they might not necessarily be wrong, if the circumstances provide an airtight case for a specific intoxication. There are too many examples of cases, however, where first impressions were not borne out by analytical results and where the light of day, decent weather, a good night's sleep, and firsthand conversations with an individual and/or individuals who are most familiar with the real facts of the case might have resulted in very different impression.

History

There is no doubt that knowledge of the actual circumstances and the realistic possibility of exposure to known toxicants are essential steps in diagnosing a suspected intoxication.[2-4] The temptation must be resisted, however, to base a diagnosis solely on a history of exposure. The post hoc fallacy, as discussed in the first article of the 2011 issue on *Ruminant Toxicology* and translated from the original Latin, says, "After the fact, therefore because of the fact."[2] Often an issue or an event temporally associated with illness or loss of animals is assumed to be causal when, in fact, this is not the case. For example, a recent delivery of feed followed by sickness or death in a herd often leads to the erroneous presumption that the feed has to be the source of the problem, even though recent animal relocation, changes in feed or water sources, acute infectious disease arising from recently introduced animals, or other information was gathered from a thorough history, such as is outlined in **Box 1**.[2-4] An another important factor to take into consideration is not only whether there has been exposure to a potential toxicant but also what was the estimated dose or dosage of the exposure.

Critical historical information to collect[2]
- Owner data
- Herd/flock health history
- Environmental data
- Patient data
- Current clinical history
- Changes in exposure
- Diet and water sources

Clinical Signs

Like the history, the observed clinical signs are extremely important to the veterinary clinician and toxicologist.[2,4] Many intoxications are associated with a characteristic toxidrome. It also is important to note the nature of the observed clinical signs and their sequence of occurrence. **Box 2** carefully outlines the types of clinical signs, which should be noted. It is especially important to note whether sudden death without any premonitory clinical signs has been observed any of the affected animals.[2]

Essential body systems to evaluate
- Sudden death without any premonitory clinical signs[2]
- Neurologic
- Cardiovascular/circulatory/hematologic
- Respiratory
- Gastrointestinal
- Hepatic/metabolic
- Renal/urinary
- Reproductive
- Dermal

Evidence of exposure to toxicant(s)
- Potential exposure of susceptible species to a given toxicant(s) as evidenced by
    Recent history of unintended/intended exposure to product containing a given toxicant
    Use of product containing a given toxicant in a species for which the product is not intended
    Junk piles/burn piles near animals
    Identification of potentially toxic plants/fungi to which animals have exposure
- Confirmed exposure to a given toxicant as evidenced by
    Presence of toxicant, including toxic plant/fungi parts in rumen contents from affected animal
    A given toxicant observed on an affected animal, especially in or around its mouth
    Witnessed or intentional toxicant exposure
    Observation of toxic plants eaten/mutilated by affected animals
    Identification of toxic plant contamination of hays + being ingested by affected animals
    Detection of toxicants in appropriate matrices using a variety of analytical techniques
- Confirmed exposure to enough of a given toxicant to cause clinical signs as evidenced by

Determination that label instructions were not followed

Calculated exposure dosage of toxicant exceeds toxic/lethal dosage for species

Chemical analyses confirming toxic concentrations of toxicant in appropriate samples

Detection of toxic concentrations of specific mycotoxins/specific feed additives in feeds

- Miscellaneous circumstances

  Other observations providing evidence of exposure to toxicant

Consistent clinical signs

- Characteristic toxidrome

  Clinical signs/clinical problems that are typical of excessive EETs

  Additional diagnostic testing procedures with typical test results for that toxicant

- Characteristic clinical pathologic changes for toxicant

  Specific clinical pathologic changes typical of excessive exposure to given toxicant(s)

- Characteristic gross/microscopic pathologic changes for toxicant

  List specific gross/microscopic changes typical of excessive exposure to given toxicant(s).

Standard diagnostic testing procedures

- Clinical pathology (complete blood cell count, serum biochemistry panel, and urinalysis)

  Anemia, hemolytic changes, basophilic stippling, methemoglobinemia

  Leukocytosis or leukopenia

  Increased liver enzyme activities, bilirubin

  Hypoglycemia or hyperglycemia

  Hypoproteinemia or

  Increased blood urea nitrogen, creatinine

  Increased muscle enzyme activities

  Serum electrolytes

  Hematuria

  Hemoglobinuria

  Specific gravity

  Crystalluria

- Anatomic pathology

  Histopathologic evaluation of biopsies or samples collected during necropsy examination

  Examine half of brain, heart, lungs, liver, kidneys, gastrointestinal/reproductive/urinary tracts

  Looking for changes consistent with characteristic toxidrome

  Necropsy samples should be collected as soon as possible after death

  Should be fixed in 10% neutral buffered formalin (NBF)

- Toxicology

  If neurologic signs, half of brain, PLUS ALWAYS rumen contents, ocular fluid, liver, kidney

  Testing rumen content pH can be a quick way to determine rumen acidosis or alkalosis.

  Ocular fluid routinely is tested for nitrate/nitrite, ammonia, sodium, calcium, and magnesium.

Half of brain can be tested for sodium or acetylcholinesterase activity.

Whole blood for lead and acetylcholinesterase activity

Serum from blood collected in royal blue–top vacutainer tube for metals

Cerebrospinal fluid, adipose tissue, and urine also can be submitted as deemed necessary.

Feed samples, source materials, and baits

Water samples, especially for cyanobacterial toxins

- Tissues and gastrointestinal contents should be fresh/refrigerated/frozen.
- Do not send samples for toxicology testing if fixed in 10% NBF.
- Ocular fluid and serum can be refrigerated or frozen, but do not freeze whole blood.
- Recommended chromatographic analyses: rumen contents (most important in acute deaths), liver, and kidneys tested using gas chromatography (GC)–mass spectrometry (MS) AND liquid chromatography (LC)-tandem MS (MS/MS) methods for detecting nonpolar (GC-MS) and more polar organic compounds (LC-MS/MS), including many environmental contaminants, pesticides, veterinary drugs, plant toxins, and mycotoxins
- Recommended inductively coupled plasma-optical emission spectroscopy or MS: serum (collected in royal blue–top tube), liver biopsies, liver, kidney, or source material for multiple metals

- Digitized images

  Digitized images of gross necropsy findings, rumen contents, suspected source material, and potentially toxic plants and harmful algal blooms should be captured and stored, especially for legal/insurance/regulatory cases and for field necropsy cases

- Microbiology, virology, serology, and molecular diagnostics as deemed necessary
- Radiographs and ultrasound, as deemed necessary

Necropsy/Postmortem Examinations

Loss of 1 or more animals in a herd or a single animal at risk is an excellent opportunity to gain additional information critical to diagnosing the cause of death in ruminant species. This type of examination also can help enhance the antemortem diagnosis and treatment of the other animals in the herd/flock.[2–4] It always is a good idea to have dead animals necropsied as soon after death as possible, especially during the heat of summer. If multiple animals die over a short period of time, a good rule of thumb is to consider necropsying at least 1 animal for every 5 animals that have died. This is important especially in legal cases and/or insurance claims or circumstances involving state or federal regulatory agencies. The samples to collect for toxicology testing are outlined in **Box 3**, with the most important asterisked. Depending on the circumstances, it might be advisable to consider sending the entire bodies of deceased ruminants or the collected and properly preserved samples from these animals to a veterinary diagnostic laboratory accredited by the American Association of Veterinary Laboratory Diagnosticians.

Note: the bare essential tissue samples to collect for diagnostic testing from ANY necropsy are brain, especially if there are neurologic signs: rumen contents, ocular fluid, liver, and kidney. If rabies is plausible, this testing should be completed before proceeding ANY further with the examination. If infectious disease is suspected, appropriate samples corresponding to the suspected sites of infection should be collected.

SUMMARY

The author has taken seriously his responsibility for writing this important article. The most critical information from the first article in the 2011 *Ruminant Toxicology* issue largely has been left intact in **Boxes 1–3** of this article, so that this information continues to be readily available, in order to provide the needed guidance for the specific types of cases for which it was originally intended.[2] The balance of this article describes the types of multifactorial cases increasingly encountered by veterinarians, with diagnostic guidelines provided that are meant to explain how collection, proper preservation, and submission of the samples described can be used to confirm a suspected intoxication and to help elucidate the etiology of observed ruminant production losses, including those that involve animal illness and/or death.

DISCLOSURE

The author has nothing to disclose.

REFERENCES

1. Evans TJ. Diminished reproductive performance and selected toxicants forages and grains. Vet Clin North Am Food Anim Pract 2011;27:345–71.
2. Osweiler GD. Diagnostic guidelines for ruminant toxicosis. Vet Clin North Am Food Anim Pract 2011;27:247–54.
3. Blodgett DJ. The investigation of outbreaks of toxicologic disease. Vet Clin North Am Food Anim Pract 1988;4:145–58.
4. Galey FD. Diagnostic toxicology for the food animal practitioner. Vet Clin North Am Food Anim Pract 2000;16:409–21.

Evaluating Mineral Status in Ruminant Livestock

Steve Ensley, DVM, PhD

KEYWORDS

• Mineral status • Toxicology • Nutrition • Ruminants

KEY POINTS

- The best choice of sample (tissue, blood, or other fluid) for mineral analysis varies with the mineral of interest and the reason for testing.
- Blood and serum samples are most often used to measure minerals and vitamins because they are easy to obtain.
- Mineral bioavailability can be affected by the chemical form of the mineral and interactions among other dietary constituents.

Determining the mineral status of production animals is important when developing an optimum health program. Nutrition is the largest expense in food animal production and has the greatest impact on health and productivity of the animals. The bioavailability of minerals in the diet is difficult to determine. Evaluating fluid or tissues from the animals themselves is the optimum method to determine the bioavailability of minerals in the diet. Evaluating the diet provides some information, but will not tell you what the animal's mineral status actually is. No matter how good your health program is, without providing the nutrition that is needed you will not get optimum health and production. Measurement of minerals and vitamins in the diet does not always provide information about bioavailability in the animal. Serum, blood, or liver from the animal needs to be analyzed to determine bioavailability of vitamin and minerals in the diet. This article reviews how to sample and the function of these particular minerals in the body of cattle.

SAMPLE TO DETERMINE MINERAL STATUS

The best choice of sample (tissue, blood, or other fluid) for mineral analysis varies with the mineral of interest and the reason for testing. Blood, urine, and serum are easy samples to collect. Many minerals are stored in the liver, so liver is considered the best overall tissue to analyze. Liver is the best sample for copper, iron, and cobalt

Anatomy & Physiology, Kansas State University, 1800 Dension Avenue, P217 Mosier Hall, Manhattan, KS 66506, USA
E-mail address: sensley01@ksu.edu

Vet Clin Food Anim 36 (2020) 525–546
https://doi.org/10.1016/j.cvfa.2020.08.009
0749-0720/20/© 2020 Elsevier Inc. All rights reserved.

concentration. Learning to biopsy livers is a technique that is easy for practitioners to learn. Liver biopsies for cattle are easily collected and there is very little risk of any adverse effects.

One of the important changes in analytical chemistry is development of the inductively coupled plasma/mass spectroscopy (ICP/MS) equipment. With the ICP/MS we can measure mineral concentrations in liver biopsy samples (usually 20–40 mg of fresh liver).[1–4] Hair samples may be used to determine a mineral toxicosis but they are not adequate to determine deficiencies. Surveys of soil, plant, and animal mineral concentrations have shown that soil and plant samples will not provide information that would be what is needed for diagnostic purposes in animals.[5]

Whole blood, serum, and plasma are the most commonly used samples to analyze for mineral concentration. Serum is most often used for analysis because it is easy to obtain. Mineral concentrations of plasma and serum have been assumed to be the same but serum contains less copper than plasma.[6] Mineral concentrations for serum or plasma samples will tell you what the mineral status of the transport pool of the mineral is. Low to deficient mineral concentrations indicate the start of a deficiency (**Fig. 1**). Whole blood can be used to measure the mineral concentration when the erythrocyte concentration of the mineral is higher than in the serum. Selenium analysis of whole blood indicates what the diet has been for the last 30 days. Serum concentration of selenium will change within days of making a feed change. Liver samples will represent what the diet has been the last 30 days.

DETERMINING HOW MANY ANIMALS TO SAMPLE FOR MINERAL EVALUATION

Determining how many animals in a population to sample depends on the variance of the mineral in the population and ultimately on the total cost of the analysis. The cost of

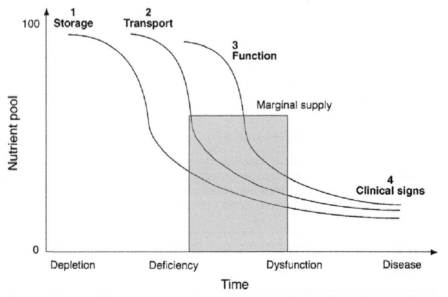

Fig. 1. Trace mineral function in animals. (*From* Underwood EJ, Suttle N. The mineral nutrition of livestock. 3rd ed. Wallingford, UK: CABI Publishing; 1999:47-66; with permission.)

the analysis versus the benefit of the data will determine what the producer will spend on doing mineral analysis.

Every analytical laboratory has their own reference ranges for mineral concentrations in the matrix they measure. There is some variation in the reference ranges between veterinary analytical laboratories, but most ranges are similar. Developing a normal range for mineral concentration in animals can be difficult. It is difficult to define what a normal group of animals are to develop a normal reference range. Most veterinary diagnostic laboratories receive samples from animals that are not normal, so these values are not helpful in determining normal ranges. Equipment varies between laboratories and methods of sample preparation are slightly different, adding another variability. Using published mineral values is also helpful to determine normal ranges. Reference ranges generated from populations of known healthy herds are not readily available, but would be the best information.

The many different terms used to describe what a low, normal, and elevated mineral concentration is problematic. Many different terms are used to describe the concentration of minerals in an animal in the different laboratories. Terms such as deficient, reference low, critically low, adequate, marginal, normal, reference high, and critically high have been used by laboratories. For some minerals, adequate concentrations in the serum, blood, or liver do not always indicate normal nutritional status. A specific mineral value that indicates a clinical deficiency is difficult to define because clinical signs of deficiency do not occur at specific mineral concentrations. There is a first number and last number to each range so 1 number below the low range is called deficient or 1 number higher than the normal range is considered elevated; thus, the term describing the data has to be used cautiously. We have to be careful with absolute diagnosis when there a 1-number change from a low to a high value.

We want to use the mineral concentration data to determine a trend within a population and the variance within the population. A clinical deficiency can be defined as the mineral concentration at which adverse clinical signs of deficiency will occur. A normal reference range is the range of mineral concentrations found in normal animals in this population. Mineral concentrations in animals are an indicator of low, normal, or elevated mineral status.

Evaluating the mineral status of a population of animals is more difficult than analyzing individual animals. Mineral concentrations in blood or serum versus liver can have much variation. Analyzing more animals in the population is always better than just measuring few individuals to determine the nutritional status of the herd. When evaluating a population's mineral concentrations, determining how many animals in the population should be analyzed and how the group data should be interpreted are important questions to answer before testing. Calculating means and standard deviations within herds and populations of herds can be helpful. It is also helpful to have the range of mineral concentrations to see what the variation is in a herd. Means provide some information, but the variance is more important.

Testing 15 to 20 animals in a herd are usually enough animals to get accurate mineral status data. This strategy is always balanced by the cost of testing. Determining how many animals to sample in a population is a difficult balance of cost and data.

New analytical instrumentation has made it cost effective to measure these minerals in serum or blood and liver. Many minerals can be analyzed at the same time verses 1 mineral at a time with an atomic absorption equipment.

MINERAL ANALYSIS

There are 16 essential trace minerals in animal diets, namely, calcium, phosphorus, potassium, sulfur, sodium, chloride, magnesium, iron, zinc, copper, manganese, iodine, selenium, molybdenum, chromium, and fluoride. In diagnostic cases I focus on these 8 trace minerals, cobalt (Co), copper (Cu), iron (Fe), iodine (I), manganese (Mn), molybdenum (Mo), selenium (Se), and zinc (Zn). The remaining 8 macro minerals are also important, calcium (Ca), chromium (Cr), phosphorus (P), potassium (K), sodium (Na), sulfur (S), chloride (Cl) and magnesium (Mg), but these minerals are not covered in this review.

Blood and serum samples are most often used to measure minerals and vitamins because they are easy to obtain. Determining the mineral concentration of the diet does not tell you what the mineral status of the animal is, because we are not able to determine bioavailability of the minerals in the diet easily. The biologic availability of minerals in the diet is highly variable. Mineral bioavailability can be affected by the chemical form of the mineral and interactions among other dietary constituents. When minerals are offered as a free choice, there is no easy method to monitor consumption. Determination of the mineral concentration in the animal is 1 method of determining an animal's mineral intake.

The use of small needle liver biopsies in cattle has made it easier to determine liver concentration of minerals. Small needle liver biopsy techniques were developed in the 1950s and have been improved upon to date. Copper (Cu), manganese (Mn), selenium (Se), and zinc (Zn) are stored in the liver. Ante mortem determination of these trace minerals in liver tissue has been found to be an accurate method to determine mineral status in animals. Measurement of the liver mineral concentration is considered the best method of measuring these minerals stored in the liver.

An alternative method of evaluating trace mineral status would be by measuring the activity of enzymes that use a particular mineral as a part of the enzyme. Determining glutathione peroxidase activity to determine selenium status or measuring ceruloplasm to determine copper status are one methods of determining mineral status. To determine cobalt or vitamin B_{12} deficiency in ruminants you can measure serum concentrations of methyl malonic acid (MMA) as a secondary marker of cobalt status in ruminants. Determining enzyme activity is a method of measuring a malfunction with an enzyme. Determining enzyme function is a more sensitive measurement of a deficient mineral status in an animal than just measuring the mineral content of serum, blood, or liver. Measuring enzymes to determine mineral deficiencies would be diagnostic, but is not commonly done. Measuring enzymes or protein products containing minerals gives information about the mineral status once the mineral is deficient. For a determination of mineral status in an animal, we want to know when the mineral is below the normal range and before there are clinical signs of adverse health.

The availability of new equipment like the ICP/MS allows multiple minerals to be measured at one time. This new technology has made this analysis very cost effective compared with previous testing methods like atomic absorption. ICP/MS is rapid, sensitive, accurate, and allows for the simultaneous measurement of a panel of trace minerals rather than 1 mineral at a time.

Underwood and Suttle[7] developed a graph (see **Fig. 1**) as a visual way to look at trace mineral function in animals. Adverse health does not occur until the storage and transport pools are depleted.

The storage and transport pools need to be depleted before the potential development of adverse health. Not all of the 8 minerals that we are discussing in this article are stored in either the serum, blood, or liver. The functional and storage pools also overlap in **Fig. 1**. The physiologic state of the animal, age and stage of production affects the mineral concentration. Animals will try to maintain homeostasis within a narrow physiologic range and this phenomenon will impact mineral storage. Adverse health can develop rapidly when minerals are not maintained in a narrow physiologic range.

COBALT
Cobalt Physiology

Cobalt is an essential component of vitamin B_{12} (cobalamin). Vitamin B_{12} is an essential vitamin in monogastrics and ruminants. Ruminants synthesize cobalamin from cobalt provided in the diet. Monogastrics need to have vitamin B_{12} added to the diet. Vitamin B_{12} requirements in ruminants are met from rumen microbes using cobalt. Cobalamin synthesis by intestinal microflora in monogastric animals occurs distal to the rumen and ileum. Monogastrics require dietary cobalt only as a constituent of preformed vitamin B_{12} and do not have a systemic cobalt requirement. Both ruminant and monogastric animals can absorb cobalt from the intestine. Cobalt can be measured in the tissues and blood of animals. Cobalt in ruminants and monogastrics is only needed as a constituent of vitamin B_{12}. Vitamin B_{12} is also essential to the metabolism of rumen microbes, and rumen function is disturbed when there is a cobalt deficiency in the diet. Vitamin B_{12} is stored in the liver is normally adequate to supply all of the animal's needs for longer than a year. Vitamin B_{12} functions in many metabolic reactions. The metabolism of carbohydrates, lipids, amino acids, and DNA all involve vitamin B_{12} as a cofactor.[8] Another reaction in which vitamin B_{12} is a required cofactor is in the metabolism of succinate into propionate. This is a reaction in energy metabolism because it is essential for the synthesis of glucose from propionate.[9] Propionate accumulates in blood when there is a vitamin B_{12} deficiency. MMA is an intermediate in the conversion of propionate to succinate and will accumulate in the blood. MMA concentrations in blood and urine can be used in the diagnosis of cobalt status in ruminants but this is not a common analysis done in veterinary diagnostic laboratories.

Cobalt Deficiency

Clinical cobalt deficiency can occur anywhere.[7] Cobalt deficiency is seen with well-drained sandy soil. Cobalt deficiency occurs more often in grass pastures than in legume pastures. Sheep are more susceptible to cobalt deficiency than cattle. High concentrate, feedlot-type diets are poor cobalt sources. The efficiency of vitamin B_{12} synthesis from available cobalt is less on high grain diets, compared with high forage diets.[10] Cobalt deficiency results in a deficiency of vitamin B_{12} in ruminants. Cobalt deficiency is associated with decreased feed intake, lowered feed conversion, reduced growth, weight loss, hepatic lipidosis, anemia, immunosuppression, and impaired reproductive function.[11] When there is severe cobalt deficiency, clinical signs include anorexia and wasting. This condition can be misdiagnosed as starvation. In advanced cases of vitamin B_{12} deficiency, anemia is severe. Young, growing animals are at greater risk than adults. Mild cases are often misdiagnosed as parasitism or poor nutrition. The clinical and pathologic signs of cobalt deficiency can be diagnosed by characteristic biochemical changes in the tissues and fluids of the body.[12] When cobalt deficiency starts, the concentrations of cobalt and of vitamin B_{12} decrease in the rumen fluid. Diagnostic laboratories commonly measure cobalt but not vitamin B_{12} because cobalt is included in the ICP/MS analysis panel.

Cobalt Toxicosis

Cobalt toxicosis is not normally observed in animals. Cobalt is not normally added at high enough concentrations in animal diets to cause a toxicosis. Misformulations may result in cobalt toxicosis. There is a 100-fold margin of safety with dietary cobalt, even then field cases of suspected cobalt toxicity in ruminants have been reported.[13]

Cobalt Status

The cobalt status of animals can be determined by measurement of serum or liver concentrations of vitamin B_{12} or cobalt. Cobalt status can be determined by measuring metabolites associated with vitamin B_{12} deficiency in blood or urine. MMA and homocysteine are metabolites.[14,15] Normal concentrations of vitamin B_{12} and cobalt in serum are low. Analysis used to measure the metabolites of vitamin B_{12} and vitamin B_{12} are not commonly measured in veterinary diagnostic laboratories. Vitamin B_{12} concentrations in serum and tissue are difficult to interpret. There are inactive cobalamin analogues in the serum that may interfere with some analysis of vitamin B_{12}.[16] There are several proteins in the serum that bind cobalamin that make it difficult to interpret serum vitamin B_{12} status. The most useful serum vitamin B_{12} assays are based on either radioimmunoassay or chemiluminescense.[17,18] Cobalt concentrations can be measured in serum or tissues with ICP/MS. Liver is the best sample because it has the highest concentration of cobalt and is the storage site for vitamin B_{12}. The analysis of cobalt is easier than the assay for vitamin B_{12}. There is a large concentration of cobalt in serum and liver that is not associated with vitamin B_{12}, making the interpretation of serum or liver cobalt concentrations difficult.

Normal bovine hepatic vitamin B_{12} concentrations are in the range of 200 to 400 nmol/kg wet tissue.[14] This liver concentration applies to growing calves and adults but not to bovine fetal and neonatal liver cobalt concentrations. Vitamin B_{12} is transported across the placenta.[19] The placenta is a selective barrier to the distribution of some of the non–vitamin B_{12}-associated serum cobalt into the fetus. Serum cobalt concentrations are difficult to interpret in relationship to vitamin B_{12} concentrations. There is not a good correlation between serum cobalt and serum vitamin B_{12} concentrations.

Normal serum vitamin B_{12} concentrations in cattle seem are 200 to 400 pmol/L or greater.[14] Vitamin B_{12} contains 4% cobalt. Serum cobalt concentrations in cattle include more than just the concentration of cobalt in vitamin B_{12}. Serum cobalt concentrations are affected by dietary cobalt intake because the bioavailability of the cobalt in cobalamin is variable. The low proportion of serum cobalt that is present in the form of cobalamin and the variable bioavailability between cobalt intake and serum cobalt concentrations makes the measurement of serum cobalt difficult when determining vitamin B_{12} status in cattle. The best method of determining cobalt status in ruminants is by measuring MMA concentrations in serum or urine. MMA accumulates when methyl malonyl coenzyme A is not converted to succinyl coenzyme A.[14] The conversion depends on the cobalamin concentration. Elevated MMA concentrations indicate cobalamin deficiency. MMA assays are not normally performed in diagnostic laboratories. There are no veterinary diagnostic laboratories that routinely offer vitamin B_{12} or MMA analysis and vitamin B_{12} deficiency remains a concern, especially with anemias. In our laboratory, we use liver and serum cobalt concentrations to determine if there is a potential cobalt deficiency in ruminants that could result in a vitamin B_{12} deficiency.

COPPER
Copper Physiology

Copper is an essential trace mineral in animals, both ruminants and monogastrics. It is a component of proteins, nucleic acids, and enzymes. Cytochrome oxidase is involved with the production of adenosine triphosphate. Superoxide dismutase is involved in immune defense and inactivates the oxygen radical tyrosinase. Lysyl oxidase is involved in connective tissue formation. There are many other enzymes containing copper that are involved in growth, immunocompetence, and the nervous system.[19] In cattle, copper deficiency is a more common condition than copper toxicosis. Copper toxicosis in adult animals is more common in sheep, but can occur in cattle. Copper toxicosis is observed more often in adult dairy cattle and neonatal dairy calves.

Copper Deficiency

Many areas in the United States are deficient in copper. The US Geological Service have maps available on line for all the minerals we measure in the laboratory. You can see what your specific geological area status is for the mineral of interest. Young grazing livestock are the most likely to be copper deficient.[20] Copper deficiency may be primary or secondary. A primary copper deficiency is a complete deficiency of copper, whereas a secondary copper deficiency involves a decreased bioavailability by the presence of copper antagonists. Forages for cattle are copper deficient if copper concentration is less than 7 ppm dry weight[21] and total rations are deficient if the concentration is less than 10 ppm.[22] Secondary copper deficiency occurs when the concentration of copper in the diet is adequate, but antagonists like molybdenum and sulfur are present that bind the available copper in the diet. These mineral antagonists will bind copper in the animal also. The nutritional copper requirements cannot be determined without knowing the molybdenum and sulfur concentrations in the diet. Dietary excesses in iron, zinc, and calcium also interfere with copper absorption.[23] These minerals may induce secondary copper deficiency by either decreasing copper absorption or by interfering with its use at the cellular level.

One clinical sign of copper deficiency is loss of hair color in dark-haired breeds of cattle called achromotrichia. Marginal copper deficiency can affect many physiologic process. A deficiency can cause a decrease in production, which is seen as an increased feed per pound of gain, decreased rate of weight gain. In addition, there can be changes in the estrous cycle length, anestrous, early embryonic loss, increased prevalence of ovarian cysts, decreased immune function, and increased incidence of disease. Increased abomasal ulceration in beef calves is also seen with copper deficiency. Copper deficiency is a common condition in beef cattle.

Copper Toxicosis

Copper toxicosis is more common in sheep than cattle because they are more sensitive to excess dietary copper. Sheep have different clinical signs of copper toxicosis than cattle. Copper toxicosis in sheep causes acute release of excess copper from the hepatocytes. Copper accumulates in the liver after being on a diet with elevated copper or a deficiency of molybdenum. The liver accumulates copper while maintaining plasma and serum copper concentrations within the normal range. Analyzing the serum copper concentration to determine liver copper concentration will not be accurate. The serum copper concentration is only increased when stressful events such as advanced pregnancy, lactation, moving animals, or weather extremes cause the lysosomes in the liver to suddenly release copper. When this release occurs, animals develop a hemoglobinuria. Hemoglobinuria results from hemolysis caused by the release of copper from the liver into the blood stream. Sheep serum copper may be elevated so that a diagnosis of copper toxicosis can be made, but this condition is for a short period of time. When copper is released from the liver it may also accumulate in the kidney, so kidney copper concentration should be measured as well when there is copper toxicosis suspected. Serum copper concentrations of greater than 3.3 µg/mL (ppm) are compatible with copper toxicosis in sheep.[24] Copper toxicosis is most often diagnosed post mortem using fresh liver and kidney samples. Elevated liver copper is often accompanied by an increased kidney copper content so that, with clinical signs or lesions, you can reach a definitive diagnosis of copper toxicosis. Copper toxicosis is seen in adult cattle and dairy steer calves. It is more common in calves than in adults in the last 5 to 7 years. Elevated liver copper is a relatively common finding in adult dairy cattle, usually caused by oversupplementation of copper in dairy diets. Feeds containing more than 100 ppm of copper can cause copper toxicosis in adult cattle.[25] Because young calves start out as monogastrics, calves are more sensitive to copper poisoning than adult ruminants. Feeds containing more than 20 ppm of copper and 1 ppm molybdenum on a dry weight basis can be toxic to calves until they become ruminants. Calves that have not developed a rumen function as monogastrics. Monogastrics accumulate copper in the liver at a higher rate than ruminants. The serum copper concentration is not helpful in diagnosing copper toxicosis in cattle either. In sheep feed, the ideal copper to molybdenum ratio is 6:1 and a ratio of greater than 10 is likely to cause chronic copper toxicosis. Sheep feed should not contain more than 20 ppm of copper and at least 2 ppm molybdenum to maintain a 10:1 copper to molybdenum ratio.

Copper Status

The long-term storage pool of copper is the liver. The liver concentration of most minerals represents what the diet has been over the last 30 days. The purpose of mineral supplementation is to have mineral concentrations within a normal range in the liver so there are no adverse health effects. A lower than normal hepatic copper concentration is the earliest sign of inadequate copper consumption and inadequate storage in the liver. Small needle liver biopsy samples are the most reliable means of evaluating copper status in an animal. Copper concentrations can be determined on liver samples as small as 20 mg of fresh tissue weight. These samples are easily obtained with many types of small needle biopsy instruments. Samples taken with most small needle biopsy needles are about the diameter of the lead in a pencil. Newer biopsy tools are spring loaded and easier to use than manually operated biopsy needles. Liver biopsy samples can be transferred directly from the biopsy needle into any test tube that is also appropriate for blood collection. Fresh refrigerated or frozen liver samples should be delivered to the laboratory as soon as possible, but sample stability is not a concern for most all minerals.

Serum copper concentrations indicate what the transport pool contains, but is also a part of the functional pool. Approximately 80% of copper in serum is present in ceruloplasm. Ceruloplasm is a protein secreted by the liver. Smaller concentrations of copper are present in association with albumin and other transport proteins.[26] The regulation of serum copper concentrations is under positive feedback control based on liver copper stores. When liver copper stores are within a normal range, serum copper concentrations remain stable. Serum copper concentrations will also be increased when there is inflammation, not just owing to copper accumulation. Ceruloplasm acts like acute phase proteins, increasing during an inflammatory response. Dietary sulfur and molybdenum are copper antagonists. These minerals can decrease serum copper concentrations and functional copper status. These minerals combine to form soluble thiomolybdates. There are mono-, di-, tri-, and tetra-thiomolybdates formed in the rumen. These insoluble copper trace mineral complexes inhibit and can block copper absorption from the rumen. Thiomolybdates can be absorbed into the bloodstream and have a copper chelating effect, mobilizing copper from tissue stores in a form that is not functional. When there are significant concentrations of circulating thiomolybdates, serum copper concentrations may be in the normal range, even though there is a copper deficiency.[5] This circumstance can create confusion with interpretation of copper concentrations in the serum and liver. Thiomolybdates in a serum sample can be removed in the laboratory by treatment with trichloroacetic acid. When copper trace mineral complexes are expected, serum copper concentrations should be evaluated both before and after trichloroacetic acid treatment of the samples. Serum is commonly used for copper assessment because it is convenient to collect and because it is a sample that may be used for multiple laboratory analyses. Plasma may be a more accurate sample for copper assessment than serum. Ceruloplasm and other copper-containing serum proteins seem to become incorporated into the clot, making plasma samples contain a higher copper concentration than serum samples from the same animal.

There is not a good correlation between liver and serum copper concentrations. Low serum copper concentrations are generally not observed until liver concentrations decrease to less than approximately 25 ppm dry weight.[27,28] Even at low hepatic copper concentrations the relationship of serum to liver values is unreliable. The only reliable sample for determining copper concentration is the liver.

IODINE
Iodine Physiology

The primary function of iodine is in maintaining normal physiology of the thyroid. The thyroid hormones regulate muscle function, thermoregulation, energy metabolism, growth, reproduction, and circulation. Iodine is a mineral that is not reviewed with enough frequency in the diagnostic laboratory. Iodine is involved with more reproduction problems that is diagnosed.

Iodine Deficiency

Iodine is deficient in many parts of the world and this has been overcome by supplementation. The clinical signs of iodine deficiency vary depending on the animal species. Fetal death can occur at any stage of gestation from iodine deficiency. Calves may be born hairless, weak, or dead.[7] Reproductive failures have been reported in both male and female cattle and sheep with iodine deficiency. Because of goitrogens in feed the iodine needed in the diet may increase 2 to 4 times the normal inclusion rates.[29] Goitrogens interfere with iodine uptake by the thyroid gland or by inhibiting thyroperoxidase. Goitrogens include thiocyanates from forages such as kale, turnips, radishes, canola seeds, white clover, and brassica seeds.[30] The brassicas have become popular fall annuals for grazing and can cause an iodine deficiency.

Iodine Toxicosis

Iodine toxicosis in cattle has typically been caused by the overuse of ethylenediamine hydroiodide in the treatment of iodine deficiency, foot rot, or the chronic bacterial disease caused by actinomycosis. Excess iodine intake in sheep has also been associated with goiter in newborns. Goiter can be caused by an excess or deficiency of iodine.

Iodine Status

Determining the iodine status is important to determine if it is involved with reproductive or production health issues. Iodine toxicity is a concern because iodine can be consumed by humans through consumption of animal products. Iodine deficiency or toxicosis can cause abortion and weak born calves. Measuring iodine status of animals is important in diagnosing problems but is not commonly done because the thyroid is not submitted. Liver or serum iodine concentrations are not reliable.

Measuring iodine concentration in animals is important because dietary requirements are not well-defined and vary depending on the environmental temperature, selenium status, and the presence of goitrogens in the diet. Iodine deficiency can be observed grossly as a goiter. Goiters may occur in utero and not be observed until birth. Congenital goiters may occur in the offspring of dams that are not affected by iodine deficiency. The tissue of choice in diagnosing iodine status in animals is the thyroid gland. The thyroid is not typically taken as a tissue to submit in a post mortem examination.

The best assessment of functional iodine status is thyroid iodine concentration. Liver concentrations are not useful in diagnosing iodine deficiency. For an ante mortem diagnosis of iodine deficiency, determining thyroid function is a way of making a diagnosis.

Measurement of serum iodine is a reliable method to diagnose iodine deficiency. Iodine in serum is either inorganic or protein-bound iodine. Determining total serum iodine, protein-bound iodine, or plasma inorganic iodine are the best diagnostic methods used to determine iodine status. The protein-bound forms represent the thyroid hormones. Protein bound iodine is mostly T4. Protein bound iodine and T4 are stable and do not reflect changes in iodine intake. Plasma inorganic iodine changes rapidly with iodine intake. Inorganic iodine is not biologically active. Inorganic iodine is the largest amount of iodine in serum. Total serum iodine and serum inorganic iodine will tell you what the current iodine consumption is in the diet. Serum iodine is a measurement of short-term iodine intake.

Having low serum total iodine concentrations does not always indicate iodine deficiency because there may be adequate thyroid iodine reserves when there is a short-term deficient intake of dietary iodine.

IRON
Iron Physiology

Iron is another essential mineral. The largest amount of iron in the body is found in hemoglobin and myoglobin. Iron is used for normal cellular function and is found in plasma (transferrin), milk (lactoferrin), and liver (ferritin and hemosiderin).[31] Iron deficiency in livestock is associated with decreased growth, poor immune function, weakness, and anemia.[7] The clinical signs of iron deficiency initially present as a decreased storage of iron present as ferritin in liver, kidney, and spleen, a depletion in serum iron concentration, an increase in serum total iron-binding capacity and a decrease in serum iron binding saturation.[32] The concentration of iron in forage plants is determined by the species of plant and type of soil in which the plants grow. Measuring serum iron is not the best method to diagnose iron deficiency.

Iron Deficiency

Iron deficiency caused by a lack of iron in the diet of production animals is not common. Iron is inexpensive and is added to most diets in different forms. Many mineral formulations contain many different forms of iron oxide combinations. Iron deficiency is most common in young animals on a milk or milk product only diet. Bacterial infection is a common cause of anemia in animals. Bacteria need iron and have various methods of obtaining iron from the animal. Severe blood loss from a parasitic infection or blood loss from other causes may produce a secondary iron deficiency. Bioavailability of iron in the diet can be varied and caused by many factors. Compounds in the diet like phytate, polyphenols, and calcium will inhibit iron availability.[33] Additional trace mineral interaction may also affect bioavailability. There are many interactions with different minerals in the diet. An excess or deficiency of 1 mineral may impact the absorption or transportation of another mineral. This can occur by possibly competing for intestinal binding sites on the mucosa.[34] For example, excessive dietary cobalt or manganese may interfere with iron availability.

Iron Toxicosis

Iron toxicosis is not a common finding in production animals because of the decreased bioavailability of iron in the diet and the decreased use of injectable iron. Systemic iron uptake is regulated closely by intestinal absorption. Iron toxicosis can occur in animals when given excessive injectable or dietary supplements that are used to prevent iron deficiencies. Iron toxicosis may occur if animals consume excessive amounts of iron over a long period. Excess dietary intake of iron results in tissue increase with large concentrations of free iron becoming elevated enough to cause oxidative damage in the liver.[7] Animals can tolerate a higher daily exposure of iron when it is consumed in feed rather than when it is provided in the water or in a fasting state. Calcium in the diet regulates iron toxicity.[35] The maximum tolerable concentration of dietary iron is 500 mg/kg for cattle and sheep. Young animals absorb iron more efficiently than older animals but have a lower tolerance. Elevated iron exposure can cause an increase concentration in liver, spleen, and bone marrow.

Iron Status

Determining liver and serum concentrations of iron can be used to diagnose iron deficiency and toxicosis. Decreased concentrations of iron in serum that occur before the development of anemia are used to diagnose iron deficiency. Hemolysis of serum will impact the measurement of iron. Hemolysis will artificially increase iron concentrations from the lysed red blood cells. Serum iron concentrations are more accurately determined by analytical methods that do not detect the iron in heme. Iron can be measured by using ICP/MS, but this method measures total iron. Additional diagnostic methods used to determine the bodies iron concentration include measuring total iron-binding capacity, the status of the complete red blood cell status in the body and serum ferritin concentration.[32] Serum ferritin concentration is the most sensitive for the determination of iron status. All serum ferritin assays are immunologically based and depend on species-specific antibodies. Generalized inflammatory diseases can alter serum and liver iron concentrations. The body defense to controlling infectious agents in the body is to limit the availability of iron to growing organisms and increase the availability of iron to the body's own immune cells. The primary iron-carrying protein in blood serum, transferrin, acts as a negative acute phase protein, with concentrations decreasing rapidly in the presence of inflammation.[36] The interpretation of the iron status in an animal should be done with consideration of the overall health of the animal.

MANGANESE
Manganese Physiology

Since the commercial development of the ICP/MS in the later 1980s, there has been more analysis of liver and serum for many different metals because it is cost effective. Previous to the ICP/MS mineral analysis, the analytical technique used was atomic absorption. Atomic absorption is a 1 mineral at a time analysis, so it was costly to do the mineral analysis panel we now do with the ICP/MS. There has been more analysis of tissue and serum for manganese done now than previously. Most of the data generated about manganese status in commercial food animal production has been within the last 20 years.

Manganese is involved in many enzyme systems in the body and the manganese concentration affects a wide variety of biochemical processes including protein, carbohydrate, and fat metabolism. Manganese is involved in proper bone development and maintenance. Manganese is required by glycosyltransferases, which are involved in the synthesis of the glycosaminoglycans and glycoproteins of bone and cartilage matrix.[37] Manganese is involved in free radical quenching and protection against oxidative tissue damage through its role in mitochondrial superoxide dismutase. Manganese is one of the least abundant trace minerals in the animal body, but is distributed widely throughout the body. Manganese is found in parts per billion in serum and liver. The liver, pancreas, and kidney contain the highest concentrations of manganese. The homeostasis of manganese is controlled by absorption and excretion. Less than 10% of manganese is absorbed from the intestine. The normal range of dietary concentrations of manganese is between 1% and 10%, so the bioavailability is influenced by the body requirements. Manganese is excreted primarily via bile. Because it is so widely distributed throughout the body, there is not a storage pool for manganese. Homeostasis is tightly regulated so animals can maintain tissue concentrations over long periods of decreased intake. There is no fetal accumulation of manganese as occurs with other minerals.[37,38] Unlike other minerals, fetal liver concentrations of manganese are typically lower or equivalent to those of the dam. Most minerals are concentrated in the fetus, but not manganese. Pasture grasses and legumes are typically good sources of manganese, but corn silage is not. Cereal grains, especially corn, are poor sources of manganese but byproducts containing substantial amounts of bran may have substantially higher concentrations than base grains from which they were derived. The availability of manganese from high phytate sources such as brans is low, especially for monogastrics. Manganese uptake in plants is inhibited by glyphosate in Round Up ready crops. The rapid increased use of Round Up ready crops has been implicated in manganese deficiency.

Manganese Deficiency

Manganese deficiency in production animals is associated with skeletal abnormalities, impaired growth, ataxia of the newborn, disturbed or depressed reproductive function, defects in lipid and carbohydrate metabolism, and productivity problems.[39] Severe manganese deficiency has also been shown to impair immunity.

Cases of well-documented manganese-responsive disorders in production animals are not common. Recently, there has been concern that congenital abnormalities of bone formation have occurred in cattle in association with manganese deficiency. In a controlled study of Holstein heifers, those fed a low manganese diet throughout growth and gestation gave birth to calves that had lower blood manganese concentrations than controls and abnormalities of bone growth, including disproportionate dwarfism, swollen joints, and superior brachygnathism.[40] This deficiency is called congenital joint laxity and dwarfism and has been associated with manganese deficiency.

In clinical observations, it has been noted that cattle of the dairy breeds seem to have generally lower tissue manganese concentrations than do cattle of beef breeds.[41] This manganese deficiency may occur because of high calcium and phosphorus concentrations in dairy rations, which can be antagonistic to the bioavailability of manganese. The National Research Council recently lowered the recommended dietary manganese concentration from 40 mg/kg to approximately 20 mg/kg, which might place some pregnant animals at risk for fetal manganese deficiency.[7]

Manganese Toxicosis

Manganese oversupplementation can produce adverse effects in cattle. Manganese is considered to be one of the least toxic of the essential elements.[42] Generally, depressed iron status and hematologic changes were the most common signs of manganese toxicosis, even in animals fed adequate iron. The chemical form of manganese can play an important role in potential toxic effects.

Manganese Status

The determination of normal manganese status is difficult. Liver, whole blood, and serum are the most frequent samples analyzed for manganese concentration. Liver and whole blood have higher manganese concentrations relative to serum. Manganese concentrations are poorly responsive to supplementation and have remained constant in the face of prolonged intake of manganese-deficient diets. Whole blood manganese concentrations of less than 20 parts per billion and liver concentrations of less than 1.0 ppm wet weight are generally considered compatible with manganese deficiency.[43] Serum seems to be the matrix most responsive to sustained intake of manganese deficient diets.[44] Careful handling in the collection and handling of serum samples for manganese analysis because red blood cells have a higher manganese concentration than serum (usually 10-fold to 20-fold).[45] Hemolysis or prolonged contact of the serum with the clot results in the increase of red cell manganese into the serum and a false increase in serum manganese concentrations. Manganese will leach from red cells quickly after sample collection, so not only should hemolysis be avoided, but serum should be separated from the clot quickly, within 2 to 3 hours of collection. Serum manganese concentrations are low and many laboratories do not offer this analysis because of inadequate sensitivity of analytical methods. ICP/MS is the analytical method of choice for serum manganese.

MOLYBDENUM
Molybdenum Physiology

Nutritional interest in molybdenum has been because of its antagonistic effect on copper availability in ruminants. Molybdenum has an essential role in xanthine oxidase and its activity depends on this metal.[46] Molybdenum is required for nitrogen fixation and for the reduction of nitrate to nitrite in bacteria.[47]

Molybdenum Deficiency

Molybdenum is essential for all production animals. The requirements are low and very few clinical signs of deficiency have been shown in few species. Molybdenum deficiency has been reported in goats with depressed growth, impaired reproduction, and death of kids and dams. Secondary molybdenum deficiency was produced in chickens fed high levels of tungsten.[48,49]

Molybdenum Toxicosis

Adverse effects on livestock owing to high dietary molybdenum are usually in association with sulfur in the diet. Cattle are the least tolerant species, followed by sheep; pigs are the most resistant.[5] The clinical signs of molybdenum toxicity also vary among species. Slow growth, weight loss, and anorexia are the most common clinical signs of molybdenum toxicosis and diarrhea is typical only in cattle.[5] Ruminants have clinical signs that look like copper deficiency if they have low concentrations of dietary molybdenum. When there is ruminal formation of thiomolybdates there is diminished copper absorption and these thiomolybdates bind systemic copper and make it nonfunctional.

Molybdenum Status

Molybdenum in the diet is readily absorbed and serum, whole blood, milk, liver, and kidney values reflect dietary intake.[50] The assessment of serum and hepatic molybdenum concentrations is useful as an indication of excessive intake with associated secondary copper deficiency.[51] Increased serum molybdenum concentrations should alert the diagnostician to the possible presence of thiomolybdates, which should affect the interpretation of serum or plasma copper concentrations.

SELENIUM
Selenium Physiology

Selenium has many physiologic functions.[52] The biologic impact of selenium was discovered because of its toxicity to livestock. Selenium deficiency is more common than selenium toxicosis. Selenium is an essential component of at least 12 enzymes. This list includes 4 glutathione peroxidases that use glutathione to break down hydroperoxides; 3 iodothyronine 50-deiodinases that catalyze the deiodination of L-thyroxine to the biologically active thyroid hormone; 3, s305-triiodothyronine; 3 thioredoxin reductases that reduce oxidized proteins; a selenophosphate synthetase 2 that is involved in selenium activation of selenocysteine synthesis; and a methionine-R-sulfoxide reductase.[53] There are 3 selenium-containing proteins: selenoprotein P, which accounts for 60% of selenium in plasma; selenoprotein W, which may be related to white muscle disease; and a 15-kDa selenoprotein that may be related to cancer.[54] Deficiencies in either selenium or vitamin E can increase viral pathogenicity by changing relatively benign viruses into virulent ones.[55]

The different forms of selenium are taken up in the small intestine. Selenocysteine and selenomethionine are absorbed via an active amine acid transport mechanism, but selenite is absorbed by simple diffusion, and selenate by sodium mediated carrier shared with sulfate.[56] There is no homeostatic control of selenium absorption. The degree to which selenium is absorbed in the body has no relationship to how well it is absorbed in the gastrointestinal tract.[57] Cattle and sheep have lower absorption of selenium with greater variation than monogastrics. High dietary sulfur, lead, alfalfa hay, and dietary calcium decrease selenium absorption in ruminants.[58]

Selenium Deficiency

In many areas of the world there is a dietary deficiency of selenium. In other areas, selenium concentrations in some plants are elevated and will result in toxicosis. The major biochemical lesions associated with selenium deficiency are low glutathione peroxidase and iodothyronine 5'-deiodinase activities.[55] Free radical damage can progress to disease. When other antioxidants like vitamins A, C, and E are deficient then this will increase the clinical signs of selenium deficiency. Selenium deficiency decreases the free radical scavenging system, which will cause clinical disease. Nutritional muscular dystrophy, white muscles disease, is a selenium-responsive disorder that mainly affects young production animals. This myopathy is associated with excessive peroxidation of lipids, resulting in degeneration, necrosis, and eventually fibrosis of skeletal and cardiac muscle fibers. This myopathy may be associated with cardiac involvement and, depending on the species, hepatic necrosis.[59] Mastitis in cattle has been shown to be selenium responsive.[58] Abortion, weak and stillborn young, testicular degeneration and impaired sperm production, infertility, and retained placenta are associated with selenium deficiency. Selenium deficiency has a negative impact on immunocompetence. Anemia is also associated with selenium deficiency and it involves a depression in glutathione peroxidase activity with Heinz body formation.[58]

Selenium Toxicosis

Selenium has the smallest safety margin of the essential trace elements. That is the reason for the legal limit of selenium that can be added to feed. Selenium is the only mineral with a legal limit. Adverse clinical signs of selenium toxicosis can result when overadministration of selenium supplements occurs and accidental acute and chronic problems have become more common.[60] Selenium toxicosis occurs in seleniferous areas of many countries, including the Great Plains of the United States and Canada. The form of the selenium determines the potential for toxicosis as well as the duration of exposure and the genotype of the animal exposed. The tolerance of grazing cattle and horses on seleniferous range is difficult to establish because selenium intakes from forages vary widely because of palatability and accessibility. Acute toxicosis, blind staggers, and chronic alkali disease have been associated with selenium toxicosis.[42] Blind staggers has never been reproduced with selenium deficiency. Blind staggers was mistakenly identified as a selenium toxicosis because of its occurrence in alkali seleniferous areas in the western United States. Blind staggers is more likely a disease caused by poisonous plant or elevated dietary sulfur. Acute selenium toxicosis is characterized by abnormal movement, respiratory distress, diarrhea, and sudden death. The clinical signs of alkali disease include emaciation, cardiac atrophy, hepatic cirrhosis, anemia, and erosion of the long bones.[42]

Selenium Status

There is not a good feedback system to regulate the amount of dietary absorption of selenium in animals. Selenium absorption depends on the concentration of selenium in the diet, the valence state of selenium, and whether it is organic or inorganic. After absorption, a large amount of selenium is transferred to the liver, which functions as the storage site for the distribution of selenium in the body.[61,62] When excess selenium is accumulated in the liver, some of the liver selenium pool is excreted in bile, but most of it is cycled back to the serum for renal excretion. Serum is the major transport pool for selenium disposal thus the concentration of selenium in serum will indicate dietary intake.[62] The half-life of selenium in the plasma compartment is 6.6 hours in humans and is similar in other animals. The kinetics of serum selenium concentration is rapid; thus, short-term changes in serum selenium occur. Increasing dietary selenium uptake in cattle results in a significant increase in serum selenium within 2 to 6 days, depending on the amount of selenium intake.[63] The major down side to using serum selenium concentration to determine dietary intake is its short-term sensitivity to dietary intake.

This factor causes rapid serum changes with small changes in dietary intake. Determining selenium status is of diagnostic interest. When selenium is analyzed in blood, selenium can be measured in whole blood or serum. Whole blood contains both the erythrocyte and serum selenium fractions. The kinetic and homeostatic patterns of each of these fractions, or pools, are different. Selenium in erythrocytes of most domestic animals is present primarily as glutathione peroxidase. The serum glutathione peroxidase concentration is affected by dietary selenium availability.[64] Glutathione peroxidase is formed at the time of erythrocyte development. This process results in a buffering effect on the rate of change in erythrocyte selenium concentrations relative to dietary intake.[65] The half-life of erythrocytes in most domestic species, including cattle, is approximately 100 days. After changes in dietary selenium occur, changes in the selenium concentration of erythrocytes will happen at a rate no faster than the rate of erythrocyte turnover. The contribution of erythrocyte selenium to whole blood selenium in cattle is roughly 60%.[66,67] The rapidly changing serum pool and the more slowly changing erythrocyte pool have an impact on whole blood selenium concentration. The combination of short-term and long-term effects makes whole blood selenium generally more accurate than serum selenium for the determination of selenium nutrition, but both measures can be used.

Variability factors other than dietary selenium concentration and availability that affect whole blood and serum selenium concentrations include gestation–lactation stage and age, at least in cattle. Selenium is preferentially partitioned to the fetus during midgestation to late gestation.[66] In late gestation, transplacental transfer decreases serum selenium concentrations in the dam, without affecting whole blood selenium concentration. The dam's low serum selenium concentrations at calving increase during at least the first month of lactation.[8,68] In the fetus, the selenium in erythrocytes is mostly in the erythrocyte pool, with a smaller amount in serum than in adult animals.[66] Newborn animals have lower serum selenium than adults, although whole blood concentrations are more similar. Serum selenium concentrations in young animals remain low during the suckling period because the selenium concentration in milk is low. Serum selenium concentrations increase after consumption of solid feed.

Liver from biopsies or postmortem samples is useful for the evaluation of selenium status. For appropriate diagnosis of selenium status, you need to know the age of the animal being sampled. Late term fetuses and early neonates have a higher normal range than adults. There is maternal movement of a significant amount of selenium to the fetus during gestation. The stored concentration in the liver helps prevent deficiency during the time period of a predominantly milk diet. An early neonate with liver selenium near the low end of the normal range for an adult likely suffers deficiency before significant grazing.

ZINC
Zinc Physiology

Zinc is the most abundant trace mineral in the body, second only to iron. Zinc is a component of many enzymes and serves catalytic, structural, and regulatory functions within the body. Zinc is important in cell division and DNA and RNA replication. Zinc is important in the regulation of appetite, growth, and immune function. It has been difficult to attribute the clinical signs of zinc deficiency to any 1 specific biochemical function.[69] Monogastric production livestock are at greatest risk of zinc deficiency because dietary phytate combination with excess dietary calcium severely decreases the availability of dietary zinc. Decreasing dietary calcium and including phytase as a dietary supplement can improve zinc availability for poultry and swine. Zinc deficiency is less of a clinical problem in ruminants because phytate is digested by rumen microbes. The risk of zinc deficiency in ruminants is generally associated with zinc-deficient forages. Consecutive cuttings of hay crops within a season are associated with lower zinc concentrations in the forage. Very mature forages, including straws generally have low zinc concentrations.[70] Cow's milk is a poor source of zinc. Ruminant and monogastric animals suffering from diarrhea are at risk of zinc deficiency, especially if the condition is prolonged. In swine, poultry, and cattle, supplementing zinc at dietary concentrations beyond those generally recognized as the nutritional requirement can result in improved growth performance and feed efficiency. Zinc homeostasis is controlled by absorption, and the efficiency of absorption is largely dependent on the zinc status of the animal.[69] Homeostasis of zinc is tightly regulated, and tissue concentrations remain relatively constant across a wide range of zinc intakes. There is no clear storage pool of zinc in the body, even though we still measure liver concentrations. Homeostasis depends on a continual pool of zinc in the intestine. When there is adequate zinc in the diet, zinc absorption is decreased and some of the absorbed amount is sequestered in the intestinal epithelium as a complex with the metal-binding protein metallothionein. This protein effectively removes zinc from the active metabolic pool and this is an important part of homeostatic regulation of zinc status.

Zinc Deficiency

The clinical signs of zinc deficiency are hoof and hair lesions, poor feed intake, and poor growth. Depressed immune function as well as reproductive performance are also observed.[71,72] Skin abnormalities generally include hair loss, skin thickening, cracking, and fissuring. Hoof integrity is also affected.

Zinc Toxicosis

Toxicosis is most commonly the result of accidental oversupplementation. Injectable zinc products, highly bioavailable organic or chelated feed grade zinc products, and water-soluble zinc can be associated with zinc toxicosis in cattle. Calves are more susceptible than adult cattle to zinc toxicosis. The clinical signs of zinc toxicosis include diarrhea, anorexia, pica, polyuria, polydipsia, pneumonia, cardiac arrhythmias, and seizures. Pathologic changes associated with toxicosis in calves include diffuse bronchopneumonia, noninflammatory pancreatitis, nephrosis, hepatosis, and adrenal cortical fibrosis.[73] The diagnosis of acute zinc toxicosis can be difficult. Serum and plasma concentrations of zinc are not always repeatable and sensitive. May factors other than dietary zinc affect zinc concentration in plasma and serum. Liver zinc concentrations are more dependable than serum or plasma.

Zinc Status

Determining zinc concentration for an animal is difficult because there is no defined storage pool of zinc in the body. Zinc can be evaluated from liver, reproductive organs (especially the testes), pancreatic tissue, and bone. Liver zinc concentrations do not always correlate with zinc intake, but liver concentrations decrease after short periods of dietary deficiency.

Serum zinc concentrations are decreased in zinc deficiency, but clinical signs such as decreases in feed efficiency may occur before a decline in serum zinc occurs. Decreased feed efficiency in cattle has been seen within 21 days after the introduction of a zinc deficient diet. A decrease in feed efficiency is observed even when serum zinc concentrations are within normal ranges.[74] Low serum zinc is significant but a normal serum zinc concentration does not rule out deficiency. Other factors than a zinc deficiency will influence serum zinc concentration. Low serum zinc can be associated with hypoalbuminemia because about two-thirds of zinc in serum is bound to albumin. Inflammation also results in decreased serum zinc concentrations. Contamination can often cause an elevated serum zinc concentration. If serum is left in contact with the clot for too long, zinc can leach from the red cells increasing serum zinc concentrations. Serum should be separated from the clot within 4 to 6 hours after collection. Rubber stoppers in many blood collection tubes are lubricated with a zinc-containing material so when serum or plasma contacts the rubber stopper there is contamination. The most accurate blood tubes for collection of serum for mineral concentration are royal blue trace mineral tubes.

The measurement of serum alkaline phosphatase activity is an indirect assessment of zinc concentration. Alkaline phosphatase is a zinc dependent enzyme so its serum activity decreases in zinc deficiency. Zinc activity is increased rather than decreased in most disease states.

SUMMARY

A variety of different samples can be tested for mineral content, but may not provide the mineral status of the animal. It is important to involve several animals in production groups when determining mineral status in animals. This evaluation should include a good clinical history, as well as ration and supplementation history. Animal responses to supplementation of minerals is a useful means of evaluating mineral status. Whole blood trace mineral concentrations can be used. Whole blood concentrations of selenium and iodine are useful. Whole blood concentrations of copper, iron, and zinc are not adequate to determine an accurate concentration. Copper, iron, and cobalt liver biopsy samples are more sensitive measures of status than are serum/whole blood concentrations. Care should be taken to use the proper sampling method. The removal of the serum from the clot within 2 hours of sample collection and minimization of hemolysis is critical for an accurate serum sample. Dietary mineral evaluation can be done as well to characterize mineral status. If the trace minerals are found to be adequate in the diet, but the animals are found to be deficient, dietary or drinking water mineral antagonism may be occurring. High sulfur or iron levels are examples of minerals that can cause deficiencies in copper and selenium, even though there are adequate concentrations of the latter in the diet.

DISCLOSURE

The author has nothing to disclose.

REFERENCES

1. Radke SL, Ensley SM, Hansen SL. Inductively coupled plasma mass spectrometry determination of hepatic copper, manganese, selenium, and zinc concentrations in relation to sample amount and storage duration. J Vet Diagn Invest 2020; 32(1):103–7.
2. Pogge D, Richter E, Drewnoski M, et al. Mineral concentrations of plasma and liver after injection with a trace mineral complex differ among Angus and Simmental cattle. J Anim Sci 2012;90:2692–8.
3. Genther O, Hansen S. A multielement trace mineral injection improves liver copper and selenium concentrations and manganese superoxide dismutase activity in beef steers. J Anim Sci 2014;92:695–704.

4. Arthington J, Moriel P, Martins P, et al. Effects of trace mineral injections on measures of performance and trace mineral status of pre-and postweaned beef calves. J Anim Sci 2014;92:2630–40.
5. Suttle N. The mineral nutrition of livestock. 4 edition. London: CABI Publishing; 2010.
6. Laven RA, Livesey CT. An evaluation of the effect of clotting and processing of blood samples on the recovery of copper from bovine blood. Vet J 2006;171: 295–300.
7. Underwood E, Suttle N. The mineral nutrition of livestock. 3rd edition. London: DABI Publishing; 1999.
8. Stabler S. Vitamin B12. In: Bowmann B, Ruseell R, editors. Present knowledge in nutrition. Washington, DC: International Life Sciences Institute; 2006. p. 302–13.
9. Kincaid RL, Socha MT. Effect of cobalt supplementation during late gestation and early lactation on milk and serum measures. J Dairy Sci 2007;90:1880–6.
10. Sutton AL, Elliot JM. Effect of ratio of roughage to concentrate and level of feed intake on ovine ruminal vitamin B 12 production. J Nutr 1972;102:1341–6.
11. Judson GJ, McFarlane JD, Mitsioulis A, et al. Vitamin B12 responses to cobalt pellets in beef cows. Aust Vet J 1997;75:660–2.
12. Somers M, Gawthorne JM. The effect of dietary cobalt intake on the plasma vitamin B 12 concentration of sheep. Aust J Exp Biol Med Sci 1969;47:227–33.
13. Dickson J, Bond MP. Cobalt toxicity in cattle. Aust Vet J 1974;50:236.
14. Stangl GI, Schwarz FJ, Muller H, et al. Evaluation of the cobalt requirement of beef cattle based on vitamin B12, folate, homocysteine and methylmalonic acid. Br J Nutr 2000;84:645–53.
15. Furlong JM, Sedcole JR, Sykes AR. An evaluation of plasma homocysteine in the assessment of vitamin B12 status of pasture-fed sheep. N Z Vet J 2010;58:11–6.
16. Herrmann W, Obeid R, Schorr H, et al. Functional vitamin B12 deficiency and determination of holotranscobalamin in populations at risk. Clin Chem Lab Med 2003;41:1478–88.
17. Zhou Y, Li HL. Determination of vitamin B12 by chemiluminescence analysis. Yao Xue Xue Bao 1989;24:611–7.
18. Kumar SS, Chouhan RS, Thakur MS. Enhancement of chemiluminescence for vitamin B12 analysis. Anal Biochem 2009;388:312–6.
19. Smith CH, Moe AJ, Ganapathy V. Nutrient transport pathways across the epithelium of the placenta. Annu Rev Nutr 1992;12:183–206.
20. Dargatz DA, Garry FB, Clark GB, et al. Serum copper concentrations in beef cows and heifers. J Am Vet Med Assoc 1999;215:1828–32.
21. Corah L, Dargatz DA. Forage analysis from cow/calf herds in 18 states. In: Health A-CfEaH, editor. Ft Collin (CO): USDA; 1996.
22. Council NR. Nutrient requirements of dairy cattle. 7th edition. Washington, DC: National Academy Press; 2001.
23. Graham TW. Trace element deficiencies in cattle. Vet Clin North Am Food Anim Pract 1991;7:153–215.
24. Osweiler G, Carson T, Buck W. Clinical and diagnostic veterinary toxicology. 3 edition. Dubuque (IA): Kendall/Hunt Publishing; 1985.
25. Perrin DJ, Schiefer HB, Blakley BR. Chronic copper toxicity in a dairy herd. Can Vet J 1990;31:629–32.
26. Prohaska J. Copper. In: Bowmann B, Russell R, editors. Present knowledge in nutrition. Washington, DC: International Life Sciences Institute; 2006. p. 458–70.
27. Claypool DW, Adams FW, Pendell HW, et al. Relationship between the level of copper in the blood plasma and liver of cattle. J Anim Sci 1975;41:911–4.

28. Mulryan G, Mason J. Assessment of liver copper status in cattle from plasma copper and plasma copper enzymes. Ann Rech Vet 1992;23:233–8.

29. Bell JM. Nutrients and toxicants in rapeseed meal: a review. J Anim Sci 1984;58: 996–1010.

30. Tripathi M, Mishra A. Glucosinolates in animal nutrition: a review. Anim Feed Sci Technol 2007;132:1–27.

31. Suttle NF. The interactions between copper, molybdenum, and sulphur in ruminant nutrition. Annu Rev Nutr 1991;11:121–40.

32. Harvey J. Iron metabolism and its disorders. 6th edition. Oxford (UK): Elsevier; 2008.

33. Hallberg L, Hulthen L. Prediction of dietary iron absorption: an algorithm for calculating absorption and bioavailability of dietary iron. Am J Clin Nutr 2000; 71:1147–60.

34. Hill C, Matrone G. Chemical parameters in the study of in vivo and in vitro interactions of transition elements. Fed Proc 1970;29:1474–81.

35. Institute of Medicine. Dietary reference intakes for vitamins and minerals. Washington, DC: National Academy Press; 2000.

36. Andrews NC. Anemia of inflammation: the cytokine-hepcidin link. J Clin Invest 2004;113:1251–3.

37. Leach R, Harris D. Manganese. In: O'Dell B, Sunde R, editors. Handbook of nutritionally essential mineral elements. New York: Marcel Dekker; 1997. p. 335–56.

38. Aschner JL, Aschner M. Nutritional aspects of manganese homeostasis. Mol Aspects Med 2005;26:353–62.

39. Keen CL, Ensunsa JL, Clegg MS. Manganese metabolism in animals and humans including the toxicity of manganese. Met Ions Biol Syst 2000;37:89–121.

40. Hansen SL, Spears JW, Lloyd KE, et al. Feeding a low manganese diet to heifers during gestation impairs fetal growth and development. J Dairy Sci 2006;89: 4305–11.

41. Hall J. Appropriate methods of diagnosing mineral deficiencies in cattle. Tri State Dairy Nutrition Conference, Grand Wayne Convention Center, Fort Wayne, Indiana, April 25-26, 2006. p. 43–50.

42. National Research Council. Mineral tolerances of animals. 2nd edition. Washington, DC: National Academy Press; 2005.

43. Hidiroglou M. Manganese in ruminant nutrition. Can J Anim Sci 1979;59:217–36.

44. Masters D, Paynter D, Briegel J. Influence of manganese intake on body wool and testicular growth of young rams and on the concentration of manganese and the activity of manganese enzymes in tissues. Aust J Agric Res 1990;39:517–24.

45. Milne DB, Sims RL, Ralston NV. Manganese content of the cellular components of blood. Clin Chem 1990;36:450–2.

46. Johnson J. Molybdenum. New York: Marcel Dekker Inc; 1997.

47. Williams RJ, Frausto da Silva JJ. The involvement of molybdenum in life. Biochem Biophys Res Commun 2002;292(2):293–9.

48. Williams R, Da Silva JF. The involvement of molybdenum in life. Biochem Biophys Res Commun 2002;292:293–9.

49. Nell JA, Annison EF, Balnave D. The influence of tungsten on the molybdenum status of poultry. Br Poult Sci 1980;21:193–202.

50. Kincaid RL. Assessment of trace mineral status of ruminants: a review. J Anim Sci 2000;77:1–10.

51. Turnlund JR, Keyes WR. Plasma molybdenum reflects dietary molybdenum intake. J Nutr Biochem 2004;15:90–5.

52. Rotruck JT, Pope AL, Ganther HE, et al. Selenium: biochemical role as a component of glutathione peroxidase. Science 1973;179:588–90.
53. Gladyshev VN, Kryukov GV, Fomenko DE, et al. Identification of trace element-containing proteins in genomic databases. Annu Rev Nutr 2004;24:579–96.
54. Brown KM, Arthur JR. Selenium, selenoproteins and human health: a review. Public Health Nutr 2001;4:593–9.
55. Beck MA. Selenium and vitamin E status: impact on viral pathogenicity. J Nutr 2007;137:1338–40.
56. Barceloux DG. Selenium. J Toxicol Clin Toxicol 1999;37:145–72.
57. Vendeland SC, Deagen JT, Butler JA, et al. Uptake of selenite, selenomethionine and selenate by brush border membrane vesicles isolated from rat small intestine. Biometals 1994;7:305–12.
58. Spears JW. Trace mineral bioavailability in ruminants. J Nutr 2003;133:1506s–9s.
59. Arthur JR. Free radicals and diseases of animal muscle. Basel (Switzerland): Birkhauser Verlag; 1998.
60. O'Toole D, Raisbeck MF. Pathology of experimentally induced chronic selenosis (alkali disease) in yearling cattle. J Vet Diagn Invest 1995;7:364–73.
61. Patterson JD, Burris WR, Boling JA, et al. Individual intake of free-choice mineral mix by grazing beef cows may be less than typical formulation assumptions and form of selenium in mineral mix affects blood Se concentrations of cows and their suckling calves. Biol Trace Elem Res 2013;155:38–48.
62. Janghorbani M, Young V. Selenium metabolism in North Americans: studies based on stable isotope tracers. Paper presented at: Third International Symposium on Selenium in Biology and Medicine, held May 27-June 1, 1984, Xiangshan (Fragance Hills) Hotel Beijing, People's Republic of China. pp. 450–71.
63. Ellis RG, Herdt TH, Stowe HD. Physical, hematologic, biochemical, and immunologic effects of supranutritional supplementation with dietary selenium in Holstein cows. Am J Vet Res 1997;58:760–4.
64. Koller LD, South PJ, Exon JH, et al. Comparison of selenium levels and glutathione peroxidase activity in bovine whole blood. Can J Comp Med 1984;48:431–3.
65. McMurry C, Davidson W, Blanchflower W. Factors other than selenium affecting the activity and measurement of erythrocyte glutathione peroxidase. Paper presented at: Selenium in Biology and Medicine, 3rd International Symposium, New York, 1984. pp. 354–9.
66. Van Saun RJ, Herdt TH, Stowe HD. Maternal and fetal selenium concentrations and their interrelationships in dairy cattle. J Nutr 1989;119:1128–37.
67. Maas J, Galey FD, Peauroi JR, et al. The correlation between serum selenium and blood selenium in cattle. J Vet Diagn Invest 1992;4:48–52.
68. Miller GY, Bartlett PC, Erskine RJ, et al. Factors affecting serum selenium and vitamin E concentrations in dairy cows. J Am Vet Med Assoc 1995;206:1369–73.
69. Cousins RJ, Liuzzi JP, Lichten LA. Mammalian zinc transport, trafficking, and signals. J Biol Chem 2006;281:24085–9.
70. White C. The zinc requirements of grazing animals. In: Robson A, editor. Zinc in soils and plants. London: Kluwer Academic Publishers; 1993. p. 197–206.
71. Fraker PJ, King LE. Reprogramming of the immune system during zinc deficiency. Annu Rev Nutr 2004;24:277–98.
72. Nagalakshmi D, Dhanalakshmi K, Himabindu D. Effect of dose and source of supplemental zinc on immune response and oxidative enzymes in lambs. Vet Res Commun 2009;33:631–44.

73. Graham TW, Holmberg CA, Keen CL, et al. A Pathologic and Toxicologic Evaluation of Veal Calves Fed Large Amounts of Zinc. Vet Pathol 1988;25: 484–91.
74. Engle TE, Nockels CF, Kimberling CV, et al. Zinc repletion with organic or inorganic forms of zinc and protein turnover in marginally zinc-deficient calves. J Anim Sci 1997;75(11):3074–81.

Water Quality for Grazing Livestock I

Merl F. Raisbeck, DVM, MS, PhD

KEYWORDS

- Selenium toxicity • Blind staggers • Alkali disease

KEY POINTS

- Water is arguably the most overlooked nutrient in domestic livestock production.
- Water quality is typically measured by analytical procedures which, although very accurate and reproducible, require some judgment to apply to situations in the field.
- Total dissolved solids is a commonly used test in water quality for human use, but is less than useful for livestock use.
- "Hardness" is another test commonly reported in potable water quality analysis, but is better suited to laundry than livestock health.

INTRODUCTION

Water is arguably the single most important nutrient for livestock. It is the most abundant component of the animal body in all phases of growth and development. Animals can survive for a week or more without food, but death is likely in a matter of days without adequate water intake. Water is involved in virtually every physiologic process essential to life: water is the medium in which all chemical reactions in the body take place; blood, which contains more than 80% water, moves oxygen and carbon dioxide to and from the tissues; it distributes nutrients, wastes, and chemical signals throughout the body; it provides the chemical base for nutrient digestion within, and uptake from, the gastrointestinal (GI) tract. Owing to water's high specific heat, it compromises an ideal temperature buffering system for the body. Restricted water intake lowers feed intake and nitrogen (ie, protein) retention, and it increases nitrogen loss in the feces. Animals may survive a loss of nearly all the fat and about one-half of bodily protein, but a loss of about one-tenth of body water results in death.

Obviously, an adequate supply of clean water is essential to the health of all animals. Under most livestock management systems, water is the cheapest and most readily available nutrient. Unfortunately, and probably because of this fact, it is also the most overlooked nutrient. Sources of dietary water include wells or surface runoff,

Department of Veterinary Sciences, College of Agriculture, University of Wyoming, 2852 Riverside, Laramie, WY 82070, USA
E-mail address: raisbeck@uwyo.edu

Vet Clin Food Anim 36 (2020) 547–579
https://doi.org/10.1016/j.cvfa.2020.08.014
0749-0720/20/© 2020 Elsevier Inc. All rights reserved.

water contained in feedstuffs (lush grass may consist of as much as 75% water), and metabolic water obtained from the oxidation of fat and protein in the body. In the arid Western United States, good quality water is a scarce commodity, and livestock are often forced to survive on what might be charitably described as less than perfect water owing to competition from urbanization, mineral extraction, and so on. In most cases, these animals do surprisingly well, but poor quality water has resulted in acute illness and death. Poor quality water also robs producers via decreased performance (growth, reproduction).

Water consumption is influenced by many factors, including genetics (species or breed), age, body size, ambient temperature and humidity, water temperature, and production level. For example, cattle (a species that has been studied extensively) consume an average of 2 to 4 L of water for each kg of dry matter consumed and an additional 3 to 5 L of water per kg of milk produced; however, this average varies dramatically with temperature, especially when the environmental temperature exceeds the thermoneutral range. For example, a 273-kg (600 lb) feeder steer drinks 22.7 L at 5°C or below; at 21°C (70°F), he needs 33 L but at 30°C (roughly 86°F) he requires 54 L or 20% of his body weight (BW) per day.[1] At 39°C (roughly 102°F), he would require 116 L.[2] Rations high in sodium, fiber, or protein also increase water requirements.[3,4] For example, horses consume twice as much water while on a hay diet compared with a high concentrate diet at the same temperature.[5] A lactating beef cow requires nearly twice as much water (64 L or about 16% of her BW) per day at 21°C as the same cow (32.9 L, 9% BW) when dry at the same temperature, and a high-producing dairy cow of similar size needs 90 L, or nearly 20% of her BW under the same conditions.[3,6,7]

The amount (dose) of any water-borne toxicant ingested by a given animal is determined both by the concentration of the substance in water and by the amount of water the animal drinks. Water intake is technically defined as free drinking water plus the amount contained in feedstuffs; however, for purposes of simplicity, I have assumed animals are consuming air-dried hay or senescent forage with a minimal (10%) water content and use the term "intake" to describe the amount of water consumed voluntarily by animals from streams, ponds, wells, and so on.

The amount an animal drinks is determined by true thirst and appetite. By definition, true thirst is the physiologic drive to consume sufficient water to meet minimum metabolic needs; however, most animals also exhibit an appetite for water and consume more than is strictly necessarily to satisfy true thirst.[8] Reasons for the latter are many, varied, and do not lend themselves to quantitative prediction. I therefore disregarded appetite in calculating doses from water intake, but instead used conservative estimates of thirst in such calculations by disregarding forage water content. Most calculations of potential toxic doses in the table at the end of this article are thus based on 273-kg (600-lb) feeder cattle that drink approximately 20% of their BW, or about 8 L/kg of dietary dry matter, per day, at 32°C (90°F). This amount may not provide adequate protection for high-producing dairy cattle or in especially high environmental temperatures, but is a reasonably conservative for range livestock (beef and sheep) and weather conditions typical of the North American high plains. Although I make note of data related to swine, virtually all modern swine are raised in intensive operations that draw water from systems (municipal, water district, etc) that are maintained according to human standards. Similarly, alternative agricultural species such as llamas and bison are not included, in part because of a scarcity of data.

Water quality is commonly evaluated by chemical methods that are designed to be very reproducible and very specific. As a result, the process of analyzing water is straightforward, and many tests are readily available commercially. Unfortunately, translating these very precise, formal, data to practical recommendations for livestock is less cut and dried. As noted by Dr Art Case, the dean of veterinary toxicologists, "sometimes the cow just didn't read the book." First, many toxicants in water act additively with the same toxicant in feedstuffs. In most such cases, the bottom line is not necessarily the concentration in water, but rather the total milligrams of toxicant ingested per kilogram of the animal's BW (commonly expressed as "mg x/kg BW"). In such cases, the recommendations in this article must be adjusted in light of the particular situation at hand.

Second, chemical water quality tests do not usually measure the specific chemical form of the toxicant present. For example, selenium as selenite or selenate behaves quite differently in the mammalian body than does selenomethionine, but the typical laboratory just reports total selenium. The recommendations are based on the chemical form most likely to be present in typical surface waters and noted any caveats that should be considered if the water source is not typical. In the absence of other data, I have assumed the free ion in water is equivalent on a milligram per kilogram of BW basis to the same chemical in feedstuffs.

Third, typical chemical tests do not differentiate between animal species. For example, some substances are more toxic in ruminants than monogastrics as a result of their unique physiology, whereas some are less. For simplicity's sake, recommendations are based on the most sensitive of the common agricultural species.

Fourth, many toxic substances interact with other toxicants and/or nutrients in the diet. I have tried to enumerate such interactions in the narrative if they are well-documented and, where possible, account for them in the bottom line calculations of acceptable water concentrations.

Finally, the rate of exposure influences the potency of many toxicants. A bolus dose of nitrate (NO_3), given via a stomach tube, is much more toxic than the same amount spread over an entire day's grazing. Under summer range conditions typical of the Great Plains, livestock drink once, or, at most, twice a day. I have, therefore, assumed all the water-borne daily dose of a given substance will be consumed during a fairly short period, once or twice a day.

Water quality constituents in this report were drawn from common water quality guidelines, prioritized according to how closely, in the author's experience, existing rangeland concentrations approached these guidelines. For example, mercury is much more toxic than many of the elements listed, but it is rarely present at detectable concentrations typical livestock water. Copper is a real problem in aquatic organisms, but copper deficiency is a much bigger problem in livestock than copper toxicity.

As noted elsewhere in this article, the interaction of water quality and animal health is considerably more complex than just x milligrams of y per liter of water. For example, many factors have been suggested to influence the palatability of water for animals. Decreased consumption owing to bad taste is potentially just as harmful as water deprivation,[4] yet the state of the art regarding palatability remains largely qualitative and anecdotal. Acid pH may mobilize toxic metals from plumbing or soil, but the particular effect of a given pH is obviously very dependent on the local situation.

Safety margins are often more a matter of judgment rather than purely objective calculations. The purpose of safety margins is to compensate for unknown, or unknowable, variables in toxicology data such as genetic variability, sex, life stage, duration of exposure, unforeseen interactions with other toxicants, and so on. The standard practice in setting human drinking water standards for noncarcinogens has been to divide the geometric mean of the no observed adverse effect level (NOAEL) and the minimum toxic dose by 10 to 1000 depending on the quality of the data. Another approach used in the past has been to set the safe limit at the upper end of the range commonly reported in natural waters where no adverse effects have been noted.

Both approaches, although unarguably safe, ignore the realities of livestock production. Water that is so perfect as to meet these theoretically desirable criteria has already been taken for other uses. In this article, I have taken the approach of presenting my best estimate of the no observed adverse effect level (ie, will not produce any measurable decrease in performance in the most sensitive class of animal) under a very conservative set of assumptions appropriate to rangelands and allowing the reader to make his or her own judgment regarding safety margins based on the narrative included.

Although there are many ways of expressing measurements regarding water quality and toxicology, I have used the following conventions. The dose of a toxicant that causes some effect is expressed in milligrams of substance per kilogram of BW or (mg x/kg BW). The concentration of a substance in water is expressed as milligrams of substance per liter of water or mg x/L. If the substance is ionized, and the ion is important in terms of its toxic effects, it will be described with the standard scientific abbreviation for the ion, for example, NO_3^-. Similarly, the concentration of a toxicant occurring in dry feedstuffs is described in terms of parts per million (ppm) dry matter.

NITRATE AND NITRITE

The nitrate (NO_3^-) and nitrite (NO_2^-) ions are intermediates in the biological nitrification cycle and the primary source of nitrogen for plants from the soil. Plants accumulate NO_3^- from soil to synthesize protein via a multistep process; excessive NO_3^- accumulation as a result of this process may cause poisoning of grazing animals.[9] Nitrate or NO_2^- may contaminate water as a result of contact with natural minerals, agricultural runoff (fertilizer, manure) or industrial processes.[9–11] Nitrate is the more stable of the two and therefore more common in surface waters.[12] Nitrite usually results from biological reduction of NO_3^-, but it may also be an industrial contaminant or exist in ground waters where pH and redox potential prevent oxidation to NO_3^-.[13] Both ions are extremely water soluble and therefore water mobile.

Although the NO_3^- ion is readily absorbed in the upper GI tract and possesses intrinsic toxicologic properties such as vasodilation, the condition referred to as nitrate poisoning actually depends on reduction of NO_3^- to NO_2^- in the upper GI tract.[9,14–16] This process may occur in human infants,[17,18] and, as such, is the basis of current human drinking water standards, but nitrate toxicity is primarily a problem in ruminant species whose rumen microflora are well-suited to reduce NO_3^-. Radiotracer studies indicate that NO_2^-, formed from NO_3^- in the rumen, may either be further reduced and incorporated via NH_3^+ into amino acids or reduced via nitric oxide to nitrogen and exhaled.[19] Unfortunately, neither of these pathways is as fast as the initial reduction to NO_2^-, and dangerous NO_2^- concentrations accumulate in the GI tract when assimilatory pathways are overloaded.[19–21] Under the proper dietary conditions (mainly adequate carbohydrates), the assimilatory pathways can adapt to high NO_3^- concentrations, and very little NO_3^- or NO_2^- escape the rumen.[10,20,22–25] Sustained exposure to moderately high NO_3^- diets results in induction of the assimilatory pathways, and this ability may be acquired by transfer of GI flora from one ruminant to another.[20,21] Once absorbed into the bloodstream, the NO_3^- ion is rapidly distributed throughout the body water and excreted via urine and saliva, whereas the NO_2^- ion is oxidized to NO_3^- via a coupled reaction with hemoglobin and eliminated as NO_3^-.[14,16,26,27]

Other differences between ruminants and monogastrics in the metabolism of the NO_2^- and NO_3^- ions, although not directly tied to the ruminal metabolism of NO_3^-, probably reflect evolutionary pressure of the constant background of NO_2^- ruminants receive from ruminal metabolism. The blood half-life of NO_2^- is similar in monogastrics and ruminants, but the elimination of NO_3^- from blood is much slower in monogastrics[16] and the normal background methemoglobin concentration is higher in monogastrics.[28] In ruminants, only a small portion of an oral dose of NO_3^- is eliminated in the urine, whereas in monogastrics most ingested NO_3^- is eliminated via urine.[10]

Some sources suggest the NO_3^- ion is more bioavailable in water than feedstuffs.[9–11] The experiments this conclusion was drawn from, however, were based on aqueous NO_3^- administered directly into the stomach versus contaminated feedstuffs offered ad *libitum*.[10] The most important determinant of NO_3^- toxicity seems to be how rapidly a given dose of NO_3^- is administered, rather than whether it is in feed or water.[10,29,30] For example, the single oral median lethal dose of $NaNO_3$ in cows was reported to be 328 mg/kg BW when given at once, but when the same dose was spread over 24 hours, the median lethal increased to 707 to 991 mg/kg.[30]

Although the most common source of NO_3^- poisoning in livestock is contaminated feedstuffs, NO_3^--contaminated drinking water has poisoned people and animals.[18,31–33] The mechanism of poisoning involves GI microbial reduction of the NO_3^- ion to NO_2^-, which is absorbed into the bloodstream where it oxidizes the ferrous iron atoms (Fe^{2+}) in hemoglobin to the ferric (Fe^{3+}) state, resulting in methemoglobin, which cannot transport oxygen from the lungs to the rest of the body. The exact mechanism by which hemoglobin is oxidized is the subject of some controversy, but it is currently thought to be a multistep autocatalytic process involving several free radicals.[27] The product of this reaction is NO_3^-, which is eliminated via urine and saliva. As might be expected, the clinical signs of acute NO_3 poisoning (cyanosis, hyperpnea, muscle tremor, weakness, collapse, and death) reflect the effects of anoxia on critical organs such as the brain and heart. Pregnant animals that survive episodes of acute NO_3 poisoning during the latter part of pregnancy may abort within 1 to 2 weeks.[32,34–37] Poisoning during earlier pregnancy does not usually result in abortion.[11,30,32,38]

Textbooks suggest that NO_3 is approximately 10-fold more toxic in ruminants than monogastric animals.[15] Burwash and colleagues[39] fed 6 mares high NO_3 (1.7%–1.85%) oat hay for 13 days. Although the serum NO_3^- concentration increased significantly, there was no change in methemoglobin concentration, no effects on blood chemistry parameters, and no clinical signs of poisoning. They concluded it is safe to feed horses diets containing 2% NO_3 and "likely much higher" concentrations. Mice exposed to drinking water containing 1000 mg NO_3^-/L for 18 months excreted more ammonium ion than controls early in the study, but did not show any signs of poisoning.[40] Seerley and colleagues[41] fed water containing 1465, 2900, or 4400 mg NO_3^-/L as $NaNO_3$ to weanling pigs for 84 days with no effect on the rate of gain, water consumption, or clinical signs of toxicity. The difference in toxicity between animal species is not nearly as pronounced for NO_2^-.[15] Although rare, monogastric animals have been acutely poisoned by the NO_2^- ion from water[42] and feedstuffs.[43]

Wright and Davison[44] reviewed the literature and concluded the median lethal dose of NO_3 in ruminants was between 700 to 985 mg NO_3/kg BW when fed as dry feed. Experimentally, sheep have been acutely poisoned by NO_3 doses as low as 300 mg/kg BW[21,23,26,45]; however, doses as large as 800 mg/kg BW have been fed without measurable effects.[21,24,25,34,45,46] Field reports have incriminated feedstuffs containing as little as 2% ppm dietary NO_3 (which would provide about 500 mg NO_3/kg BW) as causing acute lethality in sheep.[47,48] Experimentally, 3.4% dietary NO_3, fed as pigweed or oat hay killed 2 of 5 ewes. The lethal dosages, calculated from consumption data, were 660 and 730 mg NO_3/kg BW, respectively. Campagnolo and colleagues[49] reported the accidental poisoning of several animals, including sheep, by water containing 6000 mg NO_3^-/L at a county fair; however, the water contained several other substances that might also have been toxic.

Cattle have been experimentally poisoned by as little as 520 mg/kg BW NO_3 incorporated into feedstuffs,[38,44,50,51] and as little as 200 mg/kg BW may be toxic if given by gavage.[52] Several investigators[22,53,54] consistently produced sublethal toxicity with 200 to 300 mg NO_3/kg BW to test various protective strategies. Other investigators[20,55,56] failed to demonstrate toxicity at dietary concentrations as high as 0.9% (approximately 225 mg NO_3/kg BW), although one[20] reported that sustained exposure enhanced the ability of the rumen microflora to degrade NO_3^- and NO_2^-. Calves were experimentally poisoned by drinking water containing 2500 mg NO_3^-/L (250 mg/kg BW), but none were affected by 2000 mg/L or less.[35] Older texts and reviews variously describe the minimum toxic dose in cattle as 169 to 500 mg NO_3/kg BW.[11,15,57]

There are numerous anecdotal reports of acute NO_3 poisoning in cattle associated with contaminated feedstuffs. O'Hara and Fraser[58] summarized 10 episodes of acute NO_3 poisoning in New Zealand in which mortality varied from less than 1% to almost 50%. Forage concentrations associated with these cases ranged from 0.3% to 5.3% NO_3 (mean, 3.3%) with variations of 1% to 2% NO_3 between samples from the same premise. In 1 extensively investigated case, 23 of 50 calves turned into a ryegrass pasture containing 6.6% to 8.9% KNO_3 (4.0%–5.3% NO_3) died within a 12-hour period.[58] In another instance, calves died if left on a ryegrass pasture containing 3.6% NO_3 for more than 1 hour.[59] A dose of NO_3, later calculated to be 170 mg NO_3/kg BW, from contaminated hay, killed 7 of 200 heifers. The herdsman tried to dilute the toxic hay in half and killed 7 more.[60] The authors speculated that concurrent overfeeding of monensin enhanced ruminal reduction of NO_3^- to NO_2^-, thus potentiating the toxicity of the hay. Harris and Rhodes,[61] summarizing the experience of farmers during a severe drought in Victoria, Australia, reported several hundred animals were killed by plants containing "over 1.5% NO_3." Three cows fed hay containing 1% NO_3 died within 30 minutes.[51] Eleven cows aborted, and 73 of 153 died when fed sudax hay containing 1.1% to 3.1% NO_3.[62] McKenzie and associates[47] summarized several cases with acute mortalities of 16% to 44% on button grass (2.4%–7.2% NO_3) grown in nitrogen-rich soil in Queensland, Australia. Animals grazing the same grass in adjacent paddocks without the extra nitrogen were unaffected.

Although not as common as poisoning from feedstuffs, contaminated water has resulted in acute poisoning, including abortions and death. Seven of 12 cows died shortly after drinking water containing 2790 mg NO_3^-/L.[31] Several authors reported lethality as a result of fertilizer-contaminated water (1000–6000 mg NO_3^-/L).[32,49,63] Contaminated liquid whey, fed in addition to water and containing 2200 to 2800 mg NO_3^-/L, killed 17 of 360 cattle. Whey containing only 400 to 800 mg NO_3^-/L did not kill any animals, but it did result in 26 of 140 cows aborting.[32] Yong and colleagues[33] reported that water, contaminated with 4800 and 7000 mg NO_3^-/L as a result of blasting water holes, killed 16 of 100 and 4 of 90 cows in 2 separate incidents in Saskatchewan, Canada.

It is known the NO_2^- ion may react with secondary amines (common in many foodstuffs) under conditions typical of the adult human stomach (pH 1–4) to form nitrosamines.[64,65] Many nitrosamines are potent animal mutagens and carcinogens. Bacterial reduction of NO_3^- to NO_2^- does not occur under the acidic conditions necessary for nitrosamine production, or vice versa. This finding, together with the fact most herbivores have GI conditions that are relatively alkaline, suggests that cancer is not a likely sequela of NO_3 exposure in our species of interest. Elevated NO_2^- is a potential acute toxic hazard, however. Four of 4 sows were killed by drinking 1940 mg NO_2^-/L water.[42] Nitrite is reported to be 2.5 times more toxic than NO_3 in ruminants and 10 times more in monogastrics,[15] and the minimum toxic dose is reportedly between 20 and 90 mg NO_2^-/kg BW in pigs and between 90 and 170 mg NO_2^-/kg in cattle and sheep.[11,57]

Chronic NO_3 poisoning is an area of controversy. Mice exposed to 1000 mg NO_3^-/L in drinking water for 18 months (lifetime) died prematurely starting at 17.5 months. The result was of only marginal statistical significance, and no possible mechanism for the result was proposed.[40] Mice exposed to 100 mg NO_3^-/L showed no effects in any parameter measured (liver function, kidney function, serum protein, etc). Seerley and colleagues[41] fed breeding gilts $NaNO_3$ in water to provide 1320 mg NO_3^-/L for 105 days with no effect. Similar results were reported for weanling pigs.[66,67] Fan and colleagues[68] reviewed the veterinary literature on chronic NO_3 toxicity and concluded it "failed to provide evidence for teratogenic effects attributable to NO_3 or NO_2 ingestion." Bruning-Fann and colleagues[69] surveyed water from 712 swine operations in the United States and found no differences in litter size or piglet mortality attributable to well-water containing NO_3^- (1–443 mg/L).

After a widespread drought in the American Midwest in the mid-1950s, several authors summarized the experience of multiple field investigations.[68,70,71] Purportedly, feed concentrations with more than 0.5% NO_3 or water supplies containing more than 500 mg NO_3^-/L were hazardous to cattle fed poor quality rations. Other nutritional factors were not accounted for. Case[70] was first to propose that NO_3 interfered with vitamin A metabolism. The results of many controlled experiments since then have rendered this theory questionable.[9] Sheep fed 2.5% $NaNO_3$ (approximately 1.75% NO_3) diets for 135 days had slightly lower liver vitamin A concentrations than controls, and gains were depressed. A second replicate of the same experiment did not exhibit decreased vitamin A nor was there an increase in methemoglobin or signs of toxicity in either group.[46] Fourteen yearling steers were treated with various combinations of NO_3^- in drinking water, NO_2^- in drinking water, Escherichia coli, and a "thyroid depressant." Creative use of statistics demonstrated depressed carotene use, but there were no other effects. In contrast, heifers fed various amounts of NO_3 up to 0.9% NO_3 in diets containing 20% or 40% concentrate did not exhibit any difference from controls in carotene conversion or hepatic retinol concentrations.[55] Feedlot cattle fed 0.81% dietary NO_3 as $NaNO_3$ exhibited poor gains as a result of decreased feed consumption. Gains were not improved by supplementing with 12,000 IU vitamin A.[56] Emerick[72] reviewed the literature and concluded that chronic effects involving vitamin A, thyroid function, and other hypothetical chronic mechanisms only occurred at doses that were nearly lethal owing to methemoglobin formation.

Winter and Hokanson[73] fed varying amounts of NO_3 (330–690 mg/kg BW) to dairy heifers as part of their ration to maintain methemoglobin levels at either 25% to 30% or 50% for the last 6 months of pregnancy. One animal aborted, possibly as a result of NO_3 intoxication, and 2 died of acute poisoning after a diet change, but no chronic effects could be ascertained. Crowley and colleagues,[29] in what to date has been the most rigorous experimental attempt to produce chronic NO_3 poisoning in dairy cattle, fed high NO_3^- water (384 mg NO_3^-/L) for 35 months with no effects on conception rate, twinning, stillbirths, abortions, retained placenta, or a variety of production parameters. The only statistically significant effect was a slightly lower first-service conception rate in the NO_3-treated group. The authors concluded that, in a herd fed a balanced ration, "water containing up to 400 ppm NO_3 should not cause any serious problems."[29] Ensley[74] attempted an epidemiologic approach to the question of high NO_3 water for dairy cattle. In a survey of 128 Iowa dairies with water concentrations from 1 to 300 mg NO_3^-/L, he found water NO_3 concentrations positively correlated with services per conception, which agrees with the results of Crowley and colleagues,[29] but several other potentially confounding factors such as the size of the farm and other contaminants in the water were also positively correlated with NO_3 concentrations.

Other attempts to produce chronic NO_3 poisoning in ruminants have been unsuccessful. Sinclair and Jones[24] dosed ewes with 15 g KNO_3 (similar to 1.5% in forage) for 2 months and then sprayed the same dose of NO_3 on the daily hay ration for another 7 weeks. Ewes were fed diets containing 0.2% to 2.6% NO_3 as $NaNO_3$ or from natural sources for 12 weeks with no measurable effects on health or pregnancy.[34] Despite elevated serum NO_3^- concentrations, there were no effects on methemoglobin, body condition, or reproduction in the treated group. Whethers fed $NaNO_3$ in drinking water to provide 1465, 2900, or 4400 mg NO_3^-/L for 84 days did not differ from controls in gain or water consumption, and only modest increases in methemoglobin concentrations were seen at the highest dose.[41] Feeder lambs fed 3.2% dietary KNO_3 (1.9% NO_3) until slaughter differed from controls only in "carcass quality."[25] Emerick[72] reviewed the literature in 1974 and concluded that feeds containing less than 0.44% NO_3 and water with less than 440 mg NO_3^-/L were "well within a safe range for all classes of livestock."

There is no question that NO_3 contamination of drinking water can result in acute death and/or abortion in ruminant livestock. Cattle are usually reported to be more susceptible than sheep, with monogastrics such as horses and swine being relatively resistant.

The chronic toxicity of very low doses of NO_3 is controversial. Despite repeated attempts (and failures) to reproduce vitamin A deficiency, hypothyroidism, or purported forms of chronic NO_3 toxicity, experimentally it does not seem that dietary concentrations significantly less than those required for acute intoxication cause measurable ill effects in domestic ruminants. Although there is no question NO_3 can produce abortions in ruminants, the dose required seems to be very near that required for acute toxicity. The most scientifically rigorous examination of chronic NO_3 toxicity to date[29] concluded that water concentrations of less than 400 mg/L (the concentration tested) should not pose any hazard to a well-managed herd.

The lowest toxic dose of NO_3 in cattle in the experimental studies reviewed is somewhat less than 200 mg NO_3^-/kg BW, although there were several experiments that failed to produce any effect at considerably higher (as much as 800 mg/kg BW) doses. Clinical (ie, anecdotal) reports, in particular those of Yeruham and colleagues[32] and Slenning and colleagues,[60] push the minimum toxic dose down to near 100 mg NO_3/kg BW, but there are some uncertainties associated with these 2 reports. Yeruham and colleagues[32] did not specify the amount of toxic whey consumed (we assumed 20% BW when figuring a dose as it occurred in a hot climate), and there was a 2-fold variation in analytical results between samples. Slenning and colleagues[60] suggested other factors, notably overfeeding an ionophore, might have potentiated the toxicity of NO_3. The next lowest concentration reported to be acutely toxic was 1% NO_3 in Chenopodium hay, which would provide approximately 250 mg NO_3/kg BW in cattle under the assumptions outlined in the introduction. Nitrate in water is additive with NO_3 in feedstuffs, with a given dose in water being somewhat more potent than in feed because it is consumed more rapidly.

Assuming negligible forage NO_3 concentrations, a water NO_3 concentration of 500 mg NO_3^-/L (measured as NO_3^- ion) would provide a dose of 100 mg/kg BW, which is still 2- to 3-fold below the 200 to 250 mg/kg BW toxic dose. If forage concentrations are higher (not a rare occurrence in the Great Plains), the permissible water concentration should be adjusted downward.

The NO_2^- ion is commonly described as approximately 2.5-fold more toxic than the NO_3^- ion in ruminants (10-fold more toxic in monogastrics), which implies a safe threshold of about 200 mg/L. We were, however, unable to find sufficient experimental studies or well-documented field investigations upon which to base any conclusion about maximum safe concentrations. This is probably owing to the fact NO_3^- is the more stable form of the 2 in surface waters and feedstuffs, and NO_2^- is only rarely present in negligible concentrations. Garner[57] describes the minimum lethal dose of NO_2 in swine (the most sensitive species) as 40 mg/kg BW, which translates to 200 mg NO_2^-/L in drinking water under very conservative assumptions. Intravenous administration (the most potent route of exposure for most toxicants) of 12 mg NO_2^-/kg BW to cattle and 17.6 mg NO_2^-/kg BW to sheep did not produce any reported toxic effects.

Obviously, this is an area that needs further research, but, based upon the existing knowledge base, 100 mg NO_2^-/L (as the nitrite ion) should not cause poisoning in livestock.

SULFUR

Sulfur occurs in nature as free sulfur or combined with other elements as sulfides and sulfates. The most common form in water is the sulfate (SO_4^{2-}) ion, although some sulfurous wells may contain relatively high concentrations of dissolved sulfides. Sulfide concentrations do not persist for long under surface conditions, but may contribute to health problems while they are present. Sulfides in igneous and sedimentary rock are oxidized to sulfate (SO_4) during the weathering process. The resulting sulfate salts are leached from soils by runoff and may be concentrated by evaporation in playas. Some aquifers are naturally very high in SO_4^{2-}. Once SO_4^{2-} is dissolved in water, it is extremely difficult to remove. Under anerobic conditions, SO_4^{2-} may be reduced to sulfide by anaerobic organisms and precipitated in sediments, released as hydrogen sulfide (H_2S) or incorporated into organic matter.[75] Reverse osmosis, distillation, and ion exchange may be used to remove SO_4^{2-} from water; however, none of these processes is cost effective for livestock production under normal conditions. Sulfur may also be present in organic compounds synthesized by aquatic biota; however, this form is usually a relatively minor component of the total water sulfur content. In 1997, 11.5% of 454 forage/water pairs collected from around the United States yielded dietary sulfur concentrations potentially hazardous for cattle. Thirty-seven percent of these elevated pairs originated from the Western United States.[76]

Sulfur is essential for health and, in fact, comprises about 0.15% of the total body in mammals as a constituent of the amino acids methionine, cysteine, cystine, homocysteine, cystathionine, taurine, and cysteic acid. It is also a component of biotin, thiamin, estrogens, ergothionine, fibrinogen, heparin, chondroitin, glutathione, coenzyme A, and lipoic acid.[77] Calves deprived of dietary sulfur had smaller livers, spleens, and testes, and larger brains and adrenals than controls.[77] Lactating dairy cows require between 0.17% and 0.20% total dietary sulfur to remain in positive balance, because sulfur constitutes an estimated 0.78% of milk proteins.[78] The nutritional sulfur requirement of monogastrics must be provided as 2 amino acids—methionine and cystine. Ruminants can use either preformed amino acids or synthesize sulfur amino acids from inorganic sulfur; however, the efficiency of the latter process varies with other dietary conditions.[79–81]

The first step in ruminal synthesis of sulfur amino acids from inorganic sulfur is reduction of the latter to H_2S.[82] Not surprisingly, SO_4 is converted to H_2S more efficiently than preformed sulfur amino acids. Halverson and colleagues[83] examined sulfide production from various sulfur sources and found methionine produced only one-third as much sulfide as an equivalent amount of SO_4. Under normal circumstances, the reactive sulfide ion is combined with carbon by rumen microflora to create methionine, homocysteine, cystathionine, cysteine, and other sulfur amino acids. Under conditions of excessive sulfur intake, however, some of the very toxic gas escapes from the rumen into the systemic circulation resulting in poisoning.[84–87]

Excess rumen sulfide may also interact with certain trace elements, especially copper, decreasing bioavailability and result in serious nutritional deficiencies.[88–91] In ruminants, sulfur combines with molybdenum to form thiomolybdates. These, in turn, form unabsorbable complexes with copper, resulting in copper deficiency.[91] It has also been proposed that thiomolybdates interfere postabsorptively with copper incorporation into the enzymes superoxide dismutase and cytochrome oxidase, compromising mitochondrial integrity and cell function.[91–93] Of the 3 elements, copper, molybdenum, and sulfur, sulfur provides the most variation in nutritional outcomes owing to its multiplicity of metabolic pathways from the rumen. Sulfur exits the rumen principally as sulfide, but it can also leave as undegraded protein sulfur or be incorporated into microbial protein.

Dietary sulfur may also antagonize copper metabolism in the absence of excessive molybdenum. Copper deficiencies occurred in cattle fed 0.3% total dietary sulfur,[93] and 500 mg sulfur/L water was hypothesized to cause secondary deficiency as it raised dietary sulfur to 0.35%, both in the absence of excess molybdenum.[92] Sulfur inhibits the uptake of zinc. The interaction between zinc and sulfur is further magnified if animals are fed a high-fiber diet.[90] Sulfur also decreases the uptake of dietary selenium.[94,95] High dietary concentrations of sulfur are thought to reduce rumen pH, favoring the conversion of selenium to biologically unavailable selenide.[95,96] Sulfur may also reduce incorporation of dietary selenium into ruminal bacterial protein.[97] Interestingly, sulfur has been shown to protect against selenium intoxication under some circumstances.[95,98]

Monogastrics lack the ability to produce sulfur amino acids from inorganic sulfur and are thus somewhat less sensitive to the above-mentioned toxic effects of the sulfide ion. For example, the National Research Council (NRC) "maximum tolerable" sulfur concentration for range cattle is 0.5%, whereas 0.69% of diet is optimal in rats.[77] Although it is possible for a monogastric to generate toxic concentrations of H_2S after ingestion of elemental sulfur, the dosage required is much greater than in ruminants. To illustrate this, 14 horses mistakenly fed between 0.2 and 0.4 kg of flowers of sulfur (99% sulfur) resulting in a dose between 333 to 666 mg/kg BW (corresponds with 11%–22% dietary dry matter). The horses became ill within 12 hours, and 2 died after 48 hours. Post mortem examination of the 2 deceased animals revealed cranioventral consolidation of the lungs, hemorrhaging throughout the heart and GI tract, and liver congestion.[99] The toxic effect(s) of inorganic sulfur salts (eg, SO_4) in monogastric species are owing to abnormalities in water balance in the GI tract, explaining why clinical signs of toxicity differ between monogastric and ruminant mammals. In swine, SO_4 toxicity is generally manifested as watery feces and have been shown to occur when ingesting water with concentrations as low as 600 mg SO_4^{2-}/L, but more commonly require 1600 mg SO_4/L or higher.[100–102]

As with all poisons, sulfur toxicity depends on the dose, route of exposure, and the form of the element. In this article, we are most interested in ingestion (oral exposure) and SO_4^{2-}, because that is the form of sulfur commonly found dissolved in water. Between 0.3% and 0.5% of dietary dry matter is the recommended maximum tolerable limit for total daily sulfur intake for ruminant animals.[77] The amount of sulfur that water contributes to the diet total depends on the amount of water an animal drinks as well as the concentration of sulfur in the water. The former varies dramatically with environmental temperature, type of feed, and condition of the animal. In 1 published example, the amount of dietary sulfur contributed by 1000 mg SO_4^{2-}/L in drinking water varied from 0.1% to 0.27% under different environmental conditions.[103]

Toxic sulfur concentrations have been shown to reduce the feed intake, water intake, growth, and performance of animals. Cattle given water containing 1219 mg SO_4^{2-}/L in conjunction with a diet containing 0.16% sulfur (0.29% total sulfur intake), exhibited depressed dry matter intake.[104] Adding 0.72% SO_4 (0.24% dietary sulfur) to cattle diets reduced weight gains by 50% after the first 2 weeks.[105] Concentrations of 0.35% or more dietary sulfur resulted in diminished dry matter intake in lactating dairy cows.[78] Water containing 5000 mg sodium sulfate (Na_2SO_4)/L and grass hay containing "0.75% SO_4" decreased cattle's water intake by 35% and feed intake by 30%.[106] Decreases in average daily gain, feed efficiency, and dietary net energy were seen when heifers were fed 0.25% sulfur as ammonium sulfate (($NH_4)_2SO_4$).[104] Supplying heifers with water containing 2814 mg SO_4/L and hay containing "0.55% SO_4" reduced hay intake by 12.4% during the summer months.[107] Water containing 3087 mg SO_4/L decreased the average daily gain by 27%, dry matter intake by 6.2%, and water intake by 6.1 L in steers, and it increased the incidence of polioencephalomalacia (PEM).[108] Cattle on a low plane of nutrition decreased their water intake when consuming water with 1000 mg SO_4/L, and cattle on a high plane of nutrition had a slight decrease in feed intake when consuming 2000 mg SO_4/L.[109] Concentrations of sulfur greater than 0.4%, added as elemental sulfur or Na_2SO_4, decreased gains in feeder lambs.[79] Approximately 0.5% sulfur added to rations as calcium sulfate ($CaSO_4$) or Na_2SO_4 resulted in decreased feed intake and daily gains of 163 g/d and 191 g/d, respectively, compared with control lambs that gained 251 g/d[110]

In contrast, 0.75% sulfur added as $CaSO_4$ to the concentrate portion of the diet (0.477% total dietary sulfur) of 6 Hereford cattle, caused no changes in serum enzyme activity, tissue selenium concentrations, weight gains, or general health.[111] The study, however, was designed to look at sulfur–selenium interactions and lacked statistical power to examine growth, average daily gain, or other measures of performance, and one of the animals died of PEM by the end of the experiment. Cattle offered water containing 2500 mg SO_4/L showed no changes in feed or water consumption. The animals consumed an average of 3.9 kg of hay, 3.1 kg concentrate, and 33.1 kg water per day, leading the authors to suggest this level as a safe tolerable limit.[107] As with the previous study, the number of animals tested was very small. Sublimed sulfur added to the diet of steers for 10 weeks at 0.42% did not affect feed intake but did at 0.98%.[112] Qi and colleagues[113] added various amounts of $CaSO_4$ to the diet of goats and concluded that optimum feed performance occurred between 0.2% to 0.28% sulfur. Pendlum and colleagues[114] fed up to 0.3% elemental sulfur to steers without adverse effects.

The most dramatic manifestations of sulfur toxicity in ruminants are sudden death, with no lesions, and/or PEM. PEM is a neurologic disease of cattle and sheep, manifested as seizures, ataxia, blindness, and recumbency. It is usually fatal. Seven hundred of 2200 ewes grazing a pasture previously sprayed with elemental sulfur began showing abdominal discomfort within 2 hours of exposure, and 220 ewes died within 5 days. Lesions of PEM were found only in the sheep that had survived for 5 days.[115] Steers ingesting water with 4564 mg SO_4/L and feed containing 0.17% sulfur had a 47.6% incidence of PEM and a 33% mortality rate.[116] Six of 110 cows drinking 7200 mg Na_2SO_4/L water developed PEM.[117] Eighteen of 21 herds fed supplements containing 2% inorganic SO_4 developed PEM. This supplement provided approximately 0.16% sulfur beyond what was in the rest of the diet.[118] Water containing 2000 mg SO_4^{2-}/L produced PEM in 1 of 9 steers.[87] Three of 21 steers fed 3780 mg

SO_4^{2-}/L developed PEM and died. Feeding thiamin did not prevent sulfur toxicity.[119] Four steers died of PEM on a feedlot in Alberta, Canada, after consuming water with 5203 mg SO_4/L while the temperature was 30°C.[120] Four of 40 cattle developed PEM after ingesting hay with 0.39% sulfur and water containing 2250 mg SO_4/L.[121] All 10 beef calves offered water with 5540 mg sulfur/L or 7010 mg sulfur/L showed signs of PEM.[122] The incidence of death from PEM in a beef feedlot varied dramatically with environmental temperature, from none in the winter to 0.8% per month in the summer. The increase also corresponded with a 2.4-fold increase in water consumption as a result of summer weather, increasing the total dietary sulfur intake to 0.67%.[123] Cows in Canada were stricken with PEM when exposed to 3400 mg SO_4^{2-}/L water; no new cases occurred after the water was replaced. Sixty-nine animals were affected with PEM after ingesting a protein supplement containing "1.5% organosulfate" and water containing 1814 mg SO_4^{2-}/L.[124] Experimentally feeding 0.477% total dietary sulfur resulted in 1 of 12 heifers developing PEM 3 days after termination of the experiment.[111]

Sulfate-containing waters are quite unpalatable, and, when given a choice, animals will discriminate against them. A taste test was conducted between waters containing 1450 mg/L and 2150 mg/L SO_4 and tap water. The cattle discriminated against the water containing 1450 mg/L and rejected the water containing 2150 mg/L, opting for tap water instead.[107] Despite the poor palatability, if no other water is available, animals will reluctantly drink water with higher SO_4 concentrations, resulting in potential toxicity.

In ruminants, high dietary sulfur may cause acute death, PEM, trace mineral (especially copper) deficiencies, and other chronic, as yet poorly defined ailments that decrease production efficiency. All dietary sources of sulfur (water, forage, concentrates, and feed supplements) contribute to the total sulfur intake and thus to potential toxicity. The contribution of water to dietary sulfur, usually as the SO_4^{2-} ion, varies dramatically with environmental conditions as water consumption goes up and down.

From a strictly theoretic standpoint, the NRC maximum tolerable dose of sulfur for cattle is 0.5% of the total diet (0.3% for feedlot animals).[77] Great Plains grasses are reported to contain between 0.13% and 0.48% sulfur.[125] Assuming forage sulfur concentrations of 0.2% and water consumption typical of young, rapidly growing cattle at summer temperatures (30°C), a water SO_4 concentration of 1125 mg/L will meet or exceed the NRC's maximum tolerance limit for sulfur in cattle. Adult bulls, which consume one-half as much water, could theoretically be impacted by 2250 mg/L, and lactating cows would fall somewhere in between. In practice, water SO_4 concentrations as low as 2000 mg/L have caused PEM and/or sudden death in cattle. This observation is supported by many field cases investigated by the author's laboratory and other regional diagnostic laboratories since 1988. It seems to be contradicted by some of the earlier studies mentioned above, notably Digesti and Weeth, but both probability and the morbidity of poisoning increase with progressively larger SO_4 concentrations; thus, studies with small numbers of animals easily overlook marginally toxic doses. Anecdotal data also indicate that cattle are able to adapt to elevated sulfur concentrations if introduced gradually to potentially toxic waters over a period of several days or weeks. The details (ie, how rapidly dietary sulfur can change) of this process and the effect(s) of other dietary factors such as energy and protein on the process are still a matter of conjecture.

Waterborne SO_4 is reported to decrease copper uptake at concentrations as low as 500 mg sulfur/L as SO_4^{2-}.[88,93] Whether overt copper deficiency results depends on the dietary copper concentration, because excess dietary copper may compensate for some or all of the effect of SO_4^{2-}.[126] Elevated dietary sulfur also interferes with the uptake of zinc and selenium. Trace element deficiencies are multifactorial diseases that do not normally manifest themselves unless animals are exposed to other stressors, such as bacterial pathogens, bad weather, and shipping. Therefore, it is difficult, if not impossible, to settle on a single number that consistently results in deficiency or guarantees safety; however, the NRC recommends "the sulfur content of cattle diets be limited to the requirement of the animal, which is 0.2% dietary sulfur for dairy and 0.15% in beef cattle and other ruminants."[77]

Relatively low sulfur concentrations (equivalent to 500–1500 mg SO_4^{2-}/L in water) have impacted performance (eg, average daily gain, feed efficiency) in feedlot and range cattle via a variety of mechanisms not completely understood.[104,127–129] Loneragan and colleagues[87] suggested that H_2S produced from SO_4^{2-}, eructated and then inhaled, resulted in pulmonary damage and increased susceptibility to respiratory infections. Elevated SO_4^{2-} also results in decreased water intake under experimental conditions. Finally, it is possible that some, as yet unrecognized, interactions with other dietary components result in decreased use and feed efficiency. These effects have obvious implications for animal health, but they are difficult to predictively quantify under field conditions.

Monogastrics, such as horses, are at less risk of sulfur effects that involve ruminal generation of sulfide. In these species, the principle effect of elevated drinking water SO_4 seems to be diarrhea resulting from the osmotic attraction of water into the gut. The relative contributions of the SO_4^{2-} ion and its associated cation are unclear, but the literature indicates the effect (1) is transient and not life threatening and (2) probably only occurs at concentrations considerably in excess of those toxic in ruminants. Therefore, concentrations that are safe in ruminants should provide adequate protection for horses.

Assuming normal feedstuff sulfur concentrations, keeping water SO_4^{2-} concentrations of less than 1800 mg/L should minimize the possibility of acute death in cattle. Concentrations of less than 1000 mg/L should not result in any easily measured loss in in performance.

SODIUM CHLORIDE (SALT)

Sodium chloride (NaCl), or salt, was one of the first nutrients to be identified as essential to life. Although sea water contains approximately 2.68% NaCl and marine animals face the challenge of coping with excessive salt, most terrestrial animals find it difficult to obtain adequate dietary salt and have developed methods to conserve NaCl.[130–132] Sodium and chlorine are rarely found in elemental form in nature; however, most of the toxic effects of NaCl are owing to sodium.

Both sodium and chlorine are essential elements for practically all forms of life. The sodium ion (Na^+) is the major extracellular cation and Cl^- is the major extracellular anion; together, they are responsible for maintaining acid–base balance and regulating the osmotic pressure of bodily fluids.[133,134] Excitable cell membranes (ie, nerve and muscle cells) depend on tightly regulated Na^+ and Cl^- concentrations in cells and the extracellular fluid. Sodium chloride is reportedly the only mineral animals truly crave and will actually seek out.[131,135] The dietary NaCl requirement of swine is between 0.10% and 0.14%, and 0.18% sodium is needed to achieve optimal performance.[136–139] Similarly, the optimal dietary sodium concentration in horses is 0.16% to 0.18% DM[134] and for cattle is 0.08% to 0.1%.[140] Under extreme conditions, such as high temperatures, lactation, or hard work, these requirements increase owing to increased excretion of both Na^+ and

Cl^-.[140,141] The clinical signs of sodium chloride deficiency are polydipsia (extreme thirst), polyuria (extreme urination), salt hunger, pica (licking foreign materials), weight loss, and decreased productivity.[142,143] Chloride deficiencies have been produced by feeding diets with 0.10% chlorine or less and present as anorexia, weight loss, lethargy, decreased milk production, polydipsia, polyuria, and cardio-pulmonary depression as clinical signs.[144–146]

Once ingested, 85% to 95% of sodium and chlorine are absorbed from the GI tract. Large amounts of sodium and chlorine are continuously recycled into the intestinal tract via salivary, pancreatic, and intestinal epithelial secretions, as well as bile. This high intestinal Na^+ concentration is required to transport glucose, amino acids, and other nutrients across the mucosa. Chloride is also secreted into the intestine to aid in creating the low pH environment needed for proteolysis. These secretions must then be reabsorbed distad to conserve the elements.[131] Hemsley[124] reported that increased NaCl in the diet increased the rate of passage of solid digesta from the rumen, which decreased microbial degradation within the rumen and increased the amount of protein available in the small intestine. Altered ruminal fatty acid concentrations have also been related to dietary NaCl.[147–149] Dietary Na^+ and Cl^- in excess of physiologic requirements are usually efficiently eliminated from the body via the kidneys.[150]

Potassium is the main intracellular cation, Na^+ is the main extracellular cation, and Cl^- is the main extracellular anion. The relative concentrations of these 3 elements create an electrochemical gradient that is essential for nutrient transport, nerve conduction, muscle contraction, and energy generation, and they indirectly aid in maintaining pH balance. Imbalances of these elements result in a variety of disorders from decreased gains to acute death.[151–153]

The toxicity of NaCl is intimately related to the availability of water and is sometimes referred to as the "sodium ion toxicity–water deprivation syndrome"; however, if the dose of Na^+ is high enough, sodium is toxic regardless of water intake.[154] If adequate water is available, most animals tolerate relatively large doses of sodium by increasing Na^+ excretion.[150,155–158] If sufficient water is not available to excrete the excess, toxicosis results in dehydration, blindness, incoordination, convulsions, recumbency, and death.[154,159–161] The normal physiologic response to elevated dietary NaCl is increased water intake; however, if the only available water contains high NaCl concentrations, drinking results in even more NaCl intake and increases the risk of receiving a toxic dose.[158] Even when sufficient potable water is available to eliminate excess dietary sodium, every gram of NaCl excreted requires producing at least 5 mL of urine[162] at a finite metabolic cost. Thus, slight to moderately elevated Na^+ may impact growth and performance.[158,163,164]

The mechanisms underlying acute toxicity are related to cellular dehydration, or tissue shrinking, and edema. When extracellular Na^+ concentrations become elevated, water is drawn out of the cell.[131,165] Eventually intracellular Na^+ concentrations adjust to a new equilibrium with the extracellular fluid, and cells return to their normal volume. After 2 to 3 days of exposure to elevated Na^+, cells have replaced the increased intracellular Na^+ with idiogenic osmoles, hydrophilic organic molecules that compensate for the attraction of extracellular Na^+ for water.[166] Tissue shrinkage owing to elevated extracellular fluid Na^+ results in damage to the small blood vessels that supply the superficial portions of the brain. Later, after animals have adapted to elevated extracellular Na^+ concentrations (whether from excessive dietary sodium intake or water deprivation) and are allowed free access to water, the extracellular fluid becomes diluted and water is drawn back to the elevated osmolarity inside the neurons, resulting in cellular swelling and necrosis.

Acute toxicity has been observed in cattle, pigs, dogs, and rats after ingestion of extreme concentrations of NaCl. Ninety-one cattle developed muscular weakness, muscle fasciculations, and sternal and lateral recumbency, and they subsequently died, as a result of drinking water from a tank and lagoon that contained 4370 and 21,160 mg Na^+/L, respectively.[160] Cattle consuming water containing 5850 mg Na^+/L experienced decreases in feed and water intakes, with a corresponding 13.7% decrease in BW.[167] Water containing 6726 to 6826 mg Na^+/L resulted in a loss of condition, scouring, and death in 15 of 220 cattle.[168] Six cattle began showing signs of central nervous system dysfunction 4 hours after consuming 50 kg of a supplement containing 50,000 ppm NaCl (19,500 ppm sodium), despite drinking water immediately afterward.[154] A pig owner replaced a free-choice salt block with 2 handfuls of loose trace mineral salt in 30 gallons of water. Within 6 days, 4 pigs began champing jaws, frothing at the mouth, and convulsing, and 2 ultimately died.[169] Abruptly switching gilts to a diet containing 13,600 ppm NaCl resulted in feed refusal and watery diarrhea lasting several days.[170] Dosing an 11.3 to 15.9 kg (25–35 lb) pig with approximately 178.6 g NaCl (69.6 g Na^+) in 500 mL water resulted in death within 15 minutes.[171] A female dog became blind, convulsed, and eventually died after consuming seawater (26,800 mg NaCl/L) on a hot summer day.[159] Three female Boston terriers became ataxic, convulsed, and later died after drinking water contaminated with approximately 100,000 mg NaCl/L.[172] A male Airedale terrier began having seizures and eventually died after ingesting a bolus of a salt mixture clay. The concentration of NaCl in the clay was not reported; however, it was stated a minimum of 20 g NaCl remained in the dog's stomach at the postmortem examination.[165] The minimum toxic dose in canines was estimated at 2000 mg NaCl/kg BW (780 mg Na/kg BW).[173] Rats refused to drink water containing 25,000 mg NaCl/L; death occurred after several days of water refusal were followed by gorging on water.[174]

Chronic toxicity has been investigated under both field and experimental conditions. Cattle consuming water containing 12,000 mg NaCl/L (4680 mg Na^+/L) throughout the summer months did not become clinically dehydrated, but did exhibit diarrhea, a 28.2% decrease in feed intake, and a 69% increase in water intake.[175] Cattle ingesting water containing 2500 mg NaCl/L (975 mg Na^+/L) for 28 days showed increased water intake, decreased milk production, and diarrhea.[163] Steers fed diets containing 50,000 ppm NaCl (19,500 ppm sodium) for up to 175 days gained less weight and used organic matter less efficiently than controls.[147] Steers fed high grain diets containing 70,000 ppm NaCl (27,300 ppm sodium) for 126 days showed increased water intake, decreased feed intake, and altered digestion patterns.[176] Feeding lactating cows low fiber diets in conjunction with concentrate containing 60,000 ppm NaCl resulted in a 6.9% decrease in organic matter consumption and a 22% increase in water intake, but these diets had no effect on milk production.[177] Lactating heifers supplemented with 136 g NaCl/d, beginning 42 days prepartum and continuing until 10 days postpartum, showed an increased incidence of udder edema.[178] Water containing 15,000 mg NaCl/L resulted in decreased feed consumption, decreased BW, and increased water intake in sheep.[164] Drinking water containing "10,000 to 13,000" mg NaCl/L resulted in neonatal mortality and dystocia when given to twin-bearing pregnant ewes.[179] Sheep drinking water containing 15,000 mg NaCl/L for 21 days consumed less feed and more water than controls.[158] Sheep consuming water containing 20,000 mg NaCl/L for 3 days experienced a sharp decrease in feed intake. After 5 days on the water, the animals' feed consumption recovered, suggesting an adaptive response.[180] Lambs given 2 g NaCl/kg BW from an early age had significantly lower growth rates, decreased feed intakes, and diarrhea in comparison to controls.[19] Pigs consuming 15,000 mg NaCl/L water for 30 days became stiff legged and nervous, and decreased their water consumption.[181] Hypertension has been produced in rats by offering water containing 10,000 to 25,000 mg NaCl/L for 6 months or longer.[182-184] Feeding trials determined the chronic oral median lethal dose of NaCl in rats to be 2.69 g/kg BW.[185]

Toxicity has also been shown to occur when elevated dietary NaCl is coupled with water restriction. Feeding sixty 3-year-old steers a supplement containing 4.5 kg NaCl 1 day before withholding feed and water (to obtain fasting BWs) resulted in blindness, incoordination, knuckling, and recumbency in 5 animals.[161] Goats fed 30,000 ppm NaCl for 30 days showed a 20% decrease in feed intake when water was freely available and a 43% reduction when water was restricted.[186] Pigs fed NaCl at the rate of 2.4 g/kg BW with restricted water showed "extreme signs" of NaCl toxicity and ultimately died.[187] Sodium chloride poisoning was diagnosed in a herd of pigs that exhibited convulsions, unsteady gait and muscle twitching, blindness, and hyperpnea. The pigs had been without water for an undetermined amount of time, and no levels of dietary NaCl were given.[188] Swine began having convulsions and were exhibiting head pressing within 3 days of being purchased at an auction. It was determined the clinical signs developed as a result of the pigs receiving a high-salt diet before the sale and then receiving no water during the auction.[189]

There are several reports that indicate at least some sodium can be tolerated. Offering cattle water containing 4110 mg NaCl/L resulted in increased water intake and diuresis; however, no other effects on animal health were noticed.[106] Cattle consuming water with 5000 mg NaCl/L (2000 mg Na^+/L) seemed to be clinically normal throughout the course of two 30-day experiments.[157] Steers consuming 192 to 193 g NaCl/d for 84 days showed no observable negative effects when ingesting a roughage diet; however, when fed a corn silage diet, the animals consuming the high sodium diet had lesser weight gains and feed efficiencies.[148] Sheep consuming water containing 13,000 mg NaCl/L for up to 16 months increased their water intake, but they exhibited no other adverse health effects.[156,190-195] Rations with a NaCl concentration of 91,000 ppm were fed to sheep with no significant effects on breeding, gestation, lambing, or wool production.[196] Swine consuming 5150 mg NaCl/L water had a drastic increase in water intake; however, no other adverse effects were noticed.[197]

The limited data available regarding Cl^- in water seems to indicate it is primarily a palatability problem. The environmental Protection Agency's secondary water standard for human consumption suggests that more than 250 mg Cl^-/L imparts a "salty" taste.[198] Water containing 5000 mg $CaCl_2$/L offered to cattle resulted in water refusal despite lack of any other water sources. Water containing 3000 mg/L resulted in increased water consumption and urinary acidification, but no measurable effects on performance or health.[143] Rats drinking water containing 10,000 mg $CaCl_2$/L were unable to produce normal litters, and 15,000 mg $CaCl_2$/L reduced growth rates.[199] Conversely, in another study, rats consuming 15,000 mg $CaCl_2$/L adapted, grew normally, reproduced, and were able to suckle their young.[174]

The effects of sodium and chlorine are difficult to separate since neither exists in a pure state in nature, and the elements usually occur together in water. It is also difficult to separate the chronic effects of NaCl from those attributed to TDS in the literature, as the Na^+ and Cl^- ions are major constituents of salinity under normal conditions. Nevertheless, it is the Na^+ ion that seems to be responsible for most of the recognized effects of "salt" poisoning.[198] At present, there is not sufficient data to make any specific recommendations regarding Cl^- in drinking water for livestock.

The toxic effects of sodium are very dependent on the availability of fresh water. If abundant, good quality drinking water is available, animals can tolerate large doses of sodium. Despite this fact, at some point excess dietary sodium exceeds the ability of the organism to excrete Na^+, and acute poisoning results, regardless of water intake. The threshold for acute toxicity seems to be approximately 1 g Na/kg BW for swine, with cattle equal or slightly less sensitive and sheep considerably less sensitive (roughly 2.5 g Na/kg BW). Most animals will limit their consumption of NaCl to approximately 400 mg Na/kg BW/d, if possible. Beyond this dose, feed intake, water consumption, and productivity decline. Most reviews indicate horses are roughly similar in sensitivity to cattle and swine.

If the only water available is also the major source of dietary sodium, long-term impacts will occur at lower sodium dosages. Chronic health effects, mainly decreased production, have been reported at water concentrations as low as 1000 mg Na^+/L in dairy cows; however, other studies with beef heifers in cooler climates reported only minimal effects at 1600 to 2000 mg Na^+/L. Interestingly, the actual amount of sodium consumed by the cattle in all of these studies (250–400 mg Na^+/kg BW) were similar. Dosages greater than 800 mg Na/kg BW resulted in effects ranging from weight loss and diarrhea to death.

It is theoretically possible animals maintained on high-Na^+ water for prolonged periods will, if suddenly exposed to low-Na^+ water, develop acute Na^+ ion intoxication, and the author has seen such happen under field conditions. There is not sufficient quantitative information to make any recommendations about this phenomenon other than that animals should be transitioned from high to low Na^+ water sources gradually.

Assuming water consumption typical of a rapidly growing steer and only background feed sodium concentrations, the no-effect level would be about 1000 mg Na^+/L or 2500 mg NaCl/L. Serious effects, including death, become likely at 5000 mg Na^+/L. Thus, drinking water Na^+ concentrations should be kept to less than 1000 mg/L, although short-term exposure to concentrations of up to 4000 mg/L may be well-tolerated.

TOTAL DISSOLVED SOLIDS

Total dissolved solids (TDS) is defined as all inorganic and organic substances contained in water that can pass through a 2-micron filter. In general, TDS is the sum of the cations and anions in water. Ions and ionic compounds making up TDS usually include carbonate, bicarbonate, chloride, fluoride, sulfate, phosphate, nitrate, calcium, magnesium, sodium, and potassium, but any ion that is present will contribute to the total. Organic ions include pollutants, herbicides, and hydrocarbons. In addition, soil organic matter compounds such as humic/fulvic acids are also included in TDS. There are a variety of ways to measure TDS. The simplest is to filter the water sample, and then evaporate it at 180°C in a preweighed dish until the weight of the dish no longer changes. The increase in weight of the dish represents the TDS, and it is reported in milligrams per liter. The TDS of a water sample can also be estimated fairly accurately from the electrical conductivity of the sample via a linear correlation equation depending on specific conductivity. Finally, TDS can be calculated by measuring individual ions and simply adding them together.

TDS is a nonspecific, quantitative measure of the amount of dissolved chemicals present in a water sample but does not tell us anything about their nature. TDS is not considered a primary pollutant with any associated health effects in human drinking water standards, but it is rather used as an indication of the aesthetic characteristics of drinking water and as a broad indicator of an array of chemical contaminants. Although many essential elements may contribute to TDS, the measurement does not, itself, differentiate essential from toxic elements.

Interestingly, early epidemiologic studies suggested that "moderately high" TDS concentrations (high in this context being <1000 mg/L) protected people against cancer and heart disease.[200–203] Although the mechanism(s) underlying these early observations are not completely understood, it was first narrowed down to "hardness" as opposed to TDS. It now seems that certain constituents of TDS, notably magnesium, interfere with the formation of thrombi in arteriosclerosis.[202,204] Another hypothesis for the protective effect is that some components of hardness decrease leaching of toxic elements from plumbing.[201]

Saline waters may adversely impact animal health by several possible mechanisms. One of the most important biological functions of water in mammals is as a solvent for nutrients, waste products, and other substances. The presence of extraneous solutes decreases the ability of water to serve this function by decreasing its ability to dissolve additional solutes. A similar, related factor is plasma osmolarity. Solutes exert an attraction on water across membranes, and inappropriate water movement is disastrous to cells and tissues. An extreme example of this effect is water intoxication that results in death, as was the case with a young woman in California.[205] Mammals expend a considerable amount of energy maintaining the osmolar concentration of various body compartments within a narrow range. The presence of excessive solutes in drinking water adds to this burden and consumes resources that would otherwise be used for growth, reproduction, or fighting off disease. It is well-accepted that extreme drinking water TDS concentrations in the 1.5% to 3.0% range are incompatible with life[164,168,174,199,206,207]; however, the effects of lower TDS concentrations are too multifactorial, involving species, age, sex, diet, pregnancy, lactation, environmental conditions, and so on, to lend themselves to simple all-or-nothing conclusions. The fact animals may "tolerate" (in other words, survive) a particular concentration is not the same as proving they remained productive on it.

Elevated TDS adversely affects the palatability of water. In humans, taste panels rated the palatability of water with 300 mg/L TDS as "excellent," 300 to 600 mg/L "good," 600 to 900 mg/L "fair," 900 to 1200 mg/L "poor," and greater than 1200 mg/L "unusable." Earlier criteria for human health were based on this fact.[208] In livestock, decreased palatability is well-recognized as an important determinant of water consumption and, indirectly, feed consumption, and performance. Cattle given water containing 6000 to 15,000 mg/L TDS exhibited decreased water intake, feed intake, and average daily gain.[108,116,167,209–211] Five thousand milligrams per liter of decreased feed intake and gain of cattle on a high roughage diet.[212] Dairy cows given 2040 mg/L water consumed less water and produced less milk when the peak ambient temperature was 32.1°C than cows given desalinated water.[213] Similar decreases in milk production attributed to consuming saline water were seen in Arizona.[163,214] Swine subsisting on water containing 10,000 to 15,000 mg/L drank less, ate less, and performed more poorly than controls.[181] Sheep seem to be more tolerant of saline waters than most domestic species.[155,156,190–195,215,216] The only 2 references regarding saline waters in horses indicate they are reluctant to drink such water,[168] and it has been implied they can be maintained on water containing up to 9500 mg/L TDS.[217]

Even when animals drink more to compensate for poor water quality, the increased metabolic load imposed by high solute water may result in impaired performance. Water containing 1.5% NaCl (15,000 ppm), given to cattle for less than a week, resulted in a 13.7% reduction in weight, as well as decreasing feed and water intake, and marked hypernatremia.[167] In a similar, short-term experiment at cool temperatures, cattle given 15,000 mg/L TDS water drank more, ate and grew less, and showed clinical signs of dehydration.[175] Five thousand milligrams per liter of TDS for 51 days decreased gain in heifers.[211]

TDS in drinking water serve as a very poor predictor of animal health. As noted elsewhere in this article, TDS is a measure of all inorganic and organic substances dissolved in water. These individual solutes range in toxicity from relatively nontoxic substances, such as Ca^{2+}, to extremely toxic (Hg^{2+}, Se^{+4}), but tests of TDS do not differentiate between them. Several early studies suggest no significant effects in sheep at TDS concentrations up to 13,000 mg/L or cattle and swine up to 5000 mg/L, and the NRC in 1974 accepted larger concentrations as tolerable "for older ruminants and horses," yet the author has seen animals poisoned by waters in which the TDS was measured as slightly less than 500 mg/L (Raisbeck MF, Unpublished data, University of Wyoming, Department of Veterinary Sciences, 2015),[218] and there are reports of decreased productivity in dairy cattle at 2000 to 2500 mg/L. Early epidemiologic studies in people suggested high drinking water TDS decreased the incidence of cancer and heart disease in people. Later, however, the beneficial component of TDS that was negatively correlated with heart disease, was narrowed down, first to hardness, then finally to the Mg^{2+} ion concentration. In human health, the World Health Organization dropped health-based recommendations for TDS in 1993, instead retaining 1000 mg/L as a secondary standard for "organoleptic purposes." The test is just too nonspecific to be reliable. As noted by Chapman and colleagues,[219] in a study of aquatic toxicity, "Toxicity related to these ions is due to the specific combination and concentration of ions and is not predictable from TDS concentrations."

We do not recommend relying on TDS to evaluate water quality for livestock and wildlife; however, if no other information is available, TDS concentrations less than 500 mg/L should ensure safety from almost all inorganic constituents. Above 500 mg/L, the individual constituents contributing to TDS should be identified, quantified, and evaluated.

pH

The pH is defined as "the negative log of the hydrogen ion (H^+) activity," although "concentration" is often substituted for "activity" in a working definition.[220] Water with a pH of less than 7 is acidic, and water with a pH of greater than 7 is basic or alkaline. The definition of a normal water pH varies between authorities, but it is usually described as somewhere between 5.5 and 6.5, and 8 and 9. By comparison, vinegar is pH 3, colas are between 3 and 4, beer is between 4 and 5, and milk is around pH 6.4. A related measurement, namely, alkalinity, is based on the capacity of a water sample to resist a change in pH and is usually reported as mg/L of $CaCO_3$. The pH controls the solubility and thus concentrations of many elements in water. For example, many metals precipitate out of alkaline water, whereas they dissolve in acidic water.

Water pH impacts the effectiveness of various water (especially antimicrobial) treatments and palatability for animals. Acidic water tends to have a sour taste; basic is described as metallic. The taste threshold for hydrochloric acid is as low as 0.0001 mol/L.[220] Acidic water also tends to dissolve catons (metals) from plumbing and soil it contacts, further impacting palatability.

In the body, extracellular fluid is normally maintained within a very narrow range centered around pH 7.4.[220,221] Several critical physiologic processes are pH-dependent, thus any significant departure from normal.[221]

Acid–base balance in mammals represents a dynamic equilibrium between metabolic acid production and its elimination. As such, it is influenced by a number of interdependent processes, especially respiration and urine production, chemical buffering by bone and other tissues, and, to a lesser extent, several dietary elements. A comprehensive review of these processes is beyond the scope of this article, but a decrease in plasma pH from normal (acidosis) stimulates increased respiration, decreasing the blood concentration of CO_2 that would otherwise react with water to form carbonic acid (H_2CO_3). It also stimulates the kidney to produce urine that is, more acidic by increasing elimination of the H^+ ion. The net result is an active elimination of acid and an increase in plasma pH back toward normal.[220,221] The H^+ ion may also react with buffering molecules in bone, minimizing the magnitude of any pH change.[222,223]

Certain nutrients, referred to as "strong ions," although not intrinsically acidic or basic, influence animals' acid–base balance by shifting the equilibrium of internal homeostatic processes. For example, diets rich in Na^+ and K^+ tend to push the body in an alkaline direction, whereas Cl^-, as ammonium chloride (NH_4Cl), is used clinically to move the balance in an acidic direction. Dairy nutritionists have compounded rations on the basis of the strong ion difference equation ($[Na^+ + K^{+]} - [Cl^- + S_2^{-]}$)[221] to produce mild acidosis shortly before lactation, which decreases the incidence of milk fever.[224–226]

Excessively acid or basic drinking water can theoretically affect animals in 4 ways. First, extremes of pH may result in tissue damage to the mouth and oropharynx, causing irritation and refusal to drink. Second, unusual extremes of pH may dissolve materials from pipes, ditches, and so on, which are toxic and/or impart an unpleasant taste to the water. For example, copper, iron, and lead concentrations have all been shown to increase in acidic water as a result of leaching the metals from plumbing.[227–230] Consumption of acidic drinks may dissolve dental enamel and weaken teeth.[231,232] Finally, consumption of a large amount of excessively acidic or basic water could theoretically shift the body's acid–base balance.

The author was unable to find any reports describing acute damage as a result of drinking extremely acid or basic water, although he has investigated cases in which cattle drank extremely basic solutions (pH 12–14) resulting in damage to the mouth and esophagus. Acid rain, precipitation rendered acidic by atmospheric pollution, is a well-recognized problem in aquatic organisms because several toxic elements (especially aluminum) are leached from solids that come in contact with the acidic water. It is especially problematic in poorly buffered surface waters of northeastern North America.[233] Mammals are considerably less sensitive to the effects of dissolved metals than fish, but acidic water supplies have been incriminated for the presence of lead and copper in domestic drinking water, a concern for human health.[227–229] Even if not present at toxic concentrations, many dissolved elements impart a repellent taste to water.

Despite the hypothetical potential of acidic (pH < 5.5) water to cause acidosis in animals, water systems in laboratory animal colonies and, to a lesser extent, swine facilities, are commonly acidified to minimize bacterial infections.[231,234–236]

Metabolic effects have been observed in ruminants and monogastrics owing to the ingestion of acidic feed and water. Acidogenic rations are fed to dairy cattle during late pregnancy to prevent milk fever. For example, feeding a combination of 98 g each of NH_4Cl and ammonium sulfate (($NH_4)_2SO_4$) per head per day to lactating dairy cows lowered blood pH, increased blood calcium (Ca^{2+}), and increased excretion of urinary Ca^{2+} and the ammonium ion (NH^{4+}).[226] The same amount of these salts added to drinking water would result in a pH of approximately 5.5. Mineral acids (HCl and H_2SO_4) have also been fed to prevent milk fever.[237] Dairy cows given rations containing 0.65% or 1.8% hydrochloric acid (HCl) (equivalent to a pH of 2–3, respectively, if added to drinking water) had increased blood Ca^{2+}, a small (0.05) decrease in blood pH, acidic urine, and a decreased incidence of milk fever.[225]

Several experiments reported no effects when acidic water was fed, and it is commonly believed that acidifying water to approximately a pH of 3 is beneficial in rodent colonies. Rats given water acidified to a pH of 2.0 with HCl or H_2SO_4 for 6 weeks exhibited somewhat decreased feed intake and water intake, and concomitant weight loss compared with those fed pH 2.5 or pH 7.0 water; however, stomach pH values were not statistically different among treatment groups.[238] Rats experimentally fed water acidified to pH 2.5 with HCl for 6 to 11 months showed no changes in weight and "negligible" damage to tooth enamel.[232] Rats drinking pH 2 water for 21 weeks drank slightly less than controls, whereas those consuming pH 3 water showed no measurable effects in any health parameter.[239] Water with a pH of 2.5 given to rats for 30 days resulted in decreased water intake, whereas water with pH 3 given to rats produced no effect on growth.[231] Rats drinking water with a pH of 1.4 to 3.5 for 42 to 84 days showed accelerated erosion on the tooth surface; however, oral cavity pH was unchanged.[240] Mice consuming acidified water (pH 2.0) for 120 days had slightly decreased reticuloendothelial clearance rates when compared with controls, possibly as a result of decreased growth and smaller spleens.[241] It is questionable if the physiologic effects in these reports are a direct result of acidic water on acid–base status, per se. Even in the study that reported some relatively subtle effects (decreased gains) in rats at pH 2.5 or less, gastric pH was unchanged,[238] and rats and rabbits fed pH 2.3 to 2.5 water for 7 months maintained normal blood pH.[234] Rats consuming water with pH of 2.5 gave birth to and weaned more pups than control animals.[242]

SUMMARY

Existing human drinking water standards (pH 6.5–8.5) were established decades ago for aesthetic (eg, taste) reasons and to protect plumbing from corrosion, rather than on health-based criteria.[227,243] Although a number of Cooperative Extension Service Web sites suggest water below this range will produce pathologic acidosis in cattle, none offer hard evidence. Nor are there any references to direct the health effects of moderately acidic or basic water in animals. Conversely, there are a number of references to the beneficial effects of acidifying laboratory animal and swine water with mineral acids down to pH 3. The only adverse effects in these reports were relatively subtle and occurred at pH of less than 3.0. The only example of feeding a pure mineral acid to ruminants (equivalent to approximately pH of 2–3) resulted in acidified urine, but there were no adverse health effects over a period of several weeks. There are no equivalent data for basic drinking water. From a purely pathophysiologic standpoint, it seems unlikely that water with a pH between 3.0 and 7.0 would cause health problems in otherwise normally managed animals. An exception might be feedlot ruminants, which are often marginally acidotic as a consequence of the high soluble carbohydrate rations they receive, in which case, acidic water might be sufficient to trigger a crisis.

The other potential adverse effect of basic or acidic water involves mobilization of potentially toxic substances (eg, metals) from plumbing or soils. Although it seems unlikely the amounts mobilized would be sufficient to actually cause poisoning under most conditions, it is quite possible they would be large enough to cause water refusal. Because the effect of any given pH on palatability depends upon what the water contacts, there is no way to make any wide-reaching recommendation in this regard.

The author believes that the commonly touted acceptable ranges for drinking water pH (a low of 5.5–6.5 and a high of 7.5–9.0) are excessively conservative from a strictly animal health standpoint, at least on the acid side, but there are not sufficient experimental and/or clinical data to offer a specific alternative.

DISCLOSURE

This is a summary of 30 years clinical experience and literature review funded over the years by numerous small gifts from producers, and larger grants from the Wyoming DEQ and US Office of Surface Mining. I no longer have the details of all of these, and its been long ago enough that I don't feel it relevant.

REFERENCES

1. Agency for Toxic Substances and Disease Registry. Toxicological profile for fluorides, hydrogen fluoride, and fluorine. Atlanta (GA): U.S. Department of Heath and Human Services; 2003.
2. National Research Council. Water for livestock enterprises. In: Water quality criteria 1972: a report. Washington, DC: National Academy of Sciences; 1972. p. 304–60.
3. National Research Council. Vitamins and Water. In: Nutrient requirements of beef cattle. Washington, DC: National Academy of Sciences; 2000. p. 80–2.
4. National Research Council. Water. In: Nutrient requirements of dairy cattle. Washington, DC: National Academy of Sciences; 2001. p. 178–83.
5. Fonnesbeck PV. Consumption and excretion of water by horses receiving all hay and hay-grain diets. J Anim Sci 1968;27:1350–6.
6. Murphy MR, Davis CL, McCoy GC. Factors affecting water consumption by Holstein cows in early lactation. J Dairy Sci 1983;66:35–8.
7. Winchester CF, Morris MJ. Water intake rates of cattle. J Anim Sci 1956;15: 722–40.
8. Cymbaluk NF. Water balance of horses fed various diets. Equine Pract 1989; 11:19.
9. National Research Council. Nitrates and nitrites. In: Mineral tolerance of animals. Washington, DC: National Academies Press; 2005. p. 453–68.
10. Bruning-Fann CS, Kaneene JB. The effects of nitrate, nitrite, and N-nitroso compounds on animal health. Vet Hum Toxicol 1993;35:237–53.
11. Deeb BS, Sloan KW. Nitrates, nitrites, and health, vol. 750. Champaign (IL): University of Illinois Agricultural Experiment Station Bulletin; 1975. p. 1–52.
12. Mitchell RD, Ayala-Fierro F, Carter DE. Systemic indicators of inorganic arsenic toxicity in four animal species. J Toxicol Environ Health 2000;59:119–34.
13. Reddy KJ, Lin J. Nitrate removal from groundwater using catalytic reduction. Water Res 2000;34:995–1001.
14. Lewicki J, Garwacki S, Wiechetek M. Nitrate and nitrite kinetics after single intravenous dosage in sheep. Small Rumin Res 1994;13:141–6.
15. Osweiler GD, Carson TL, Buck WB, et al. Nitrates, nitrites, and related problems. In: Osweiler GD, Carson TL, Buck WB, et al, editors. Clinical and diagnostic veterinary toxicology. Dubuque (IA): Kendall Hunt; 1985. p. 460–7.
16. Schneider NR, Yeary RA. Nitrite and nitrate pharmacokinetics in the dog, sheep, and pony. Am J Vet Res 1975;36:941–7.
17. Comly HH. Cyanosis in infants caused by nitrates in well water. J Am Med Assoc 1945;129:112–6.
18. Johnson CJ, Bonrud PA, Dosch TL, et al. Fatal outcome of methemoglobinemia in an infant. J Am Med Assoc 1987;257:2796–7.
19. Wang LC, Garcia-Rivera J, Burris RH. Metabolism of nitrate by cattle. Biochem J 1971;81:237–42.

20. Cheng KJ, Pillippe RC, Kozub CC, et al. Induction of nitrate and nitrite metabolism in bovine rumen fluid and the transfer of this capacity to untreated animals. Can J Anim Sci 1985;65:647–52.
21. Killingmo O, Luthman J. Toxicity of fertilizer grade calcium nitrate. Acta Agr Scand 1968;18:80–6.
22. Burrows GE, Horn GW, McNew RW, et al. The prophylactic effect of corn supplementation on experimental nitrate intoxication in cattle. J Anim Sci 1987;64: 1682–9.
23. Emerick RJ, Embry LB, Seerley RW. Rate of formation and reduction of nitrite-induced methemoblogin in vitro and in vivo as influenced by diet of sheep and age of swine. J Anim Sci 1965;24:221–30.
24. Sinclair KB, Jones DIH. The effect of nitrate on blood composition and reproduction in the ewe. Br Vet J 1964;120:78–86.
25. Sokolowski JH, Carrigus US, Hatfield EE. Effects of inorganic sulfur on KNO_3 utilization by lambs. J Anim Sci 1961;20:953.
26. Sar C, Mwenya B, Pen B, et al. Effect of ruminal administration of Escherichia coli wild type or a genetically modified strain with enhanced high nitrite reductase activity on methane emission and nitrate toxicity in nitrate-infused sheep. Br J Nutr 2005;94:691–7.
27. Titov VY, Petrenko YM. Proposed mechanism of nitrite-induced methemoglobinemia. Biochem 2005;70:575–87.
28. Bartik M. Certain quantitative relations of nitrate and nitrite metabolism in farm animals with special regard to the origin and development of methaemoglobinemia caused by nitrites and the diagnosis of poisonings. I. Methods for determining nitrate, nitrite and methaemoglobin in the blood. Normal methaemoglobin content in the blood of farm animals. Folia Vet 1964;8:83–94.
29. Crowley JW, Jorgensen NA, Kahler LW. Effect of nitrate in drinking water on reproductive and productive efficiency of dairy cattle. Technical Report WIS WRC74-06, Water Resources Center. Madison (WI): University of Wisconsin; 1974.
30. Gangolli SD. Nitrate, nitrite, and N-nitroso compounds. In: Ballantyne B, editor. General and Applied toxicology. London: Macmillan; 1999. p. 2111–43.
31. Campbell JB, Davis AN, Myhr PJ. Methaemoglobinaemia of livestock caused by high nitrate contents of well water. Can J Comp Med 1954;18:93–101.
32. Yeruham I, Shlosberg A, Hanji V, et al. Nitrate toxicosis in beef and dairy cattle herds due to contamination of drinking water and whey. Vet Hum Toxicol 1997; 39:296–8.
33. Yong C, Brandow RA, Howlett P. An unusual cause of nitrate poisoning in cattle. Can Vet J 1990;31:118.
34. Davison KL, McEntee K, Wright MJ. Responses in pregnant ewes fed forages containing various levels of nitrate. J Dairy Sci 1965;48:968–77.
35. Dollahite JW, Rowe LD. Nitrate and nitrite intoxication in rabbits and cattle. Southwest Vet 1974;27:246–8.
36. Johnson JL, Grotelueschen D, Knott M. Evaluation of bovine perinatal nitrate accumulation in western Nebraska. Vet Hum Toxicol 1994;36:467–71.
37. Malestein A, Geurink JH, Schuyt G, et al. Nitrate poisoning in cattle 4. The effect of nitrite dosing during parturition on the oxygen capacity of maternal blood and the oxygen supply to the unborn calf. Vet Q 1980;2:149–59.
38. Sonderman JP. Nitrate intoxication in ruminants: effects on pregnancy and corpus luteum function and analytical methods for nitrates. Ph.D. Dissertation. Fort Collins (CO): Colorado State University; 1993.

39. Burwash L, Ralston B, Olson M. Effect of high nitrate feed on mature idle horses. Proc Annu Symp Equine Sci Soc 2005;19:174–9.

40. Mascher F, Marth E. Metabolism and effect of nitrates. Cent Eur J Public Health 1993;1:49–52.

41. Seerley RW, Emerick RJ, Emery LB, et al. Effect of nitrate or nitrite administered continuously in drinking water for swine and sheep. J Anim Sci 1965;24:1014–9.

42. Gibson R. An outbreak of nitrite poisoning in sows. Vet Rec 1975;96:270.

43. Wiese WJ, Joubert JP. Suspected nitrite poisoning in pigs caused by Capsella bursa-pastoris (L.) Medik. ('herderstassie', shepherd's purse). J S Afr Vet Assoc 2001;72:170–1.

44. Wright MJ, Davison KL. Nitrate accumulation in crops and nitrate poisoning in animals. Adv Agron 1964;16:197–247.

45. Setchell BP, Williams AJ. Plasma nitrate and nitrite concentration in chronic and acute nitrate poisoning in sheep. Aust Vet J 1962;38:58–62.

46. Hoar DW, Embry LB, Emerick RJ. Nitrate and vitamin A interrelationships in sheep. J Anim Sci 1968;27:1727–33.

47. McKenzie RA, Rayner AC, Thompson GK, et al. Nitrate-nitrite toxicity in cattle and sheep grazing Dactyloctenium radulans (button grass) in stockyards. Aust Vet J 2004;82:630–4.

48. Neilson FJA. Nitrite and nitrate poisoning with special reference to 'grassland tama' ryegrass. N Z Vet J 1974;22:12–3.

49. Campagnolo ER, Kasten S, Banerjee M. Accidental ammonia exposure to county fair show livestock due to contaminated drinking water. Vet Hum Toxicol 2002;44:282–5.

50. Kocar BD, Garrot RA, Inskeep WP. Elk exposure to arsenic in geothermal water-sheds of Yellowstone National Park. Environ Toxicol Chem 2004;23:982–9.

51. Ozmen O, Mor F, Unsal A. Nitrate poisoning in cattle fed Chenopodium album hay. Vet Hum Toxicol 2003;45:83–4.

52. Buxton JC, Allcroft R. Industrial molybdenosis of grazing cattle. Vet Rec 1955;67:273–6.

53. Horn GW, Burrows GE, Lusby KS. Preliminary studies on the effect of yeast culture supplementation on nitrate/nitrite induced methemoglobinemia in lambs and steers. Vet Hum Toxicol 1984;26:309–13.

54. Van Dijk S, Lobsteyn AJH, Wensing T, et al. Treatment of nitrate intoxication in a cow. Vet Rec 1983;112:272–4.

55. Wallace JD, Raleigh RJ, Weswig PH. Performance and carotene conversion in Hereford heifers fed different levels of nitrate. J Anim Sci 1964;23:1042–5.

56. Weichenthal BA, Embry LB, Emerick RJ, et al. Influence of sodium nitrate, vitamin A and protein level on feedlot performance and vitamin A status of fattening cattle. J Anim Sci 1963;22:979–84.

57. Garner RJ. Nitrates and Nitrites. In: Clarke EG, Clarke ML, editors. Veterinary toxicology. London: Bailliere, Tindell & Cassell; 1967. p. 108–12.

58. O'Hara PJ, Fraser AJ. Nitrate poisoning in cattle grazing crops. N Z Vet J 1975;23:45–53.

59. Low ICS. Nitrite poisoning of calves grazing 'Grasslands Tama' ryegrass. N Z Vet J 1974;22:60–1.

60. Slenning BD, Galey FD, Anderson M. Forage-related nitrate toxicoses possibly confounded by nonprotein nitrogen and monensin in the diet used at commercial dairy heifer replacement operation. J Am Vet Med Assoc 1991;198:867–70.

61. Harris DJ, Rhodes HA. Nitrate and nitrite poisoning in cattle in Victoria. Aust Vet J 1969;45:590–1.

62. Carrigan MJ, Gardner IA. Nitrate poisoning in cattle fed sudax (Sorghum sp. hybrid) hay. Aust Vet J 1982;59:155–7.
63. Villar D, Schwartz KJ, Carson TL, et al. Acute poisoning of cattle by fertilizer-contaminated water. Vet Hum Toxicol 2003;45:88–90.
64. DeRoos AJ, Ward MH, Lynch CF. Nitrate in public water supplies and the risk of colon and rectum cancers. Epidemiology 2003;14:640–9.
65. Walker R. Nitrates, nitrites and N-nitrosocompounds: a review of the occurrence in food and diet and the toxicological implications. Food Addit Contam 1990;7: 717–68.
66. Anderson DM, Stothers SC. Effects of saline water on young weanling pigs. Proceedings, Western Section, American Society of Animal Science 1972;23: 133–8.
67. Anderson DM, Stothers SC. Effects of saline water high in sulfates, chlorides and nitrates on the performance of young weanling pigs. J Anim Sci 1978;47: 900–7.
68. Fan AM, Willhite CC, Book SA. Evaluation of the nitrate drinking water standard with reference to infant methemoglobinemia and potential reproductive toxicity. Regul Toxicol Pharmacol 1987;7:135–48.
69. Bruning-Fann C, Kaneene JB, Miller RA, et al. The use of epidemiological concepts and techniques to discern factors associated with the nitrate concentration of well water on swine farms in the USA. Sci Total Environ 1994;153:85–96.
70. Case AA. Some aspects of nitrate poisoning in livestock. J Am Vet Med Assoc 1957;130:323–9.
71. Garner GB. Learning to live with nitrate. Mo Agr Exper Sta Bull 1958;708:1–8.
72. Emerick RJ. Consequences of high nitrate levels in feed and water supplies. Fed Proc 1974;33:1183–7.
73. Winter AJ, Hokanson JF. Effects of long-term feeding of nitrate, nitrite or hydroxylamine on pregnant dairy heifers. Am J Vet Res 1964;25:353–61.
74. Ensley SM. Relationships of drinking water quality to production and reproduction in dairy herds. Ames (IA).: Ph.D. Dissertation. Iowa State University; 2000.
75. Fleck M, Shurson GC. Effects of sulfate in drinking water for livestock. J Am Vet Med Assoc 1992;201:487–92.
76. Gould DH, Dargatz DA, Garry FB, et al. Potentially hazardous sulfur conditions on beef cattle ranches in the United States. J Am Vet Med Assoc 2002;221: 673–7.
77. National Research Council. Sulfur. In: Mineral tolerance of animals. Washington, DC: National Academies Press; 2005. p. 372–85.
78. Bouchard R, Conrad HR. Sulfur metabolism and nutritional changes in lactating cows associated with supplemental sulfate and methionine hydroxy analog. Can J Anim Sci 1974;54:587–93.
79. Albert WW, Garrigus US, Forbes RM, et al. The sulfur requirement of growing-fattening lambs in terms of methionine, sodium sulfate and elemental sulfur. J Anim Sci 1956;15:559–69.
80. Block RJ, Stekol JA. Synthesis of sulfur amino acids from inorganic sulfate by ruminants. Proc Soc Exp Biol Med 1950;73:391–4.
81. Johnson WH, Goodrich RD, Meiske JC. Metabolism of radioactive sulfur from elemental sulfur, sodium sulfate, and methionine by lambs. J Anim Sci 1971; 32:778–83.
82. Anderson CM. The metabolism of sulphur in the rumen of the sheep. N Z J Sci Technol 1956;37:379–94.

83. Halverson AW, Williams GD, Paulson GD. Aspects of sulfate utilization by the microorganisms of the ovine rumen. J Nutr 1968;95:363–8.

84. Dougherty RW, Mullenax CH, Allison MJ. Physiological phenomena associated with eructation in ruminants. In: Dougherty RW, editor. Physiology of digestion in the ruminant. Washington, DC: Butterworths Inc.; 1965. p. 159–70.

85. Evans CL. The toxicity of hydrogen sulphide and other sulphides. Q J Exp Physiol 1967;52:231–48.

86. Gould DH, McAllister MM, Savage JC. High sulfide concentrations in rumen fluid associated with nutritionally induced polioencephalomalacia in calves. Am J Vet Res 1991;52:1164–9.

87. Loneragan GH, Gould DH, Wagner JJ, et al. The effect of varying water sulfate content on H2S generation and health of feedlot cattle. J Anim Sci 1997; 75(Supplement 1):272.

88. Gooneratne SR, Olkowski AA, Klemmer RG. High sulfur related thiamine deficiency in cattle: a field study. Can Vet J 1989;30:139–46.

89. Gould DH. Update on sulfur-related polioencephalomalacia. Vet Clin North Am Food Anim Pract 2000;16:481–96.

90. Krasicka B, Gralak MA, Sieranska B, et al. The influence of dietary sulphur loading on metabolism and health in young sheep fed low fibre and high starch diet. Reprod Nutr Dev 1999;39:625–36.

91. Suttle NF. The interactions between copper, molybdenum, and sulphur in ruminant nutrition. Annu Rev Nutr 1991;11:121–40.

92. Mason J. The relationship between copper, molybdenum and sulphur in ruminant and non- ruminant animals: a preview. Vet Sci Commun 1978;2:85–94.

93. Smart ME, Cohen R, Christensen DA, et al. The effects of sulphate removal from the drinking water on the plasma and liver and copper and zinc concentrations of beef cows and their calves. Can J Anim Sci 1986;66:669–80.

94. Ivancic JJ, Weiss WP. Effect of dietary sulfur and selenium concentrations on selenium balance of lactating Holstein cows. J Dairy Sci 2001;84:225–32.

95. Pope AL, Moir RJ, Somers M, et al. The effect of sulphur on Se absorption and retention in sheep. J Nutr 1979;109:1448–55.

96. Cummings BA, Gould DH, Caldwell DR, et al. Ruminal microbial alterations associated with sulfide generation in steers with dietary sulfate-induced polioencephalomalacia. Am J Vet Res 1995;56:1390–5.

97. Saiki MK: A field example of selenium contamination in an aquatic food chain. Proceedings of the Annual Symposium on Selenium in the Environment - Fresno, CA June 10–12, 1986 1:67-76.

98. Halverson AW, Monty KJ. An effect of dietary sulfate on selenium poisoning in the rat. J Nutr 1960;70:100–2.

99. Corke MJ. An outbreak of sulphur poisoning in horses. Vet Rec 1981;109:212–3.

100. Gomez GG, Sandler RS, Seal JE. High levels of inorganic sulfate cause diarrhea in neonatal piglets. J Nutr 1995;125:2325–32.

101. Paterson DW, Wahlstrom RC, Libal GW, et al. Effects of sulfate in water on swine reproduction and young pig performance. J Anim Sci 1979;49:664–7.

102. Veenhuizen MF, Shurson GC, Kohler EM. Effect of concentration and source of sulfate on nursery pig performance and health. J Am Vet Med Assoc 1992;201: 1203–8.

103. Olkowski AA. Neurotoxicity and secondary metabolic problems associated with low to moderate levels of exposure to excess dietary sulphur in ruminants: a review. Vet Hum Toxicol 1997;39:355–60.

104. Loneragan GH, Wagner JJ, Gould DH, et al. Effects of water sulfate concentration on performance, water intake, and carcass characteristics of feedlot steers. J Anim Sci 2001;79:2941–8.
105. Sadler WC, Mahoney JH, Puch HC, et al. Relationship between sulfate and polioencephalomalacia in cattle. J Anim Sci 1983;57(Supplement 1):467.
106. Weeth HJ, Hunter JE. Drinking of sulfate-water by cattle. J Anim Sci 1971;32: 277–81.
107. Weeth HJ, Capps DL. Tolerance of growing cattle for sulfate-water. J Anim Sci 1972;34:256–60.
108. Patterson HH, Johnson PS, Patterson TR, et al. Effects of water quality on performance and health of growing steers. Proc West Section, Am Soc Anim Sci 2002;53:217–20.
109. Harper GS, King TJ, Hill BD, et al. Effect of coal mine pit water on the productivity of cattle. II. Effect of increasing concentrations of pit water on feed intake and health. Aust J Agric Res 1997;48:155–64.
110. Johnson WH, Meiske JC, Goodrich RD. Influence of high levels of two forms of sulfate on lambs. J Anim Sci 1968;27:1166.
111. Khan AA, Lovejoy D, Sharma AK, et al. Effects of high dietary sulphur on enzyme activities, selenium concentrations and body weight of cattle. Can J Vet Res 1987;51:174–80.
112. Rumsey TS. Effects of dietary sulfur addition and synovex-s ear implants on feedlot steers fed an all- concentrate finishing diet. J Anim Sci 1978;46:463–77.
113. Qi K, Lu CD, Owens FN. Sulfate supplementation of growing goats: effects on performance, acid-base balance, and nutrient digestibilities. J Anim Sci 1993; 71:1579–87.
114. Pendlum LC, Boling JA, Bradley NW. Plasma and ruminal constituents and performance of steers fed different nitrogen sources and levels of sulfur. J Anim Sci 1976;43:1307–14.
115. Bulgin MS, Lincoln SD, Mather G. Elemental sulfur toxicosis in a flock of sheep. J Am Vet Med Assoc 1996;208:1063–5.
116. Patterson HH, Johnson PS, Epperson WB. (2004). Effect of total dissolved solids and sulfates in drinking water for growing steers. Research Report, South Dakota State University, Brookings, SD, 2004. Paper 6.
117. Hamlen H, Clark E, Janzen E. Polioencephalomalacia in cattle consuming water with elevated sodium sulfate levels: a herd investigation. Can Vet J 1993;34: 153–8.
118. Raisbeck MF. Is polioencephalomalacia associated with high-sulfate diets? J Am Vet Med Assoc 1982;180:1303–5.
119. Ward EH, Patterson HH. Effects of thiamin supplementation on performance and health of growing steers consuming high sulfate water. Proc West Section, Am Soc Anim Sci 2004;55:375–8.
120. Harries WN. Polioencephalomalacia in feedlot cattle drinking water high in sodium sulfate. Can Vet J 1987;28:717.
121. Beke GJ, Hironaka R. Toxicity to beef cattle of sulfur in saline well water: a case study. Sci Total Environ 1991;101:281–90.
122. Niles GA, Morgan S, Edwards WC, et al. Effects of dietary sulfur concentrations on the incidence and pathology of polioencephalomalacia in weaned beef calves. Vet Hum Toxicol 2002;44:70–2.
123. McAllister MM, Gould DH, Raisbeck MF, et al. Evaluation of ruminal sulfide concentrations and seasonal outbreaks of polioencephalomalacia in beef cattle in a feedlot. J Am Vet Med Assoc 1997;211:1275–9.

124. Hemsley JA. Effect of high intakes of sodium chloride on the utilization of a protein concentrate by sheep. I. Wool growth. Aust J Agric Res 1975;26:709–14.

125. Hamilton JW, Gilbert CS. Composition of Wyoming range plants and soils. Univ Wyo Agr Exper Sta Res J 1972;55:1–14.

126. Raisbeck MF, Siemion RS, Smith MS. Modest copper supplementation blocks molybdenosis in cattle. J Vet Diagn Invest 2006;18:566–72.

127. Olkowski AA, Rousseaux CG, Christensen DA. Association of sulfate-water and blood thiamine concentration in beef cattle: field studies. Can J Anim Sci 1991; 71:825–32.

128. Wagner JJ, Loneragan GH, Gould DH, et al. The effect of varying water sulfate concentration on feedyard performance and water intake of steers. J Anim Sci 1997;75(Supplement 1):272.

129. Zinn RA, Alvarez E, Mendez M, et al. Influence of dietary sulfur level on growth performance and digestive function in feedlot cattle. J Anim Sci 1997;75: 1723–8.

130. Morris JG, Delmas RE, Hull JL. Salt (sodium) supplementation of range beef cows in California. J Anim Sci 1980;51:722–31.

131. National Research Council. Sodium chloride. In: Mineral tolerance of animals. Washington, DC: National Academies Press; 2005. p. 357–71.

132. Vincent IC, Williams HL, Hill R. Effects of sodium intake on lactation and Na levels in body fluids of Blackface sheep. Br J Nutr 1986;56:193–8.

133. Coppock CE, Fettman MJ. Chloride as a required nutrient for lactating dairy cows. Feedstuffs 1978;50:20–2.

134. National Research Council. Nutrient requirements, deficiencies and excesses. In: Nutrient requirements of horses. Washington, DC: National Academy of Sciences; 1989. p. 2–31.

135. Fraser D, Reardon E. Attraction of wild ungulates to mineral-rich springs in central Canada. Holarctic Ecol 1980;3:36–9.

136. Hagsten I, Perry TW. Evaluation of dietary salt levels for swine. I. Effect on gain, water consumption and efficiency of feed conversion. J Anim Sci 1976;42: 1187–9.

137. Hagsten I, Perry TW. Evaluation of dietary salt levels for swine. II. Effect on blood and excretory patterns. J Anim Sci 1976;42:1191–5.

138. Honeyfield DC, Froseth JA. Effects of dietary sodium and chloride on growth, efficiency of feed utilization, plasma electrolytes and plasma basic amino acids in young pigs. J Nutr 1985;115:1366–71.

139. Honeyfield DC, Froseth JA, Barke R. Dietary sodium and chloride levels for growing- finishing pigs. J Anim Sci 1985;60:691–8.

140. Silanikove N, Maltz E, Halevi A, et al. Metabolism of water, sodium, potassium, and chlorine by high yielding dairy cows at the onset of lactation. J Dairy Sci 1997;80:949–56.

141. Shalit U, Maltz E, Silanikove N, et al. Water, sodium, potassium and chlorine metabolism of dairy cows at the onset of lactation in hot weather. J Dairy Sci 1991;74:1874–83.

142. Jones G. Salt deficiency in dairy cattle. Clinical Report. Mod Vet Pract 1982;63: 810–1.

143. Whitlock RH, Kessler MJ, Tasker JB. Salt (sodium) deficiency in dairy cattle: polyuria and polydipsia as prominent clinical features. Cornell Vet 1975;65: 512–26.

144. Fettman MJ, Chase LE, Bentinck-Smith J, et al. Nutritional chloride deficiency in early lactation Holstein cows. J Dairy Sci 1984;67:2321–35.

145. Fettman MJ, Chase LE, Bentinck-Smith J, et al. Effects of dietary chloride restriction in lactating dairy cows. J Am Vet Med Assoc 1984;185:167–72.
146. Neathery MW, Blackmon DM, Miller WJ, et al. Chloride deficiency in Holstein calves from a low chloride diet and removal of abomasal contents. J Dairy Sci 1981;64:2220–33.
147. Croom JWJ, Harvey RW, Amaral DM, et al. Growth, carcass, ruminal and metabolic parameters of fattening steers fed elevated levels of sodium chloride and limestone. J Anim Sci 1983;57(S1):11–2.
148. Harvey RW, Croom JWJ, Pond KR, et al. High levels of sodium chloride in supplements for growing cattle. Can J Anim Sci 1986;66:423–9.
149. Hemsley JA, Hogan JP, Weston RH. Effect of high intakes of sodium chloride on the utilization of a protein concentrate by sheep. II. Digestion and absorption of organic matter and electrolytes. Aust J Agric Res 1975;26:715–27.
150. Mason GD, Scott D. Renal excretion of sodium and sodium tolerance in the pig. Q J Exp Physiol Cogn Med Sci 1974;59:103–12.
151. Golz DI, Crenshaw TD. Interrelationships of dietary sodium, potassium and chloride on growth in young swine. J Anim Sci 1990;68:2736–47.
152. Masters DG, Rintoul AJ, Dynes RA, et al. Feed intake and production in sheep fed diets high in sodium and potassium. Aust J Agric Res 2005;56:427–34.
153. Tucker WB, Hogue JF. Influence of sodium chloride or potassium chloride on systemic acid- base status, milk yield and mineral metabolism in lactating dairy cows. J Dairy Sci 1990;73:3485–93.
154. Sandals WCD. Acute salt poisoning in cattle. Can Vet J 1978;19:136–7.
155. Potter BJ. The effect of saline water on kidney tubular function and electrolyte excretion in sheep. Aust J Agric Res 1963;14:518–28.
156. Tomas FM, Jones GB, Potter BJ, et al. Influence of saline drinking water on mineral balances in sheep. Aust J Agric Res 1973;24:377–86.
157. Weeth HJ, Lesperance AL, Bohman VR. Intermittent saline watering of growing beef heifers. J Anim Sci 1968;27:739–44.
158. Wilson AD. The tolerance of sheep to sodium chloride in food or drinking water. Aust J Agric Res 1966;17:503–14.
159. Baird AC. Salt poisoning in the dog. Vet Rec 1969;85:756.
160. Hibbs CM, Thilsted JP. Toxicosis in cattle from contaminated well water. Vet Hum Toxicol 1983;25:253–4.
161. Trueman KF, Clague DC. Sodium chloride poisoning in cattle. Aust Vet J 1978; 54:89–91.
162. Berger LL. Salt for beef cattle. In: Berger LL, editor. Salt and trace minerals for livestock, poultry and other animals. Fairfax (VA): Salt Institute; 1993. p. 7–13.
163. Jaster EH, Schuh JD, Wegner TN. Physiological effects of saline drinking water on high producing dairy cows. J Dairy Sci 1978;61:66–71.
164. Peirce AW. Studies of salt tolerance of sheep. I. The tolerance of sheep for sodium chloride in the drinking water. Aust J Agric Res 1957;8:711–22.
165. Khanna C, Boermans HJ, Wilcock B. Fatal hypernatremia in a dog from salt ingestion. J Am Anim Hosp Assoc 1997;33:113–7.
166. Strange K. Regulation of solute and water balance and cell volume in the central nervous system. J Am Soc Nephrol 1992;3:12–27.
167. Weeth HJ, Lesperance AL. Renal function of cattle under various water and salt loads. J Anim Sci 1965;24:441–7.
168. Ohman AFS. Poisoning of cattle by saline bore water. Aust Vet J 1939;15:37–8.
169. Sautter JH, Sorenson DK, Clark JJ. Symposium on poisoning - Part I. Case 1 - Salt poisoning in swine. J Am Vet Med Assoc 1957;130:12–3.

170. Pretzer SD. Diarrhea in gilts caused by excessive dietary sodium chloride. Swine Health Prod 2000;8:181–3.

171. Fountaine JH, Gasche JDG, Oehme FW. Experimental salt poisoning (water deprivation syndrome) in swine. Vet Toxicol 1975;17:5–8.

172. Hughes DE, Sokolowski JH. Sodium chloride poisoning in the dog. Canine Pract 1978;5:28–31.

173. Barr JM, Kahn SA, McCullough SM, et al. Hypernatremia secondary to home-made play dough ingestion in dogs: a review of 14 cases from 1998 to 2001. J Vet Emerg Crit Care 2004;14:196–202.

174. Heller VG. Saline and alkaline drinking waters. J Nutr 1932;5:421–9.

175. Weeth HJ, Haverland LH. Tolerance of growing cattle for drinking water containing sodium chloride. J Anim Sci 1961;20:518–21.

176. Croom JWJ, Harvey RW, Linnerud AC. High levels of sodium chloride in beef cattle diets. Can J Anim Sci 1982;62:217–27.

177. Amaral DM, Croom JWJ, Rakes AH, et al. Increased concentration of sodium chloride on milk production of cows fed low fiber diets. J Dairy Sci 1985;68: 2940–7.

178. Nestor KE, Hemken RW, Harmon RJ. Influence of sodium chloride and potassium bicarbonate on udder edema and selected blood parameters. J Dairy Sci 1988;71:366–72.

179. Potter BJ, McIntosh GH. Effect of salt water ingestion on pregnancy in the ewe and on lamb survival. Aust J Agric Res 1974;25:909–17.

180. Wilson AD. Observations on the adaptation by sheep to saline drinking water. Aust J Exper Agric Anim Husbandry 1967;7:321–4.

181. Heller VG. The effect of saline and alkaline waters on domestic animals. Okla Agric Exp Sta Bull 1933;217:4–23.

182. Koletsky S. Role of salt and renal mass in experimental hypertension. Arch Pathol 1959;68:11–22.

183. Koletsky S. Hypertensive vascular disease produced by salt. Lab Invest 1958;7: 377–86.

184. Sapirstein LA, Brandt WL, Drury DR. Production of hypertension in the rat by substituting hypertonic sodium chloride solutions for drinking water. Proc Soc Exp Biol Med 1950;73:82–5.

185. Boyd EM, Abel MM, Knight LM. The chronic oral toxicity of sodium chloride at the range of the LD50 (0.1L). Can J Physiol Pharmacol 1966;44:157–72.

186. Rossi R, Del Prete E, Rokitzky J, et al. Effects of a high NaCl diet on eating and drinking patterns in pygmy goats. Physiol Behav 1998;63:601–4.

187. Medway W, Kare MR. The mechanism of toxicity associated with an excessive intake of sodium chloride. Cornell Vet 1959;49:241–51.

188. Lames HS. Salt poisoning in swine (water deprivation syndrome). Vet Med Small Anim Clin 1968;63:882–8.

189. Gudmundson J, Meagher DM. Sodium salt poisoning in swine. Can Vet J 1961; 2:115–6.

190. Peirce AW. Studies on salt tolerance of sheep. III. The tolerance of sheep for mixtures of sodium chloride and sodium sulfate in the drinking water. Aust J Agric Res 1960;11:548–56.

191. Peirce AW. Studies on salt tolerance of sheep. IV. The tolerance of sheep for mixtures of sodium chloride and calcium chloride in the drinking water. Aust J Agric Res 1962;13:479–86.

192. Peirce AW. Studies on salt tolerance of sheep. VI. The tolerance of wethers in pens for drinking waters of the types obtained from underground sources in Australia. Aust J Agric Res 1966;17:209–18.

193. Peirce AW. Studies on salt tolerance of sheep. II. The tolerance of sheep for mixtures of sodium chloride and magnesium chloride in the drinking water. Aust J Agric Res 1959;10:725–35.

194. Peirce AW. Studies on salt tolerance of sheep. V. The tolerance of sheep for mixtures of sodium chloride, sodium carbonate, and sodium bicarbonate in the drinking water. Aust J Agric Res 1963;14:815–23.

195. Potter BJ, Walker DJ, Forrest WW. Changes in intraruminal function of sheep when drinking saline water. Br J Nutr 1972;27:75–83.

196. Meyer JH, Weir WC. The tolerance of sheep to high intakes of sodium chloride. J Anim Sci 1954;13:443–9.

197. Berg RT, Bowland JP. Salt water tolerance of growing-finishing swine. Feeder's Day Report, vol. 39. Edmonton (Canada): Univ. of Albert; 1960. p. 14–6.

198. Thompson LJ. Sodium chloride. In: Gupta RC, editor. Veterinary toxicology - basic and clinical principles. New York: Elsevier; 2007. p. 461–4.

199. Heller VG, Larwood CH. Saline drinking water. Science 1930;71:223–4.

200. Burton AC, Cornhill JF. Correlation of cancer death rates with altitude and with the quality of water supply of the 100 largest cities in the United States. J Toxicol Environ Health 1977;3:465–78.

201. Craun GF, McCabe LJ. Problems associated with metals in drinking water. J Am Water Works Assoc 1975;67:593–9.

202. Monarca S, Donato F, Zerbini I, et al. Review of epidemiological studies on drinking water hardness and cardiovascular diseases. Eur J Cardiovasc Prev Rehabil 2006;13:495–506.

203. Schroeder HA. Relation between mortality from cardiovascular disease and treated water supplies. J Am Med Assoc 1960;172:1902–8.

204. Sauvant M-P, Pepin D. Drinking water and cardiovascular disease. Food Chem Toxicol 2002;40:1311–25.

205. CBC News: Water drinking contest blamed in death of California woman. 2007. Available at: http://www.cbc.ca/world/story/2007/01/14/water-intoxication.html. Accessed February 2, 2007.

206. Moule GR. Salt poisoning of sheep following evaporation of saline waters. Aust Vet J 1945;21:37.

207. Weeth HJ, Haverland LH, Cassard DW. Consumption of sodium chloride water by heifers. J Anim Sci 1960;19:845–51.

208. World Health Organization. Total dissolved solids in drinking water. In: Guidelines for drinking water quality. Geneva (Switzerland): World Health Organization; 2007. p. 223.

209. Challis DJ, Zeinstra JS, Anderson MJ. Some effects of water quality on the performance of high yielding cows in an arid climate. Vet Rec 1987;120:12–5.

210. Ray DE. Interrelationships among water quality, climate and diet on feedlot performance of steer calves. J Anim Sci 1989;67:357–63.

211. Saul GR, Flinn PC. Effects of saline drinking water on growth and water and feed intakes of weaner heifers. Aust J Exp Agric 1985;25:734–8.

212. Ray DE. Limiting the effects of stress on cattle. Utah Agric Exp Bull, Logan, UT 1986;512:17–26.

213. Solomon R, Miron J, Ben-Ghedalia D, et al. Performance of high producing dairy cows offered drinking water of high and low salinity in the Arava Desert. J Dairy Sci 1995;78:620–4.

214. Wegner TN, Schuh JP. Effect of water quality and season on milk production and water metabolism in Holstein cows. J Dairy Sci 1988;71(supplement 1):185.

215. Ahmed MH, Farid MFA, Shawket SM, et al. Effects of water deprivation on feed utilization and mineral balances in sheep drinking natural saline well water. J Arid Environ 1989;16:323–9.

216. Peirce AW. Studies on salt tolerance of sheep. VII. The tolerance of ewes and their lambs in pens for drinking waters of the types obtained from underground sources in Australia. Aust J Agric Res 1968;19:577–87.

217. Ramsay AA. Waters suitable for livestock. Analyses and experiences in New South Wales. Agric Gaz N S W 1924;35:339–42.

218. Idaho Mining Association. Interim surface water survey report. Table 3-3. Belleview (WA): Montgomery Watson; 1998.

219. Chapman PM, Baley H, Canaria E. Toxicity of total dissolved solids associated with two mine effluents to chironomid larvae and early life stages of rainbow trout. Environ Toxicol Chem 2000;19:210–4.

220. Ganong WF. Review of Medical physiology. Canada: Lange Medical Publications; 1971.

221. National Research Council. Minerals and acid-base balance. In: Mineral tolerance of animals. Washington, DC: National Academies Press; 2005. p. 449–52.

222. Bushinsky DA, Smith SB, Gavrilov KL, et al. Chronic acidosis- induced alteration in bone bicarbonate and phosphate. Am J Physiol Renal Physiol 2003;285: F532–9.

223. Swan RC, Pitts RF. Neutralization of infused acid by nephrectomized dogs. J Clin Invest 1955;34:205–12.

224. Ender F, Dishington IW, Helgebostad A. Parturient paresis and related forms of hypocalcemic disorders induced experimentally in dairy cows. Acta Vet Scand 1962;3(Supplement 1):3–52.

225. Goff JP, Horst RL. Use of hydrochloric acid as a source of anions for prevention of milk fever. J Dairy Sci 1998;81:2874–80.

226. Wang C, Beede DK. Effects of ammonium chloride and sulfate on acid-base status and calcium metabolism of dry Jersey cows. J Dairy Sci 1992;75:820–8.

227. DeZuane J. Handbook of drinking water quality: standards and controls. 1st edition. New York: Van Nostrand Reinhold; 1990.

228. Nordberg GF, Goyer RA, Clarkson TW. Impact of effects of acid precipitation on toxicity of metals. Environ Health Perspect 1985;63:169–80.

229. Sharpe WE, DeWalle DR. Potential health implications for acid precipitation, corrosion, and metals contamination of drinking water. Environ Health Perspect 1985;63:71–8.

230. Wood JM. Effects of acidification on the mobility of metals and metalloids: an overview. Environ Health Perspect 1985;63:115–9.

231. Ritskes-Hoitinga J, Meijers M, van Herck H. Bacteriological quality and intake of acidified drinking water in Wistar rats is pH-dependent. Scand J Lab Anim Sci 1998;25:124–8.

232. Tolo KJ. (397) and Erichsen S: Acidified drinking water and dental enamel in rats. Z Versuchstierkd 1969;11:229–33.

233. Environmental Protection Agency. Acid rain. 2009. Available at: https://www.epa.gov/acidrain. Accessed December 10, 2019.

234. Tober-Meyer BK, Bieniek HJ, Kupke IR. Studies on the hygiene of drinking water for laboratory animals. 2. Clinical and biochemical studies in rats and rabbits during long-term provision of acidified drinking water. Lab Anim 1981;15:111–7.

235. van der Wolf PJ, van Schie FW, Elbers AR. Administration of acidified drinking water to finishing pigs in order to prevent Salmonella infections. Vet Q 2001; 23:121–5.
236. Wu L, Kohler JE, Zaborina O, et al. Chronic acid water feeding protects mice against lethal gut-derived sepsis due to Pseudomonas aeruginosa. Curr Issues Intest Microbiol 2006;7:19–28.
237. Ender F, Dishington IW, Helgebostad A. Calcium balance studies in dairy cows under experimental induction and prevention of hypcalcaemic paresis. Z Tierphysiol Tierernahr Futtermittelkd 1971;28:233–56.
238. Hall JE, White WJ, Lang CM. Acidification of drinking water: its effects on selected biologic phenomena in male mice. Lab Anim Sci 1980;30:643–51.
239. Clausing P, Gottschalk M. Effects of drinking-water acidification, restriction of water-supply and individual caging on parameters of toxicological studies in rats. Z Versuchstierkd 1989;32:129–34.
240. McClure FJ. The destructive action, in vivo, of dilute acids and acid drinks and beverages on the rats' molar teeth. J Nutr 1943;26:251–9.
241. Hermann LM, White WJ, Lang CM. Prolonged exposure to acid, chlorine, or tetracycline in the drinking water: effects on delayed-type hypersensitivity, hemagglutination titers, and reticuloendothelial clearance rates in mice. Lab Anim Sci 1982;32:603–8.
242. Les EP. Effect of acidified-chlorinated water on reproduction in C3H-HeV and C57BL-5J mice. Lab Anim Care 1968;18:210–3.
243. Yiasoumi B. pH in water. 2003. Available at: http://www.ricecrc.org/reader/water-quality-supply/ac2-ph.htm. Accessed May 1, 2007.

Water Quality for Cattle
Metalloid and Metal Contamination of Water

Merl F. Raisbeck, DVM, MS, PhD

KEYWORDS

- Water quality • Arsenic • Barium • Fluoride • Molybdenum • Selenium

KEY POINTS

- Arsenic interacts with many other dietary factors, resulting in either increased or decreased toxicity.
- Livestock should not be fed water containing more than 10 mg Ba^{2+}/L even for short periods. Until there are better data, it is impossible to make any recommendations regarding chronic exposure.
- The effects of fluoride in feedstuffs and water are additive; what counts is the total dose of biologically available fluoride ion ingested by the animal.

ARSENIC

Arsenic (As) is a metalloid that occurs naturally in water and soil. It is also released from several human activities, including mining, petroleum and natural gas extraction, wood preservation, and burning coal.[1–6] Although As is rare in nature as a pure element, both inorganic and organic forms of As are commonly found in several different oxidation states, of which 2 (+3 and +5) occur in soil, water, and vegetation. Inorganic forms of As^{III} (ie, the arsenite ion) may be found under reducing conditions; however, As^V (ie, the arsenate ion) predominates in surface waters containing considerable dissolved oxygen.[7] Organic arsenical compounds have also been used as herbicides, insecticides, and drugs.

As was one of the first drugs to be used successfully against the syphilis organism in humans. Until recently, the organic arsenical roxarsone (4-hydroxy-3-nitrobenzenearsonic acid) was used to control coccidia in poultry and swine. More recently, arsenic trioxide (As_2O_3) has been suggested for treatment of promyelocytic leukemia and multiple myeloma.[8]

Most of what was known about the toxicity of As before the 1980s was based on the direct cytotoxic effects of As.[9] More recently, chronic consumption of low-level As-contaminated drinking water has become associated with several chronic maladies

Department of Veterinary Sciences, College of Agriculture, University of Wyoming, 2852 Riverside, Laramie, WY 82070, USA
E-mail address: raisbeck@uwyo.edu

Vet Clin Food Anim 36 (2020) 581–620
https://doi.org/10.1016/j.cvfa.2020.08.015
0749-0720/20/© 2020 Elsevier Inc. All rights reserved.
vetfood.theclinics.com

in people.[2,10–12] In contrast, some reports[13,14] suggest a hormetic (beneficial) effect of As at very low doses. So far, most of the evidence for chronic effects in humans consists of epidemiologic studies, but mechanistic, toxicologic explanations are appearing in the literature. The latter are important because they suggest these effects (and therefore dosages) are not likely relevant to our species of interest (discussed later).

The nomenclature of the arsenicals is often bewildering. In this article, the following metabolites are discussed: the trivalent, methylated metabolites monomethylarsonous acid (MMA^{III}) and dimethylarsonous acid (DMA^{III}), the pentavalent metabolites monomethylarsonic acid (MMA^V) and dimethylarsinic acid (DMA^V), and the inorganic ions such as arsenite (iAs^{III}) and arsenate (iAs^V).

Although the physiologic functions of As remain unknown, experiments with As deprivation in some species suggest As may be an essential element.[15] For example, rats maintained on a diet containing 30 ppb As showed decreased growth rate, rough hair coats, and decreased hematocrit levels compared with controls supplemented with 4.5 ppm As.[16] Lactating goats consuming a diet containing less than 10 ppb As had decreased growth rates, decreased milk production, lower birth weights, and a higher mortality compared with controls.[17] Female miniature pigs on a low-As diet produced smaller piglets, and only 62% were reported to give birth compared with pigs supplemented with 350 ppb As.[17] The results of experimentally induced deprivation in both in vivo and in vitro experiments suggest As plays a role in the methylation of both proteins and genetic molecules.[15] Although this and other similar research is scientifically interesting, As deficiency has never been shown in nature, probably because the apparent nutritional requirements are considerably less than common background concentrations.

It is commonly accepted that, with the possible exception of the trivalent methylated metabolites (MMA^{III} and DMA^{III}), inorganic forms of As are considerably more toxic in mammals than organic arsenicals.[10,11,18–20] Because the inorganic forms are also by far the most common water contaminants under field conditions and because MMA^{III} and DMA^{III} are too unstable to persist for any length of time under natural conditions, this article focuses on exposure to the inorganic forms of As^{III} and As^V.

Arsenate is absorbed from the gut by a 2-stage process. First, it is concentrated in mucosal cells and then, as protein-binding sites become filled, it moves down the resulting concentration gradient into the portal circulation.[15] The absorption mechanism of iAs^{III} is less completely understood, but it is commonly accepted that iAs^{III} is even more readily absorbed than iAs^V because of its greater water solubility.[7] Once absorbed, As is transported to various tissues via blood. In general, plasma concentrations increase relative to red cell concentrations as the dose increases, and trivalent As has a higher affinity for erythrocytes than As^V, resulting in slower clearance. Humans, rats, and mice have higher erythrocyte binding than other domestic mammals, resulting in slower elimination,[7,17] and thus greater potential for chronic effects.

The metabolism and excretion of As varies significantly between genotypes within humans.[17,21–23] These genetically mediated differences in metabolism are important in the pathogenesis of As intoxication. In general, inorganic As is methylated in vivo via a series of sequential reduction and oxidative-methylation reactions. Inorganic As^V is reduced in a linked reaction with oxidation of reduced glutathione to iAs^{III}, which is then methylated to MMA^V by reaction with S-adenosylmethionine. MMA^V is, in turn, reduced and methylated to DMA^V and so forth.[12] These metabolites are more readily excreted than inorganic As. In many, but not all, mammalian species, this process proceeds to DMA^V or the trimethyl arsenic metabolite trimethylarsine oxide; however, in human beings, significant amounts of MMA^{III} and DMA^{III} apparently escape methylation and react with critical tissue components. The rate of methylation and physiologic site of metabolism are thus important determinants of the rate of elimination and the potential for chronic effects at very low doses.[12,19]

As interacts with many other dietary factors, resulting in either increased or decreased toxicity. As has been known to minimize the toxicity of selenium (Se) for many years.[24–27] Simultaneous administration of Zn lessened the toxicity of As-spiked drinking water, possibly by induction of metallothionein, a metal-binding protein.[12,28] Folate can affect As methylation, and both folate deficiency and excess As induce fetal malformations in rats, thus a dietary deficiency of folate potentiates As toxicity.[12,29]

The acute toxicity of inorganic As has been attributed to the generation of reactive oxygen species and oxidative stress,[8,10,28] to the denaturation of critical protein moieties, and to interfering with phosphate metabolism.[7,30] In virtually all models, iAs^{III} is reported to be several-fold more toxic than iAs^V.[3,18,20,30] Trivalent iAs^{III} exerts its toxic effects by binding with specific functional groups (thiols and vicinyl sulfhydryls) on proteins.[4,7,17,31] For example, mitochondrial respiration is blocked by the reaction between As^{III} and the dihydrolipoic acid cofactor required for substrate oxidation.[30] As cited by Thomas and colleagues,[32] in 1966 Webb listed more than 100 enzymes that were inhibited by As^{III}. In contrast, pentavalent As^V displaces phosphate from certain biochemical reactions (eg, oxidative phosphorylation), resulting in depletion of ATP,[4,30–33] but may also be converted to As^{III} in the rumen.[33] Clinical signs associated with acute toxicity in virtually all species include diarrhea, vomiting, abdominal pain, weakness, staggering gait, myocardial degeneration, and death.[7,15,20,31,33]

Most acute As toxicity results from accidental exposure as a result of improper handling, use, and/or storage of arsenical compounds.[1,33] Cattle began staggering and showing signs of abdominal pain, diarrhea, anorexia, and recumbency shortly after ingesting forage that had been sprayed with sodium arsenite ($NaAsO_2$). Analysis of the grass performed several days later revealed it contained 2 ppm As, but the author noted concentrations were probably higher immediately after spraying.[34] Cows and calves became recumbent and showed a rapid weak pulse, intermittent clonic convulsions, and paddling movements after drinking fluid from a dipping vat containing 200 mg As/L.[35] A herd of approximately 275 cattle allowed to graze a road right of way recently sprayed with sodium arsenate (Na_2HAsO_4) sickened within hours, and 80 died within 4 days. Samples of grass taken at the onset contained 10,500 ppm As.[5] Selby and colleagues reported a similar scenario in Missouri in which the toxic vegetation contained 440 ppm As.[36] Cattle that consumed water containing 6 to 20 mg As/L and silage contaminated with 140 ppm As became progressively weaker, emaciated, and recumbent, and eventually died.[37] Nine adult cattle developed acute hemorrhagic diarrhea, and 2 died after consuming a dairy premix containing 5.50 ppm As; however, the As concentration of gastrointestinal (GI) contents suggested the exposure may have been considerably higher.[38] Heifers became weak, recumbent, and dysenteric, and died after ingesting vegetation containing approximately 2000 ppm As from herbicide contamination.[39] Approximately 12 hours after consuming pellets containing 27,000 ppm As and 20 ppm metaldehyde, cattle developed ataxia, profuse diarrhea, and muscle fasciculations.[40] The investigators suggested that most of the toxic effects were caused by As because the predominate clinical signs did not fit metaldehyde.

The toxicity of the herbicide lead arsenate ($PbHAsO_4$) is thought to be caused by the As content rather than lead (Pb).[41–43] After licking bags containing $PbHAsO_4$, cattle showed rapid pulse and respiration, oral mucosal erosions, diarrhea, and decreased milk production. As toxicity was confirmed when stomach contents were found to contain 175 ppm As.[42] Yearling cattle showed severe colic, diarrhea, and death after consuming an undetermined amount of a powder containing 39% Pb and 10% As. Rumen contents from the animals contained 478 to 531 ppm As.[44] Five calves began showing lethargy, ataxia, anorexia, decreased heart rates, and diarrhea after consuming powder containing 700,000 ppm As_2O_3. Four of the animals eventually died.[45] Cattle receiving 67 g of As_2O_3 and calves receiving 17 g of As_2O_3 as a topically applied medication became depressed and showed bloody diarrhea and a staggering gait soon after treatment. By 20 hours after treatment, 94 of 101 animals were dead.[46] Depression, ataxia, weakness, recumbency, diarrhea, abdominal pain, and tachycardia developed in 15 cattle that ingested ash from As-preserved wood. The ash was found to contain 780 ppm As.[47] After 260 heifers were moved to a new pasture containing an abandoned cattle dip, they became restless and belligerent and began showing signs of profuse salivation and watery diarrhea. More than 50% of the herd showed convulsions and became comatose, and 67 eventually died. The soil around the dip contained 10 to 150 ppm As and 50 to 500 ppm toxaphene. The investigators suggested that, because tissue As concentrations were not diagnostically significant, the combination of As and toxaphene caused the mortality.[48] Experimentally, 4 of 5 cattle died within 10 days of being dosed with 10 mg As/kg body weight (BW)/d as monosodium methanearsonate (As^V).[49] More than 650 of 1000 sheep developed diarrhea and died after consuming vegetation that had been sprayed with a $PbHAsO_4$ solution containing 0.58% As.[50] The condition was reproduced by dosing lambs with 12 mg As/kg BW.[50] Lambs showed signs of lethargy, abdominal pain, salivation, and diarrhea after ingesting forage containing 62 to 95 ppm As because of contamination with a cotton defoliant; 172 of 923 lambs died.[51] Six doe white-tailed deer were found dead after eating soil and vegetation contaminated by aerial spraying of an arsenical herbicide at the rate of 0.73 kg As per 4047 m^2 (1.6 lb per acre). Later analysis of a combined soil and vegetation sample yielded 2.4 ppm As, and water samples yielded 0.36 to 0.48 mg As/L.[52] However, the application rate calculates to a forage concentration of approximately 368 ppm or a dose of approximately 11 mg As/kg BW in an animal consuming 3% BW daily. These numbers are more consistent with reported tissue concentrations (18–19 ppm As) in the dead deer than the soil and water analysis.

As poisoning has also been reported in monogastrics. Nine thoroughbred racehorses died after showing signs of extreme distress, weakness, colic, rapid, weak pulse, hyperemic mucous membranes, and watery diarrhea. It was discovered that roughly 225 g (8 oz) of arsenical rat poison had spilled into their corn bin. Postmortem chemical analysis discovered significant amounts of As in the stomach and liver of 2 horses.[53] Working backward from the numbers presented, the authors estimate the horses received a dose of between 1 and 10 mg As/kg BW. GI cramps, vomiting, diarrhea, electrocardiogram changes, and liver disruption developed in a 27-year-old woman after she ingested 9000 mg of As_2O_3.[54] Furr and Buck[55] poisoned cats with a commercial ant bait. Doses of As (as Na_2HAsO_4) greater than 8 mg/kg BW were lethal; the threshold of toxic signs was 2 mg/kg BW, and the no-effect level was 1.5 mg/kg BW.

In swine, arsanilic acid has been used as a growth promotant and as a treatment of swine dysentery.[56] In several cases, excessive doses or prolonged treatment periods have resulted in a chronic syndrome characterized by apparent blindness caused by degeneration of the optic nerve and optic chiasma.[57–63] The toxic mechanism and toxicity of this class of arsenical drugs are distinct from and less than inorganic As and therefore are not considered further here.

At present, despite convincing epidemiologic evidence that very low concentrations of As in drinking water can cause chronic disease, especially cancer, in human beings, there are no animal models that reliably duplicate these toxic effects without resorting to high doses and/or pharmacologic and genetic manipulation to render them more sensitive.[9,23] The current belief, derived from in vitro studies and specialized laboratory animal models, is that small amounts of DMA[III] and MMA[III] escape the methylation process in people and, over prolonged periods, cause cellular damage that results in diseases such as cancer.[4,11,14,22,30,32] DMA[V] and MMA[V] are the main urinary metabolites of As excreted in most mammals; however, the trivalent As metabolites, dimethylarsinous acid (DMA[III]), and MMA[III] have been reported in fresh urine of As-poisoned human patients.[11] The glutathione conjugate of DMA[III] was more toxic to cells in vitro than inorganic As,[64] and DMA[III] causes single-strand breaks in DNA in vitro.[11,65] These processes are apparently limited to human beings and specialized laboratory models; thus, based on known differences in metabolism, this class of disease and dosages does not seem relevant for livestock.

Developmental studies of orally administered MMA[V] and DMA[V] (the metabolites of inorganic As in most nonhuman mammals) in rats and rabbits determined that the threshold of fetal damage was similar to that for maternal toxicity, or about 36 and 48 mg/kg BW, respectively.[66] Administration of As by gavage to pregnant rats and mice did not produce morphologically evident teratogenesis at non–maternally toxic dosages, although there was some evidence of behavioral changes in pups born to dams consuming drinking water with slightly less As[III] than the lowest maternally toxic dose.[67] In contrast, Domingo[68] reported that As[III], via the oral route of exposure, was much less teratogenic in several species. This finding indicates that dietary limits safe for a dam should also provide adequate protection for her fetus.

There are few reports of chronic toxicity in nonrodent species. Because of the rapid excretion of As in cattle, sheep, dogs, and so forth, these species are able to clear less-than-acutely toxic doses of As before they cause much of a problem.[15,69] Reports of chronic toxicity involve dosages similar to those reported for acute or subacute poisoning. Female beagles fed 4 to 8 mg of NaAsO$_2$ (2.3–4.6 mg As)/kg BW/d for 183 days showed decreased weight gains caused by decreased feed consumption and slightly increased liver enzyme levels.[70] Beagle dogs were fed varying concentrations of As as either As[III] or As[V] for 2 years. At 50 ppm and less, there were no measurable effects. At 125 ppm dietary As, the dogs lost weight and several died with lesions of inanition.[71] Three of 4 sheep given 88 mg PbHAsO$_4$/kg BW once per month died within 24 hours of the seventh dose. Other sheep in that study, given 22 and 44 mg of PbHAsO$_4$ (4.9 and 9.7 mg As/kg BW), survived 11 doses with no clinical signs.[41] One of 2 lambs dosed with 1.5 mg As/kg BW/d as PbHAsO$_4$ died after 35 days; the other survived until the study was stopped at 94 days.[50] Sheep fed a mean daily dose of 1.4 mg As/kg (As species unspecified) for 3 weeks remained in good condition for the duration of the study.[72] Bucy and colleagues[73] fed potassium arsenite to feedlot lambs at doses as high as 3.26 mg As/kg BW/d for 8 weeks without adverse effects. In a later study, 1.75 mg/kg BW/d was not toxic, but higher doses caused feed refusal and clinical signs of toxicity.[74] Peoples[69] added arsenic acid to dairy rations at 1.25 ppm, a dose of approximately 0.48 mg As/kg BW/d for 7 weeks with no effects. Virtually all of the ingested As was eliminated as quickly as it was eaten.

It has been proposed that elk in the Madison-Firehole watershed of Yellowstone National Park have shorter lifespans because of naturally increased As levels in water and feedstuffs.[75] Exposure was estimated to be greater than 1.25 mg/kg BW/d based on tissue concentrations and extrapolation from bovine studies and between 0.01 and 6.2 mg/kg BW/d based on forage and water analysis. The difference in longevity may be caused by other environmental differences between the Madison-Firehole area and the control site.[75] Forsberg[76] showed slight but measurable inhibition of normal rumen fermentation in vitro with As concentrations as low as 5 mg/L of rumen fluid, but did not provide any data as to how this concentration related to dietary intake. Assuming that the rumen fluid concentration is equivalent to the combined concentrations in feed and water, the concentration would be equivalent to a dose of roughly 1 mg As/kg BW.

Recommendations in this article are based on the most toxic form of water-soluble As, specifically inorganic As[III], as the arsenite ion. Routine water quality analysis available to livestock producers does not distinguish between As species, and, although the less toxic pentavalent forms of As are more likely to occur in surface waters, trivalent As is seen frequently enough in specialized surveys to justify the assumption.[77,78] It is suggested that ruminant animals are less susceptible to As than monogastrics.[15,79] However, with the exception of laboratory rodents, I was not able to confirm this, thus I have assumed that horses and ruminants are equally sensitive to As.

Chronic poisoning of the type (cancer, blackfoot disease, and so forth) that prompted lowering the human drinking water standard from 0.05 to 0.01 mg As/L does not apparently occur in livestock species, as shown by the ongoing search for an appropriate animal model to study the human condition. The mechanisms putatively involved in the pathogenesis of chronic damage in people (ie, chemical attack by methylated As[III] metabolites on cellular macromolecules) do not seem to be relevant in livestock. In domestic livestock, as opposed to people, most As is excreted via urine as DMA[III].[23] Together with the shorter observed half-life in these species, this suggests that little trivalent As escapes methylation and excretion to cause cancer. Chronic poisoning in livestock species involves mechanisms similar to acute poisoning and requires dosages very similar to acute poisoning.

Given the accumulating evidence that As is a human carcinogen, the question of residues arises. Can food animals consuming As from water accumulate dangerous amounts of As in edible tissues without themselves showing signs of toxicity? The literature to date suggests cattle, sheep, and so forth eliminate As too quickly for this to be a concern, and a study completed in 2007 by the University of Minnesota (Murphy MJ, Professor of Veterinary Toxicology, University of Minnesota, personal communication, 2007)[80] failed to find any evidence of As accumulation in milk or edible tissues from dairy cattle watered from As-contaminated (140 μg/L) wells.

The threshold toxic dose in domestic ruminants seems to be between 1 and 2 mg/kg BW. This dose is in general agreement with the National Research Council (NRC),[15] which recommended 30 to 50 ppm dietary As as a maximum tolerated dose and with other reviews.[33,79,81,82] It differs from the European Union recommendation of 2 ppm dietary As, for which I have not discovered any published justification. Sufficient quantitative data were not found to estimate a similar threshold for horses, but this dose is similar to that reported in another monogastric species (dogs),[70] and previous reviews suggest horses are similar to cattle in sensitivity and/or less frequently affected than cattle under similar field conditions.[81,83] Therefore, it seems reasonable that limits that are safe for cattle should be protective for horses. Assuming legible As in feedstuffs, 5 mg As/L in drinking water provides the minimum toxic dose of 1 mg As/kg BW to grazing animals in warm weather. Obviously, if animals are receiving any As from other sources, less will be required to achieve a toxic dose.

Assuming a no observed adverse effect level (NOAEL) of 0.5 mg/kg BW/d and allowing for small forage concentrations, I recommend drinking water for livestock not exceed 1 mg As/L.

BARIUM

Barium (Ba), an alkaline earth element, oxidizes easily when exposed to air, and is mainly present as the Ba^{2+} ion in water. Ba found in surface water and groundwater is predominantly derived from weathered rock and minerals. Commonly occurring Ba minerals are insoluble barite (barium sulfate, $BaSO_4$) and the more soluble witherite (barium carbonate, $BaCO_3$), whereas the Ba^{2+} ion is most common in natural waters.[84] Ba concentrations in water are likely to be higher near drilling platforms than natural background concentrations.[85] In water, soluble Ba may precipitate out of aqueous solution as insoluble salts (eg, $BaSO_4$ and $BaCO_3$). At pH less than 9.3, the formation of $BaSO_4$ limits the Ba^{2+} concentration in natural waters. Ba has a variety of uses: $BaSO_4$ is used in patients for digestive tract imaging and for oil drilling, and $BaCO_3$ is used in rodenticides.[85–87]

Ba absorbed from the GI tract is primarily deposited in bones and teeth and excreted via feces and urine.[88,89] The bioavailability of various Ba compounds given orally varies widely (0.7%–85%) depending on the chemical form, species, age, and fasting status of the animal.[90–92] In general, more soluble forms of Ba such as barium chloride ($BaCl_2$) are more readily absorbed. Young rats absorb approximately 10-fold more than adults.[91] Ba disappears from blood and milk with a half-life measured in days[88,93]; however, Ba deposited in bone has a half-life measured in years, and disappearance from bone generally depends on bone turnover.[94] These observations, together with the divalent cationic nature of Ba and the fact that Ba is known to bind calcium (Ca)-dependent enzyme systems in cells, suggest that Ba metabolism uses Ca transport systems in the body.

Water-soluble forms such as $BaCl_2$ and, to a lesser extent, $BaCO_3$ are generally the most toxic. $BaSO_4$ is insoluble and is not considered hazardous to people or other monogastric animals. The specific mechanism of Ba toxicity is a blockade of passive transmembrane potassium (K^+) conductance in excitable cells by the ion.[86,87,95,96] Ba also competes with and/or mimics the functions of Ca in muscle contraction and in second messenger pathways.[86,95] The characteristic systemic effect of Ba poisoning is "violent contraction of smooth, striated, and cardiac muscle."[96,97] Clinically, this effect is manifested as arterial hypertension and premature supraventricular and ventricular contractions, followed by skeletal muscle contraction, salivation, vomiting, colic, and diarrhea.[86,87,95,96,98,99] Death results from arrhythmias and cardiac failure.[90,99,100] The hypokalemia seen in Ba poisoning is thought to result from blockade of passive K channels and intracellular sequestration, because Ba has no proven activity on the $Na^+K^+ATPase$ pump.[87,96,101]

Data on the toxicity of Ba in grazing animals are limited. Two ruminally fistulated dairy goats were infused with 5 mM $BaCl_2$ at a rate of 60 mL/h. The ruminal fluid $BaCl_2$ ion concentration was estimated to be 0.4 mM assuming no absorption or precipitation occurred. After receiving Ba^{2+} for 6 hours, the animals showed weakness and paralysis, and died later that night. The resulting oral lethal dose of $BaCl_2$ in the goat was determined to be less than 4.6 mg Ba^{2+}/kg BW.[102] This Ba dose equates to approximately 23 mg/L in drinking water under the conditions outlined at the beginning of this article. Ba poisoning occurred during 2 successive years in cattle that were trailed through an abandoned Pb/silver mine site containing a Ba-contaminated pond.[103] Six of 30 animals died the first year and 16 of 20 the second. Liver and kidney tissues from affected animals contained increased Ba concentrations, and other metals (Pb, As, Se, and so forth) were within normal limits. Pond water contained 2.2 mg Ba^{2+}/L; however, clay found in both the abomasum of the dead cattle and in the pond contained 69,000 ppm Ba. The amount of Ba, if any, absorbed from the clay is unknown. Radiograph diffraction analysis of the clay indicated that the Ba in clay was primarily present as insoluble $BaSO_4$, with lesser amounts of $BaCa(CO_3)_2$ and $BaCO_3$. Reagor (Reagor JC, Toxicologist, Texas Veterinary Medical Diagnostics Laboratory, Personal communication, 2011) fed $BaCO_3$ to steers at 0.4% and 0.8% of the dry matter diet to steers (0.28% and 0.56% Ba respectively). All 3 receiving the high dose died after a single feeding; all 3 receiving the lower concentration remained healthy for the duration of the experiment. Clinical signs in the steers were similar to those reported in monogastrics.

Malhi and colleagues[104] investigated the optimum concentration of $BaCO_3$ for a rodenticide and concluded that 1.5 g of $BaCO_3$ per 100 g BW (or 15,000 mg/kg) was the most efficient rat poison. There was no attempt to determine a minimum lethal dose. Mattila and colleagues[105] administered $BaCl_2$ via the marginal ear vein of 6 rabbits instrumented with an electrocardiograph. From 3 to 5 mg Ba^{2+}/kg BW caused dysrhythmias with and without convulsions. Rabbits receiving 3 mg Ba^{2+}/kg BW survived, despite convulsions. Roza and Berman[99] observed anesthetized dogs after infusing them with 0.66 to 2.64 µmol Ba (as $BaCl_2$)/kg/min to identify mechanisms of Ba-induced hypokalemia and hypertension and to study the Ba-K interaction on the heart in vivo. Rates greater than 4 µmol $BaCl_2$/kg/min ($\sim$362 µg Ba^{2+}/kg/min) were fatal within a few minutes because of respiratory paralysis.

Gosselin and colleagues[97] described the oral lethal dose in humans as 1 to 15 g. A research chemist attempted suicide by ingesting a teaspoon (approximately 13 g) of $BaCl_2$. He was rushed to a hospital and survived after intensive therapy. In another case, a 26-year-old man consumed 1 can of Magic Shave containing 12.8 g of Ba^{2+} ion and 3 g of sulfide.[106] He developed respiratory paralysis, severe respiratory acidosis, and hypokalemia. He survived after intensive therapy.

Several studies have examined the chronic oral toxicity of low-concentration $BaCl_2$ in drinking water to people because of Ba's recognized cardiac toxicity. Wones and colleagues[107] concluded that drinking water concentrations of 5 and 10 mg Ba^{2+}/L did not affect any known cardiovascular risk factors. Eleven healthy men were given $BaCl_2$ in their drinking water for 6 weeks. For the first 2 weeks of the experiment, no $BaCl_2$ was added to their water. $BaCl_2$ was then added at rates of 2 to 5 mg/L for the next 4 weeks and 10 mg Ba/L for the last 4 weeks. The investigators discovered no apparent changes in modifiable cardiovascular risk factors, but there was a trend toward slightly increased total blood Ca. Brenniman and Levy[108] conducted an epidemiologic study to determine whether mortality and morbidity rate were significantly increased in human populations drinking increased (2–10 mg/L) Ba levels compared with populations with little or no Ba exposure. They found higher cardiovascular mortalities in communities consuming increased levels of Ba, but there were also several confounding variables. There were no significant differences in blood pressure, hypertension, stroke, and heart or kidney disease.

The single oral LD_{50} (dose that is lethal for 50% of a test sample) of $BaCl_2$ in rats was estimated to be approximately 264 mg Ba/kg BW.[109] Short-term (1–10 day) oral exposure to $BaCl_2$ at daily doses up to 138 mg Ba/kg BW produced no significant adverse health effects. Because of the link with cardiovascular disease in people, most chronic laboratory animal studies focus on cardiac effects. Barium acetate, $Ba(CH_3COO)_2$, added to drinking water at 5 mg Ba^{2+}/L and fed to rats over their lifespan had little or no effect on growth, carcinogenesis, or longevity.[110] Rats drinking water with 100 mg Ba^{2+}/L as $BaCl_2$ for 16 months showed significant but varying increases in systolic blood pressure.[111] In a similar study, the average systolic pressure increased significantly after exposure to 100 mg Ba^{2+}/L for 1 month and after 10 mg Ba^{2+}/L for 8 months. After 16 months, rats exposed to 100 mg Ba^{2+}/L had depressed heart rates and decreased cardiac function.[112,113] Another experiment examined the effect of $BaCl_2$ in drinking water for 92 days on serum electrolytes, BW, behavior, and fertility in rats and mice.[114] The NOAEL for Ba, based on depressed BW gain and renal, fertility, and lymphoid lesions, was estimated to be 1120 mg Ba^{2+}/L. Mortality was attributed to kidney damage. Tardiff and colleagues[115] studied acute oral and sub-chronic toxicity of Ba as $BaCl_2$ in rats. The acute oral LD_{50} for weanling rats was 220 mg Ba/kg BW and for adults was 132 mg Ba/kg BW. Drinking 250 mg Ba^{2+}/L for up to 13 weeks resulted in less water consumption than controls, but it did not cause any clinical signs of toxicity, nor was BW affected. McCauley and colleagues[116] found no significant lesions in rats exposed to up to 250 mg Ba/L drinking water for 68 weeks, nor were there measurable electrocardiographic changes when measured at 5 months.

Chronic Ba exposure causes nephropathy in rodents. Male rats drinking 5 ppm Ba as the acetate salt in a lifetime study developed proteinuria.[110] McCauley and colleagues[116] identified kidney lesions in rodents administered 1000 mg Ba/L in drinking water for 16 weeks. Dietz and colleagues[114] identified kidney lesions in male and female mice receiving doses of 436 to 562 mg Ba^{2+}/kg BW/d via drinking water for 92 days. Rats receiving the same water drank less, receiving only about one-quarter of the dose and had much milder renal lesions. In a subsequent 2-year cancer bioassay, female and male rats receiving 75 and 60 mg Ba^{2+}/kg BW/d, respectively, in drinking water gained less than controls but did not show any Ba-related clinical signs. Mice in the same 2-year study drank up to 160 (male) or 200 (female) mg Ba^{2+}/kg BW/d and had significantly greater premature mortality caused by kidney disease than did controls.[117]

The acutely toxic effects of Ba are similar in monogastrics and ruminants, which argues that (1) Ba is a valid water quality concern for livestock, and (2) subacute and chronic effects are probably similar, if not identical, between these species. The putative toxic mechanisms of the Ba^{2+} ion in rodents and human beings involve physiologic mechanisms that are highly conserved (ie, very similar) throughout terrestrial mammals; therefore, any species-specific differences in toxicity logically derive from species-specific differences in the toxicokinetics of Ba. In monogastric mammals, the oral toxicity of Ba compounds correlates with their water solubility. Less soluble forms of Ba (notably $BaSO_4$) are poorly absorbed and are thus considerably less toxic than more soluble salts such as $BaCl_2$, barium nitrate $[Ba(NO_3)_2]$, or barium hydroxide $[Ba(OH)_2]$.[92] There are no equivalent data in ruminants. Theoretically, reduction of the SO_4 salt to sulfide by rumen microflora might result in increased bioavailability of the Ba^{2+} ion. However, as a practical matter, this theoretic effect would be significant only in solid feedstuffs because insoluble forms of Ba (ie, $BaSO_4$) are presumably not present in drinking water in any significant concentration.

The long-term effects of Ba, especially on reproduction, have been incompletely investigated in any species. A single Russian report of Ba inhalation toxicity describes reproductive lesions in both male and female rats,[118] whereas more recent rodent studies did not note alterations in reproductive tissues or reproductive function following acute, intermediate or chronic exposure to Ba.[114,116,117] Kidney damage was observed in laboratory rodents following 2-year exposure to 200 mg Ba/kg BW and in long-term (91-day) oral exposure to 450 mg Ba/kg BW, but it was not seen after administration of 250 mg Ba/kg BW for 36 to 46 weeks.[116,117]

The only quantitative data available in ruminants indicates that 138 mg Ba/kg BW, as $BaCO_3$, in dry feedstuffs was acutely toxic to steers, whereas 69 mg Ba/kg BW was not (Reagor JC, toxicologist, Texas Veterinary Medical Diagnostics Laboratory, personal communication, 2011). Assuming water consumption of 20% of BW, this translates to 690 mg Ba^{2+}/L in drinking water as being acutely toxic or 345 mg Ba^{2+}/L as the NOAEL. This finding contrasts with the report of Richards and colleagues[103] that 2 mg soluble Ba^{2+}/L water, plus some undetermined amount of Ba from sediment, was immediately toxic to cows and calves. It is also much higher than the toxic dose reported in goats, where 7 mg/kg BW $BaCl$[119] (4.6 mg Ba/kg BW) was lethal.[102] It is likely that $BaCO_3$ in feed is not as bioavailable as the Ba^{2+} ion in water. The acutely lethal dose in the goat study translates to 23 mg Ba^{2+}/L under the assumptions outlined at the start of this article.

Obviously, much more research needs to be done with Ba in ruminants, but, given the current state of knowledge, soluble Ba^{2+} concentrations should be held to much less than 23 mg/L to avoid acute toxicity. There are no data on chronic Ba^{2+} ion toxicity in any livestock species. In addition to the limited and conflicting data from chronic studies in other animals, this makes it impossible to postulate a long-term safe level of the Ba^{2+} ion in drinking water for domestic livestock species with any degree of certainty.

Livestock should not be fed water containing more than 10 mg Ba^{2+}/L even for short periods. Until there are better data, it is impossible to make any recommendations regarding chronic exposure.

FLUORIDE

Fluorine (F) is the most electronegative and reactive of known elements. It rarely occurs freely in nature, usually combining with other elements to form fluorides. Mineral forms of F include cryolite (Na_3AlF_6), fluorite (CaF_2), and fluorapatite [$Ca_5(PO_4)_3F$]. Vegetation can accumulate fluoride from soil, water, and the atmosphere.[120] In aqueous environments, F occurs as the free fluoride ion (F^-) and is mobile, especially in alkaline waters.[84] Unless surface waters are contaminated by a F^- source, groundwater tends to have higher concentrations.

Fluoride is readily absorbed by the stomach, rumen, and small intestine. The efficiency of absorption depends on the solubility of the specific F compound; other dietary components; and the species, sex, and age of the animal.[121,122] Conditions that result in very low pH favor the formation of hydrogen fluoride (HF), which is lipophilic and thus diffuses easily across lipid membranes. The F^- ion is absorbed in the small intestine via a pH-independent process.[121] Soluble fluorides (ie, the F^- ion in water) are almost 100% absorbed. Less soluble sources, such as F compounds in bone meal, are poorly absorbed. Dietary Ca, magnesium (Mg), aluminum (Al), sodium chloride (NaCl), and lipid are known to depress F uptake.[121,123]

Two mechanisms are responsible for removal of F^- from the systemic circulation: renal excretion and deposition in calcified tissues. After absorption, most F^- circulates in plasma as ionic F^-. To a lesser extent, it circulates as CaF_2 or HF, or it is bound to protein.[123–125] Circulating F^- represents a small portion of the total body burden but is the form most easily exchanged with other tissues and/or eliminated via renal filtration.[124,125] Urinary excretion is the primary route of elimination and is directly related to urinary pH.[123,126] Under normal circumstances, roughly 50% of ingested F^- is eliminated immediately, and the remainder is incorporated into bony tissues[121]; however, these percentages may be dramatically modified by physiologic factors such as age and sex. Calcified tissues such as teeth and bone have a great affinity for F^-, incorporating it as fluorapatite in place of hydroxyapatite in the calcified matrix.[121,126] To a certain extent, bone deposition represents a form of detoxication by decreasing the F^- exposure of other tissues. However, fluorapatite crystals are less soluble than the hydroxyapatite they replace and thus (1) persist for long periods in bone, and (2) interfere with normal turnover (remodeling) of bone. Thus, bone F^- interferes with normal physiologic processes such as growth and healing. Because F^- deposition in skeletal tissues is related to the turnover of bone minerals, young, rapidly growing animals are more likely affected.[121]

In the past, forages contaminated by smelters or grown in naturally high-F soils, rock phosphate nutritional supplements, and/or consumption of naturally high F^- water have resulted in fluorosis.[121,122,127–129] Large doses of soluble F^- can form corrosive HF, interfere with excitable cells, and/or precipitate divalent cations from serum.[130,131] Acute fluorosis is manifested as gastroenteritis, cardiac arrhythmias, and/or collapse.[130] Chronic or subchronic exposure to lower doses results in kidney damage,[130,132,133] neurologic damage, or reproductive failure.[134–136,] The most sensitive (ie, occur at the lowest dose) clinical manifestations of F^- toxicosis in livestock under real-world conditions are tooth and bone deformities.[122,137–142] These bony lesions result in difficulty grazing, reduced feed intake, ill thrift, and decreased performance.[122,140,142] Alternating periods of high and low F^- exposure are more toxic than a continuous intake of the same average amount. Nutritional status and the age when exposed to F^- also influence tolerance.[143]

Rats exposed in utero and as pups to F^- had sex-specific and dose-specific behavioral deficits.[144] Males were most sensitive to prenatal exposure; females were more sensitive to weanling and adult exposure. Drinking water containing 125 mg F^-/L resulted in reduced growth, and 175 mg F^-/L was lethal. Both 30 and 100 mg F^-/L in the drinking water produced subtle brain damage, indicating oxidative stress in rats.[145] Paul and colleagues[146] administered sodium fluoride (NaF) by oral intubation daily at 20 or 40 mg/kg BW to adult female rats for 60 days. This treatment suppressed spontaneous motor activity and tissue and serum protein concentrations in a dose-dependent manner. Wang and colleagues[147] found decreased total phospholipid concentrations and ubiquinone in rat livers, which they attributed to oxidative stress after 7 months of consuming water containing 30 or 100 mg F^-/L.

Rats were offered drinking water containing 225 mg F^-/L as NaF for 60 days.[148] A second group was additionally gavaged with calcium carbonate ($CaCO_3$). NaF treatment resulted in decreased food and water intake, reduced BW, and impaired nervous function. Fluoride-induced dental lesions, inhibition of acetylcholinesterase and N^+K^+ATPase activity, and hypoproteinemia improved after NaF withdrawal. Concurrent Ca treatment lessened the impact of F by decreasing serum F concentrations.[148] Rats given drinking water with either 30 or 100 mg F^-/L as NaF for 7 months had decreased kidney proteins and BW gains, and dental fluorosis.[132] Either 10 or 30 mg F^-/L administered to male rats via drinking water for 3 to 6 months did not cause any overt clinical effects but did produce biochemical indications of liver damage.[149] Oral administration of NaF in water at 5 or 10 mg (2.25 or 4.5 mg F^-)/kg BW/d for 30 days to adult male rats resulted in reduced BW and sperm count.[134] Heindel and colleagues[150] studied fetal development in rats and rabbits fed up to 300 or 400 mg NaF (135 or 180 mg F^-)/L drinking water during gestation. Although there were no teratogenic effects at any dose, dams lost weight after drinking water with concentrations greater than 150 mg NaF/L (rat) or 200 mg NaF/L (rabbit).

Certain elements are known to interfere with the uptake of F, a fact some clinicians have attempted to exploit therapeutically. Rats were offered water with equivalent amounts of F as either aluminum fluoride (AlF_3, 0.5 mg/L) or NaF (2.1 mg/L) for 52 weeks to evaluate the interaction of Al with F.[151] AlF_3 reduced the neuronal density of the brain neocortex compared with the NaF and control rats. Brain and kidney Al concentrations were higher in both AlF_3-treated and NaF-treated groups than in controls. Rabbits were fed drinking water containing various combinations of either

F⁻ (1–50 mg/L as NaF) or Al (100–500 mg/L as AlCl₃) for 10 weeks. Although none of the treatments resulted in significant weight loss, Al treatment decreased F⁻ accumulation in bone. Surprisingly, F⁻, by itself, increased bone Al concentrations, suggesting Al or an Al-F complex plays a role in osteofluorosis.[152] Kessabi and colleagues[153] gavaged sheep with 0, 1.9, or 4.7 mg F⁻/kg BW, with or without 13.5 mg Al/kg, for 33 months. In all treated animals, the general health status declined, and osteodental signs appeared while F levels increased in teeth, bones, and organs. In the sheep given 4.7 mg F⁻/kg BW, lesions were observed in kidney and liver. Aluminum sulfate [(Al₂(SO₄)₃] alleviated some, but not all, of the effects of 1.9 mg F⁻/kg BW.

Rats and mice were treated with NaF in drinking water at 11, 45, or 79 mg F⁻/L for up to 2 years in a carcinogenesis bioassay.[154] Body weights and survival rates of ⁻animals treated with F⁻ were similar to controls. Osteosarcomas occurred in a small, statistically and historically insignificant number of male rats at the highest dose, whereas there was no evidence of carcinogenic activity in female rats or mice of either sex. Rats on the highest 2 dosages also showed some increased osteofluorosis and dental fluorosis.[154] Deer mice captured and fed 38, 1065, 1355, or 1936 ppm dietary F⁻ for 8 weeks lost weight and many died at the highest dose.[155]

Osteodental fluorosis was observed in cattle, buffalo, sheep, and goats from several villages in India where the mean F⁻ concentration in drinking water was 1.5 to 4.0 mg/L.[139] The prevalence and severity of skeletal fluorosis increased with increasing F⁻ concentration and age. Cattle and buffalo near a phosphate plant in India developed dental and bony lesions caused by fluorosis.[156] Lesions were more common in older animals than in younger and in buffalo than in cattle. Environmental F⁻ concentrations were 534 mg F⁻/kg in fodder, 1.2 mg F⁻/L in pond water, and 0.5 mg F⁻/L in groundwater, which, assuming standard consumption of forage and water, would have provided approximately 14 mg F⁻/kg BW. Two ranches, 1 with drinking water containing up to 10.5 mg F⁻/L, the other with 3 mg/L, were compared in Argentina.[157] Although both had similar forage F⁻ values (~15–25 ppm), cattle from the former showed excessive dental erosion. Neeley and Harbaugh[158] studied a Texas dairy herd drinking 4 to 5 mg F⁻/L before and after management changes resulted in increased F⁻ intake from 0.52 mg/kg BW to 1.69 mg/kg BW, primarily as a result of increased water consumption. Most animals showed dental fluorosis both before and after the change, but productivity increased after the change, probably as the result of better nutrition and management. Rand and Schmidt[159] followed several Arizona herds drinking water containing 16 mg F⁻/L and consuming forage containing up to 25 ppm F⁻. They concluded that 1 mg F⁻/kg BW can be tolerated for 5 to 10 years with only minor cosmetic effects, but 2 mg F⁻/kg BW results in accelerated tooth wear. After the Lonquimay volcano erupted in Chile, animals were exposed to water concentrations less than 2 mg F⁻/L and as much as 48 ppm F⁻ in forage. Two years later, cattle were still developing fluorosis.[160] Cattle fed a contaminated supplement that provided between 0.7 and 1.6 mg F⁻/kg BW/d for a year developed bone lesions and dental fluorosis.[161]

Merriman and Hobbs[162] conducted an extensive 5-year study of the interactions between soil and water F⁻ ion and nutrition in cattle. Cattle on pastures with average forage concentrations of 143 ppm F developed dental fluorosis. Fluoride in soil, water, and grasses reportedly did not affect gain, but the experimental design was too small to reliably detect differences in performance. Suttie and colleagues[163] fed dairy calves 1.5 or 3 mg F⁻/kg BW, either continuously or in a 6-month rotation, for 6 years. Bone F was related to total intake and urinary F⁻ remained high during the off period, but dental lesions were related to the F⁻ concentration when teeth were being formed. None of the treatments affected growth or reproduction, but only a small number of animals was studied. The physiologic effects of forage contaminated by fumes from an Al smelter and NaF-treated forage were examined in cattle.[164] Gains were significantly less on diets containing more than 200 ppm F⁻ as NaF. Cattle receiving 70 to 100 ppm F⁻ showed decreased reproductive efficiency indirectly attributed to dental fluorosis.

Cattle were fed 134 ppm dietary F⁻ as soft phosphate or CaF_2, or 67 ppm F⁻ as NaF for 91 days to compare the bioavailability and toxicity of the different sources of F. Feed consumption, average daily gains, and feed conversion were not influenced by source of F⁻ [11,165]; however, the study was too short to detect dental effects, and no controls were included. Shupe and colleagues[166] summarized 30 years of experimental and observational studies in cattle, sheep, horses, deer, elk, and bison exposed to differing F⁻ concentrations. They concluded that excessive dietary F⁻ during tooth formation damages teeth, and the abnormal wear of these teeth results in impaired performance. Offspring from animals damaged by F⁻ showed no signs of fluorosis. Short-term exposure of dairy heifers to 2.5 mg F⁻/kg BW during 13 to 15 or 16 to 18 months of age resulted in severe dental fluorosis, even though the total F intake was not excessive.[167] Eckerlin and colleagues[168] and Maylin and colleagues[169] described a farm where F⁻-contaminated concentrate contributed approximately 12.8 to 56 ppm F⁻ to the diet. Cows had depressed milk production, and their calves showed dental fluorosis and osteofluorosis and had severely stunted growth.

Holsteins raised and maintained for 7.5 years on forage containing 12, 27, 49, or 93 ppm F⁻ as NaF initially showed no effect on feed intake, digestion coefficients, or nutrient absorption.[170] However, after the cows had been through 2 lactations, cattle consuming the higher 2 F⁻ diets consumed and digested less. The tolerance level for dietary F was concluded to be between 27 and 49 ppm of the total diet. McLaren and Merriman[171] monitored beef cattle maintained on high-F (125 ppm) or low-F (37 ppm) pastures and good (80%–100% of NRC recommendations) or poor nutrition in a 2 × 2 factorial experiment. They concluded that neither F⁻ concentrations nor plane of nutrition had any effect on the general health of the animals. Sixteen dairy heifers were fed hay containing 10 or 62 ppm F⁻ or 10 ppm hay supplemented with CaF_2 at 69 ppm F⁻ or NaF at 68 ppm F⁻ for 588 days.[172] These diets resulted in doses of 1.14, 1.32, or 1.29 mg F⁻/kg, respectively. Calcium fluoride was less toxic than contaminated hay or NaF. Fluoride caused no adverse effects on soft tissues but did cause significant damage to teeth and bones. Cows were fed 5 to 12 mg F⁻/L in drinking water, with or without superphosphate, through 4 breeding seasons.[173] By the second season, the 8 and 12 mg F⁻/L groups showed prolonged postparturition anestrus, and fertility declined in those 2 groups during the third season. By the fourth season, toxic effects were apparent in the 5-mg F⁻/L group as well.[173]

Sheep were maintained on 2, 5, or 10 mg F⁻/L drinking water from natural sources for 4 years.[174] The highest dose affected wool production, probably as a result of limited food consumption caused by dental fluorosis. Pregnant ewes drinking 10 mg F⁻/L water did not transmit toxic quantities of F⁻ to the fetus or to the lamb through milk. Sheep fed a commercial, nondefluorinated, rock phosphate lick to provide 2 mg F⁻/kg BW showed signs of fluorosis.[175] Thirty-seven percent of the commercial flock was affected, as opposed to only 17% of the breeding animals of the same age that were in better nutritional condition. Cattle and sheep raised on South African farms where water F⁻ ranged from 4 to 26 mg/L and forage from 5.3 to 22.4 ppm experienced severe osteodental fluorosis.[176] Assuming normal consumption of forage and water, the dose received was between 2 and 4 mg F⁻/kg BW. A New Mexico ranch experiencing dental fluorosis was discovered to have water sources varying from 0.09 to 3.32 mg F⁻/L. Interestingly, the higher concentrations occurred in wells only used during part of the year, and a child drinking from the highest well had dental fluorosis as well.[177]

Horses and swine are thought to be less susceptible to fluorosis than cattle and sheep, but there are few clinical and no experimental data to support the contention.[121] Horses grazed in areas contaminated with F^- developed similar fluorotic signs as cattle and sheep.[178] Swine were fed 200 or 1000 ppm dietary F^- as NaF for 45 days in an experiment to determine the effects of F^- on bone growth.[179] The higher concentrations of F^- produced dose-related decreases in bone growth, feed consumption, and overall growth. Bones from pigs treated with F^- were less dense and showed growth plate abnormalities.

Fluoride toxicosis was diagnosed in elk, deer, and bison from lesions and F^- concentrations in teeth and bones collected by hunters in Utah, Wyoming, and Idaho. Vegetation and water samples collected from areas where fluorotic animals were discovered contained 5.5 to 430 ppm F^- and 0.5 to 24 mg F^-/L, respectively.[180] Suttie and colleagues[181] studied deer near a new Al smelter where forage concentrations ranged from 1 to 30 ppm F^-. All deer had increased dental F^- and some mild cosmetic fluorosis, but none showed excessive tooth wear. Tissue F^- concentrations in deer diagnosed with fluorosis from dental lesions near an Al smelter were similar to those reported for cattle.[182] Suttie and colleagues[183] fed 25 or 50 ppm F^- as NaF to whitetail deer fawns. Fluorotic lesions were similar to those in cattle fed the same amount, but cattle seemed to develop more bony lesions and fewer dental lesions than deer. Vikoren and colleagues[184] surveyed several hundred jawbones from moose, red deer, and roe deer near Al smelters where forage concentrations averaged 30 ppm F^-, and also studied a small number of sheep in the same area. Although the overall incidence of fluorosis was low, tissue concentrations were similar in sheep and cervids, and the threshold bone F^- concentration for disease in cervids was similar to what was previously reported in domestic species.

Fluoride generates considerable controversy in human health, largely as a result of the common practice of fluoridating municipal water supplies. However, there are no convincing experimental studies that suggest that the dramatic effects associated with acute exposure to high doses of F carry over to low-level, long-term exposure. Although there are a few reports of dental fluorosis in people at slightly lower concentrations, the current primary drinking water standard for human consumption is 4 mg F^-/L; the secondary standard, apparently based on cosmetic dental effects, is 2 mg F^-/L.

A search of the literature pertaining to fluorosis in animals yielded similar results. There were no reports of toxic effects in livestock that occurred at lower F dosages than those that cause osteodental fluorosis. Thus, as a practical matter, maximum tolerable concentrations of F^- in water for livestock should be based on dental and bone effects.

The effects of F in feedstuffs and water are additive; what counts is the total dose of biologically available F^- ion ingested by the animal. Most of the reports reviewed, when reduced to mg F^-/kg BW, indicate the threshold dose for chronic osteodental fluorosis in cattle is approximately 1 mg F^-/kg BW. This finding is in agreement with the NRC,[121] which indicates that 30 to 40 ppm dietary F^- (which translates to 0.75–1.0 mg F^-/kg BW) is the tolerance level for the more sensitive (ie, during dental development) classes of cattle.

Numerous studies have shown the susceptibility of wild ungulates (deer, elk, and so forth) to fluorosis; however, there has been only 1 controlled experiment[183] from which dose-response data can be extrapolated. A few epidemiologic studies provide sufficient data to form rough estimates of the amount of F^- required to produce signs of fluorosis in wild ruminants. Taken together, these indicate that such animals are approximately as sensitive to the toxic effects of F^- as cattle. Sheep seem to be slightly less sensitive than cattle, although 1 Australian report indicated that long-term exposure to as little as 10 mg F^-/L drinking water in Queensland decreased wool production.[174] Given temperatures in that region, water consumption probably resulted in 1 to 2 mg F^-/kg BW for much of the year. The sole report that included any data on horses suggested horses are 2-fold more tolerant than cattle, but it goes on to describe situations in which ruminants and horses, sharing a pasture and water supply, were similarly affected.

Assuming North American forages normally contain less than 10 ppm F, a water concentration of 3.75 mg F^-/L would be required to achieve the 1 mg F/kg BW necessary to cause fluorosis in sensitive aged cattle, and water containing less should not cause measurable production problems.

Water for cattle should contain less than 2.0 mg/L F^-. By extension, these waters should also be safe for sheep, and probably horses.

MOLYBDENUM

Molybdenum (Mo) is an essential trace element required for nitrogen fixation and the reduction of nitrate to nitrite in plants and bacteria, and is widely distributed in nature.[185] Geochemical surveys in the United Kingdom found that Mo content in soil and sediment corresponds closely to underlying black shales.[186] Other sources of Mo in the environment include industrial contamination by metal alloy manufacturing, copper (Cu) mining, and coal mining.[187–192] Mo occurs predominately as the molybdate (MoO_4^{2-}) ion in natural water sources, and concentrations are typically very low (<2–3 μg/L), unless contaminated by an outside source, in which case they can reach 25 mg Mo/L.[193,194] In forage, Mo concentrations vary dramatically and depend on the Mo concentration, moisture content, and the pH of the soil.[193,195] Alkaline environments greatly increase the bioavailability of Mo to plants, and thus increase the likelihood of Mo toxicity in grazing animals.[193,196] Surveys have identified extensive areas of forage containing potentially toxic concentrations of Mo (10–20 ppm) in at least 5 western states.[197]

Mo is essential for mammals as a cofactor in aldehyde oxidase, sulfite oxidase, and xanthine oxidase,[185,198] where it is responsible for catalyzing the oxidation or metabolism of sulfur (S)-containing amino acids, purines, pyrimidines, and aldehydes. Dietary requirements are so low (about 100 ppb dry matter); however, that deficiency is very rare under natural conditions.[198]

Once ingested, Mo is absorbed in the stomach and throughout the small intestine. In the small intestine, MoO_4^{2-} is actively transported across the mucosal epithelium via the same carrier-mediated transport mechanism that transports sulfate (SO_4^-).[199] The administration of SO_4 to monogastric diets rich in Mo decreases blood Mo concentration and increases excretion, potentially alleviating toxicity.[199–203] In contrast, dietary S increases the toxicity of Mo in ruminants, presumably as a result of thiomolybdate formation in the rumen. Mo is transported in mammalian blood as MoO_4^{2-}, where it is distributed to tissues for integration into enzyme systems. Excretion is primarily via urine; however, feces and milk can also serve as important routes of removal.[80,185,204–206] The rate of absorption differs among species, age groups, and sexes. For example, after orally administering Mo to swine and cattle, Mo peaked in the blood of swine after 2 to 4 hours, whereas it took 96 hours to peak in cattle.[204] Water-soluble forms of Mo, such as ammonium molybdate [$(NH_4)_6Mo_7O_{24}$], sodium molybdate (Na_2MoO_4), and Mo from forage, are more readily absorbed than their organic counterparts.[185]

The ruminal interaction between Mo, SO4, and Cu is responsible for the greater sensitivity of ruminants to Mo. In the rumen, S compounds (mostly SO_4^{2-}) are reduced to sulfide by rumen microbes. Sulfide then combines with MoO_4^{2-} to form either tri-thiomolybdates or tetrathiomolybdates (TMs).[185,207,208] Thus, in ruminants, little Mo or S reaches the small intestine to be absorbed as such. In the rumen, TMs bind irreversibly to the solid phase of digesta and act as powerful chelators of Cu, retaining it in the gut. As a result, Cu absorption from the GI tract is decreased as much as 88%.[209–213] Trithiomolybdates can also enter the circulation,[213,214] where they bind cooperatively with Cu to albumin, resulting in decreased bioavailability of Cu.[210,213,215–217] As a consequence of binding to albumin, biliary excretion of Cu is enhanced, less Cu is incorporated into enzymes, and less Cu is stored in tissues. The decreased availability of Cu for enzyme synthesis has dramatic effects on several physiologic processes, including immune function and bone and elastin formation.[210,212,218–229] Trithiomolybdates bound to albumin are relatively stable; however, once unbound, TMs are rapidly hydrolyzed to MoO_4^{2-} and SO_4.[214,215,230]

Despite Mo being intrinsically (ie, without metabolism to TM) toxic,[210,231,232] secondary Cu deficiency is the most common pathogenesis underlying molybdenosis under field conditions. The form of Mo ingested and, more importantly, the Cu/Mo ratio are critical determinants of toxicity.[233–235] Cu/Mo ratios of 2:1 or less result in clinical signs, and effects are exacerbated by high dietary S.[235] Various authorities have recommended Cu/Mo ratios of 4:1 or greater as the minimum safe ratio.[185,235,236] Signs of acute Mo toxicity include GI irritation, diarrhea, liver and kidney damage, and ultimately death.[219,235,237] Diarrhea seems to be a direct effect of Mo on the intestinal mucosal cells, rather than Cu deficiency.[210] Anorexia and weight loss are the initial clinical signs of chronic toxicity, followed by diarrhea, anemia, achromotrichia, ataxia, and bone and joint deformities.[185,235,237–240] Decreased reproductive function, including decreased libido and fertility, has also been associated with molybdenosis.[234,241–244]

Acute to subacute toxicity has been shown experimentally and occurs naturally in cattle, buffalo, and mule deer. The accidental addition of Na_2MoO_4 at the rate of 19,000 ppm (estimated Mo concentration 7400 ppm) to cattle rations resulted in decreased feed intake, hind limb ataxia, profuse salivation and ocular discharge, diarrhea, liver and kidney damage, rough hair coat, and death.[237] Feeding 1.36 g of Mo per head per day to 5 cows for an unspecified amount of time produced extreme scouring and loss of condition in 3 animals.[245] After consuming a ration containing 10.5 ppm Cu and 140 ppm Mo for 3 to 4 days, Holstein-Friesian lactating cows and steers developed hemorrhagic diarrhea and front limb lameness, and they died.[246] Mo-contaminated grazing pastures with forage concentrations between 16 and 24 ppm Mo and 6 to 11 ppm Cu resulted in acute diarrhea, loss of condition, and posterior stiffness in cattle.[190] Feeding 2000 ppm Mo as $(NH_4)_6Mo_7O_{24}$ for 3 days resulted in diarrhea and feed refusal in cattle.[247] After grazing a pasture contaminated with used motor oil containing Mo bisulfide for 2 weeks, cattle showed diarrhea, anemia, decreased milk production, achromotrichia, and hind limb weakness.[248] Four male buffalo were given 5 mg Na_2MoO_4 (2.35 mg Mo)/kg BW/d for 180 days; by 2 weeks, clinical signs included diarrhea, decreased weight gains, incoordination, swelling of hind fetlocks, and irregular hoof wear.[89] Including 2500 ppm Mo as Na_2MoO_4 (equivalent to approximately 62.5 mg Mo/kg BW) or more in the diets of mule deer for 33 days resulted in diarrhea and feed refusal; smaller doses were without apparent effect.[249]

Chronic toxicity has been investigated both in field studies and experimentally in cattle, sheep, and ruminant wildlife. Forage containing 24 to 28 ppm Cu and 14 to 126 ppm Mo that had been contaminated by a metal alloy manufacturing plant resulted in emaciation and diarrhea in cattle beginning 4 weeks after introduction to the affected pasture.[188] Cattle grazing pasture contaminated by Al alloy plants at a concentration of 77.5 ppm Mo showed severe scouring, loss of condition, decreased milk production, and achromotrichia.[192] Cattle grazing pastures containing 1 to 20 ppm Mo showed diarrhea, listlessness, and abnormal hair color compared with animals grazing pastures containing less than 1 ppm Mo with no clinical signs.[187] Feeding 2 male calves, with average BWs of 209 kg (460 lb), 4.0 g Na_2MoO_4/d resulted in diarrhea, discolored hair, weight loss, anemia, and decreased libido.[234] Cattle consuming a diet containing 4 ppm Cu and 5 ppm Mo showed decreased weight gain, decreased feed intake, and abnormal hair texture and color after 16 to 20 weeks.[231] Pastures containing 25.6 ppm Mo produced severe diarrhea, emaciation, anemia, faded hair color, salt craving, and death in grazing cattle.[249] Yearling steers given 1.5 mg Mo/kg BW for 150 days and grazed on pasture containing 0.32% S developed diarrhea, inflammation of the sheath, rough hair coat, and anemia.[250]

Grazing forage containing 4 to 14 ppm Cu and 95 to 460 ppm Mo and drinking water with 14 µg Cu/L and 7200 µg Mo/L for 11 weeks resulted in watery diarrhea, rough hair coats, and a stiff shuffling gait in 50% of cow-calf pairs.[251] Forage contaminated with 2 to 220 ppm Mo caused diarrhea, roughening and discoloration of the hair coat, and weight loss in grazing cattle.[252] Forage concentrations of 16.5 to 23.5 ppm Mo and 2 to 25 ppm Cu resulted in diarrhea, weight loss, and achromotrichia in cattle.[253] Feeding 100 ppm Mo to heifers for 11 months resulted in anemia, scouring, achromotrichia, and weight loss. Five of 16 died 2 weeks after termination of the experiment.[254] Heifers receiving diets containing 100 ppm Mo and 0.3% S as SO_4 became emaciated and diarrheic after 1 month at this treatment level. Heifers given 5 to 20 ppm Mo with 0.3% S or 50 ppm Mo without added S did not show any signs of illness, but they did have decreased tissue Cu compared with controls.[255] Weight loss and scouring were evident in cows ingesting 173 ppm Mo for 2 months. Diets containing 53 and 100 ppm Mo did not produce clinical signs but did interfere with Cu metabolism.[256] Forage containing 6 to 36 ppm Mo resulted in emaciation in cattle with severe diarrhea, anemia, achromotrichia, and swollen genitals.[257] Water containing 50 ppm Mo induced signs of secondary Cu deficiency in 5-week-old calves.[258]

Sheep grazing pastures containing 5.5 to 33.5 ppm Mo and 6.0 to 8.7 ppm Cu for 76 weeks developed hemorrhaging around the femoral heads, tuber sacrales, and psoas muscles. Exostoses were frequent on humeri and femurs, and the periosteum appeared to have lifted from the bone surface.[196] Feeding ewes 1-kg commercial grass cubes with 5 ppm Cu and supplemented with Na_2SO_4 and $(NH_4)_6Mo_7O_{24}$ to provide 10 g of SO_4 and 50 mg of Mo, respectively, until 1 month before lambing resulted in incoordination of front and hind limbs and a marked ataxia in lambs within 60 days of birth.[259] Sheep grazing pastures containing 20 ppm Mo and 5 to 7 ppm Cu developed connective tissue lesions, including lifting of the periosteum and hemorrhaging in periosteum and muscle insertions.[260] Drenching goats daily with $(NH_4)_6Mo_7O_{24}$ to provide 50 ppm dietary Mo for 235 days caused general debility, depigmentation of hair coat, and weight loss.[261]

Notwithstanding the previous, several studies have failed to produce any adverse health effects after Mo ingestion. Grazing cattle on pastures containing 13 ppm Mo and supplementing with 17 ppm Cu for 6 months resulted in no signs of adverse effects.[262] Cattle grazing a reclaimed mine tailing site containing 21 to 44 ppm Mo and 13 to 19 ppm Cu for 3 consecutive summers showed no signs of Mo toxicity.[191,263,264] No adverse effects were noticed in a cannulated steer consuming sun-cured hay containing 49.68 ppm Mo and 19.09 ppm Cu.[265] In each of these studies, low S in both the diet and water was offered as being a possible explanation for the lack of clinical signs observed.

Like most monogastric animals, horses are very resistant to the effects of Mo compared with ruminants. Cattle are commonly cited as more susceptible to molybdenosis than sheep, possibly because they are more sensitive to Cu deficiency. Therefore, drinking water Mo concentrations that are safe for cattle are probably also safe for horses and other classes of livestock. Although there is variability in the reports summarized earlier, and some (large) amount of dietary Mo may cause poisoning regardless of Cu status, the bottom line seems to be that total dietary Cu/Mo ratios of less than 2 to 4 can result in chronic toxicity and decreased production in cattle, especially if dietary S is higher than necessary.

As with many substances, the effects of forage and water Mo concentrations are additive, and, in some areas, forage Mo concentrations are already toxic or nearly toxic. Under these conditions, any additional Mo intake contributed by drinking water is potentially dangerous. However, in these areas, producers are likely already aware of the problem and feeding supplemental Cu. A more normal situation is cattle grazing typical forage containing 7 ppm Cu (or supplemented to that level) and negligible Mo (~1 ppm). Under such conditions, the critical safe 4:1 ratio would be exceeded whenever drinking water contains 375 µg Mo/L.

In the absence of other specific data on forage concentrations, drinking water for livestock should contain less than 0.3 mg/L. If dietary Mo is higher, which is common in some regions, water Mo concentrations should be adjusted downward accordingly.

SELENIUM

Se, a metalloid that shares many chemical properties with S, is predominantly present in cretaceous rocks, volcanic material, seafloor deposits, and glacial drift, especially in the Great Plains.[266] It can be present in soil at levels sufficient to cause toxicity or low enough to result in deficiency in grazing animals. Either outcome represents serious economic losses to livestock producers. Normal soil concentrations range from 0.1 to 2.0 µg total Se per gram of soil; however, in seleniferous areas, soils can contain as much as 324 µg Se per gram of soil.[267] Plants grown on such soils tend to accumulate Se and, depending on the species, may bioconcentrate Se to concentrations in excess of 10,000 ppm.

Water in contact with seleniferous soils (eg, irrigation wastewater) may also accumulate Se.[268,269] The most common form of Se in surface waters of the Great Plains is the selenate (SeO_4^{2-}) ion. Normal surface water is described as containing less than 2 µg Se/L,[269] and it is thus not normally a major source of Se for livestock and mammalian wildlife; however, poisoning as a result of seleniferous water has occurred in horses and sheep (Raisbeck MF, Department of Veterinary Sciences, University of Wyoming, unpublished data, 2015).[270,271] Dissolved Se becomes concentrated in successive levels of the aquatic food chain and is a major concern for waterfowl that depend on aquatic biota for food[269,272,273]; however, aquatic bioconcentration does not seem to pose a hazard to grazing herbivores (eg, cattle) under normal conditions because their intake of algae and aquatic organisms is very small. Interestingly, bioconcentration of Se in the aquatic food chain removes Se from the water column,[269,274] thus decreasing the risk to livestock; however, forages irrigated with seleniferous water contain increased Se concentrations and pose a risk to grazing animals.[268,269,274] Although each of the preceding sources is important, this article is concerned specifically with the hazard posed to livestock by Se in drinking water and focuses on that source.

Se is an essential trace element. Most authorities agree that, worldwide, deficiency is a more common problem than toxicity, and, thus, for the last 50 years, more research has focused on the effects of inadequate dietary Se than on too much. Se is a component of several enzyme systems, most involved in catalyzing oxidation-reduction reactions.[275,276] The selenoprotein thought to be most critical in deficiency situations is glutathione peroxidase.[267,277] Se deficiency results in white muscle disease, a degenerative condition in muscle resulting from oxidant stress.[277–279] The US Food and Drug Administration permits 0.3 ppm Se (total ration) as a feed additive, up to 0.7 and 3 mg Se per head per day as a feed supplement for sheep and beef cattle, respectively, and in fortification mixtures up to 90 and 120 ppm Se for sheep and cattle, respectively.[280] Deficiency is rarely a problem in northern Great Plains states.[281,282]

Selenomethionine is the predominant form of Se in common forages, even though it is not a major component of accumulator plant species.[283–285] However, it constitutes most of the ingested Se under range conditions, because accumulator plants are highly unpalatable and are usually avoided to the point of starvation.[286] Waterborne Se, usually selenite (SeO_3^{2-}) or selenate (SeO_4^{2-}) ions, normally comprises a small portion of large herbivores' total exposure; however, (1) water concentrations sufficient to cause poisoning have been recorded in several western states[287,288]; (2) poisoning has occurred in livestock as a result of Se water contamination associated with mineral extraction; and (3) Se-contaminated water has the potential to add to the already high background forage concentrations common to many parts of the Great Plains and intermountain West.

Inorganic Se is absorbed from the small intestine in both ruminant and monogastric species. Selenocysteine and selenomethionine are transported across the intestinal epithelium by active amino acid transport mechanisms.[289] Selenite is absorbed passively by simple diffusion, but SeO_4^{2-} is accumulated via a sodium (Na)-mediated carrier with SO_4^{2-}.[275,290,291] To date, there is no evidence for homeostatic control of Se absorption because neither dietary concentration nor Se status affect absorption efficiency.[292,293] Se bioavailability is influenced by animal species and the form of Se ingested. Selenomethionine, the predominant form of Se in forages, is absorbed more efficiently than inorganic forms of Se, at least when the comparison is based on tissue concentrations.[294] Selenate is better absorbed than SeO_3^{2-}, at least in laboratory rodents, and both are more efficiently absorbed than elemental Se.[275] Ruminants reduce Se to insoluble selenides in the rumen and are to some degree protected against poisoning. It is common to see selenosis in pastured horses while cattle on the same pasture remain unaffected.[282] Because the reduction of Se by rumen microflora is heavily influenced by other dietary factors, ruminants also show greater variation in Se absorption than monogastrics (Raisbeck MF, Department of Veterinary Sciences, University of Wyoming, unpublished data, 2015).[295]

Following absorption, Se becomes associated with plasma proteins, mainly albumin and selenoprotein-P, for transport to tissues.[296] Selenomethionine is nonspecifically substituted for methionine in protein[293] and only becomes available for either toxicity or nutrition as the protein turns over. Other forms are incorporated into essential selenoproteins and/or methylated to dimethylselenide or trimethylselonium ion for elimination.[297] Both elimination and protein incorporation seem to involve metabolic activation to a reactive intermediate, which, when cellular defenses become saturated, is responsible for most of the toxic effects of Se.[275] Under normal conditions, Se is eliminated via urine and, to a lesser extent, bile, but, as tissue concentrations increase to toxic levels, an increasing proportion is eliminated via respiration as dimethylselenide.[275] Increased (ie, potentially toxic) dietary Se level also results in a shift of the distribution of Se between various proteins and body compartments,[269,294,298] although both the physiologic and toxicologic significance of this observation is not yet known.

Se interacts with several other common dietary constituents, primarily at the pharmacokinetic level. These interactions modulate both the nutritional and toxic properties of Se. As decreases Se toxicity by decreasing tissue Se concentrations.[24,289] Mercury decreases the toxicity of Se in birds[25,290] and possibly mammals.[269] S is thought to alleviate Se toxicity.[299] When sheep were given 2 mg of Se as Na_2SeO_4, those receiving 0.05% dietary S showed greater Se toxicity than sheep given 0.11%, 0.17%, or 0.24% dietary S, mostly as added SO_4.[300] Dietary SO_4 decreased the Se balance in dairy cows fed Na_2SeO_4, reduced the true availability of nutritional levels of Se, and increased its excretion via feces in dairy cattle. Added dietary SO_4 (0.29%) resulted in a 20% growth increase in rats fed 10 ppm Se, 0.58% SO_4 caused a 40% growth increase, and 0.87% SO_4 ameliorated liver damage caused by Se intoxication.[301] However, the interaction between SO_4 and Se is not universal; 3000 mg SO_4^{2-}/L in drinking water failed to alter the uptake of sublethal dietary concentrations of sodium selenite (Na_2SeO_3) or selenomethionine in mallard ducks,[302,303] and more research is needed to elucidate the conditions under which the protective interaction occurs. Cyanogenic glycosides block uptake of Se and ameliorate Se toxicity[212,304] and have been investigated as a means of protecting livestock against selenosis. Cu and cadmium have also been shown to reduce Se toxicity, although the mechanisms are not known.[305,306] Increased dietary protein reduces the severity of poisoning.[307] The type of feedstuff (alfalfa vs grass hay) may influence the bioavailability of Se.[212] Even being Se deficient predisposes animals to Se toxicity.[308]

Although essential, Se shows a narrow margin of safety. Toxic effects have occurred in livestock at dietary concentrations only 40 to 100 times larger than deficiency.[277] The form of Se administered influences tissue accumulation and thus toxicity.[309–313] The chemical species most common in water are the inorganic ions SeO_3^{2-} and SeO_4^{2-}. Se toxicity can be manifested in 2 forms: acute or chronic. Acute toxicity usually results in GI, liver, kidney, and heart damage, shock, and death.[286,310,314] Se has also been implicated as a cause of hypertension and cardiac damage.[175] Reproductive problems, including teratogenesis and embryonic mortality, occur in egg-laying species[269,272,311,315]; however, there is little evidence that Se is teratogenic in mammals.[316–318] Se may compromise reproduction in mammals.[319,320] Chronic selenosis (alkali disease) in ungulates is manifested most apparently as epithelial damage (hair loss and cracked hooves) as a result of necrosis of the keratinocytes[310,321] and ill thrift.

A single subcutaneous dose of 2 mg Se/kg BW given to pigs caused death after 4 hours.[322] Three-hundred and seventy-six of 557 calves injected with a Na_2SeO_4 solution that contained 100 mg of Se (0.5 mg/kg BW), rather than the 12 mg of Se that was intended, died within 5 weeks.[323] Intramuscularly injecting 2 mg Se/kg BW as Na_2SeO_3 into 4 calves caused shock within 3 hours and death in 12 hours.[324] Ewes injected intramuscularly with doses from 0.4 to 1.0 mg Se/kg BW showed dyspnea, anorexia, colic, and a seromucoid nasal discharge. Doses less than 0.6 mg/kg BW were not lethal within 192 hours. The calculated LD_{50} was determined to be 0.7 ± 0.035 mg/kg.[325] Injecting sheep intramuscularly with 0.68 mg Se/kg BW as Na_2SeO_3 produced death within 20 hours. Smaller doses took longer to be lethal, or they only caused reduced feed consumption and transient signs of intoxication.[325] There were no clinical signs in ewes given 90 μg Se/kg BW intramuscularly as Na_2SeO_4; however, 350 μg Se/kg BW was lethal in some. Barium selenate ($BaSeO_4$), given similarly at rates of 0.225, 0.454, 0.908, 1.816, or 4.9 mg/kg BW, produced no signs other than irritation at the injection site.[207]

Se fed as Na_2SeO_3 at 22.3, 33.5, or 52.1 ppm Se in diet to rats for 359 days resulted in the deaths of 5 of 9, 8 of 9, and all 9 rats in the 3 treatment groups, respectively, as well as decreased fertility and anemia in the population as a whole.[326] An experiment focused on Se as a causative factor of tooth decay offered drinking water containing 3 mg Se/L as Na_2SeO_3 to rats for 4 weeks. Two of 15 rats died, and the others showed significantly reduced feed consumption, water intake, and BW.[327] Rations containing 6.4 ppm Se, as seleniferous wheat or Na_2SeO_3, resulted in significantly decreased growth and enlarged spleens in rats. Lower concentrations were without measurable effects. Higher concentrations resulted in decreased organ weights and anemia and were lethal in some rats.[328]

In one of the earliest reported Se dose-response experiments, Miller and Williams[326] reported that the single oral minimum fatal doses (which they defined as a dose large enough to kill 75% of the test group) were 0.68 mg Se/kg BW for horses and mules, 1.1 to 2.2 mg Se/kg BW for cattle, and 2.2 to 3.6 mg Se/kg BW for swine, all given as Na_2SeO_3. Although the experimental protocol was not up to modern standards, more recent reports in cattle and horses usually place the doses within 2-fold to 5-fold. Depression, anorexia, hind limb ataxia, and sternal recumbency developed in 256 pigs in a commercial piggery after the pigs were exposed to feed containing 84 ppm Se.[329] Feed containing 8.1 ppm Se resulted in decreased feed consumption and paralysis in 54 feeder pigs.[330] Rations containing 14.75 ppm and 26.65 ppm Se caused hair loss, reddening of skin, and hind limb ataxia in 80 of 160 pigs. Higher concentrations resulted in feed aversion.[331] Porcine diets fortified with approximately 25 ppm Se as Na_2SeO_3 resulted in hair and hoof lesions and weight loss. Higher concentrations produced feed aversion and poliomyelomalacia.[331] Corn, naturally contaminated with 10 ppm Se, fed for 5 months, resulted in 2 of 5 pigs developing alopecia and hoof lesions.[332] Pelleted rations containing 26.6 or 31.7 ppm Se, fed as Na_2SeO_3 or the Se accumulator *Astragalus bisulcatus*, respectively, and fed for several weeks, resulted in reduced feed consumption, alopecia, cracked hooves, and posterior paresis in pigs.[309]

A single dose of 5 mg Se/kg BW, given orally as Na_2SeO_3, was acutely toxic in lambs.[333] Drenching 190 lambs with 6.4 mg Se/kg BW resulted in the death of 180 within 15 days.[334] Twenty lambs, 4 to 14 days of age and averaging 4.5 kg, were mistakenly given 10 mg of Na_2SeO_3 (2.2 mg Se/kg BW) orally to prevent white muscle disease; 7 died within 17 hours, and 8 more experienced diarrhea as a result of acute toxicosis. As a follow-up experiment, an additional ewe was injected with 0.45 mg Se/kg BW, which resulted in death within 8 hours.[335] Glenn and colleagues[316] fed ewes increasing dosages of Na_2SeO_4 for 100 days and concluded that the minimum lethal dosage was 0.825 mg Se/kg BW/d. One of a group of 12 adult ewes and their lambs, pastured in an area of seleniferous forage and water, died after 14 days; other animals were unaffected when removed after 4 weeks. The exposure from the combination of contaminated forage and water was calculated to be 0.26 mg Se/kg BW/d.[270] Sheep were lethally poisoned after grazing high-Se forage (<49 ppm Se DM) and drinking high-Se water (340–415 μg Se/L) for 4 weeks; however, a similar group on a neighboring pasture with forages less than 13 ppm Se and normal water were unaffected.[270]

Steers gavaged with doses varying between 0.25 and 0.5 mg Se/kg BW as Na_2SeO_3 showed inappetence, depression, and death. Two of 8 died within 8 weeks, and 4 more died within 14 weeks.[336] Feeding 0.28 and 0.8 mg Se/kg BW (approximating 10 ppm and 25 ppm dietary Se, respectively, under range conditions) as selenomethionine or 0.8 mg/kg BW as Na_2SeO_3 to yearling steers for 4 months resulted in overt clinical signs of alkali disease in 1 steer and histologic lesions of dyskeratosis in several more.[312] Primary antibody response was significantly impaired in the same dose groups.[337] A dose of 0.15 mg/kg BW (approximating 5 ppm Se in diet), fed as either selenomethionine or Na_2SeO_3, and 0.28 mg/kg BW as Na_2SeO_3 in the same experiments were without measurable effects.[312,332] Dosing calves with 0.25 mg Se/kg BW as Na_2SeO_3 via bolus for 16 weeks resulted in hair and hoof lesions typical of chronic selenosis and indications of increased oxidant stress.[338] Decreased growth and anemia occurred in preruminant calves fed 10 ppm as Na_2SeO_4 for 40 days, but no measurable effects occurred in calves fed 0.2 to 5.0 ppm Se.[339]

There is a paucity of quantitative data in horses, although horses are the species most commonly diagnosed with selenosis in the author's laboratory. Ponies dosed via stomach tube with 6 or 8 mg Se/kg BW as Na_2SeO_3 developed signs of acute selenosis within 6 hours; ponies given 2 or 4 mg Se/kg BW remained clinically normal for the 14-day experiment.[306] A 4-year-old gelding accidentally given 25 mg of Se (0.055 mg Se/kg BW) orally as Na_2SeO_4 for 5 consecutive days developed a straw-colored exudate on its lips, prepuce, and anus. Within 3 weeks, its hooves had separated from the coronary band, and alopecia was present on the mane and tail.[340] This report did not investigate the Se content of the rest of the diet. Chronic Se toxicosis was diagnosed in 7 horses consuming hay containing between 0.49 and 58 ppm Se (mean 22 ppm) in combination with a mineral supplement that contained 1.9 ppm Se.[341,342] Eight of 20 horses developed alkali disease after being fed alfalfa hay that contained 5.9 to 17 ppm (mean 11.9 ppm) Se for several weeks (Galey FD, Veterinary Toxicologist, California Veterinary Laboratory System, personal communication, 1996). Several horses were diagnosed with alkali disease in southeastern Idaho after being turned into a pasture where the only water supply contained approximately 0.5 mg Se/L (Talcott PS, Professor of Veterinary Toxicology, Washington State University, personal communication, 2006). Assuming water consumption of 10% BW, this works out to 0.05 mg/kg BW, but there was probably some additional Se from forage in the pasture. Feeding horses oats containing 96 ppm added Se (19.2 ppm of total ration) as Na_2SeO_3 for several months resulted in listlessness, loosening of hair, softening of the horny wall of hoof, and ultimately death.[343] A 9-year-old gelding developed a swollen prepuce, vesicles on its nostrils and mouth, and hoof lesions of alkali disease after receiving 153.4 mg Se per day in his feed (16.4 ppm dry matter) for several days.[344] In Queensland, Australia, horses and sheep were diagnosed with chronic and acute Se toxicity after grazing areas with vegetation containing 200 to 3038 ppm Se and corresponding soil concentrations of 64 to 128 ppm Se.[345]

In goats, daily oral doses of 5 to 160 mg Se/kg BW administered via bolus were uniformly lethal within 31 days. Daily doses of 0.11 to 0.45 mg Se/kg BW were given for 225 days with no toxic effects.[119] Increased levels of Se in the soil (1.45–2.25 ppm Se) and forage (40.32–80.64 ppm Se) in West Bengal, India, have been blamed for a gangrenous condition (Deg Nala) in grazing buffaloes showing hoof cracks, malaise, abdominal pain, laminitis, and edema on the tails and ear tips.[346] Feeding captive pronghorn antelope grass hay that contained 15 ppm Se for 164 days did not result in any overt clinical signs but did decrease primary antibody response to a challenge with hen egg albumin.[347]

The foregoing notwithstanding, feeding steers seleniferous wheat, seleniferous hay, or a control diet with supplemental Na_2SeO_4 to supply 12 ppm dietary Se (65 µg Se/kg BW/d) for 100 days did not produce any obvious evidence of selenosis.[298,348] Ellis and colleagues[349] fed adult Holstein cows up to 50 mg Se/head/d (approximately 87 μg Se/kg BW/d) as Na_2SeO_3 for 90 days, followed by 100 mg Se/head/d (approximately 175 μg Se/kg BW/d) for another 28 days with no apparent health effects. Ewes tolerated 24 ppm dietary Se from Na_2SeO_3 or 29 ppm Se from *A bisulcatus* for 88 days[183] or 10 to 15 ppm dietary Se through 2 pregnancies.[350] Cristaldi and colleagues[351] fed wethers Na_2SeO_3 at dietary Se concentrations up to 10 ppm for 1 year with no effect on rate of gain, serum enzymes, or disease and concluded that less than or equal to 10 ppm dietary Se as selenite is not toxic. The same research group fed 4, 8, 12, 16, and 20 ppm dietary Se as Na_2SeO_3 to adult ewes for 72 weeks with no effect on BW or other evidence of poisoning.[352]

Although the NRC[277] suggests that horses are about as sensitive to oral Se as cattle, sheep, and goats, research and field experience by this author and others indicates that species sensitivity is horses > cattle > sheep and goats. Experience at several regional diagnostic laboratories indicates that horses may be poisoned, whereas ruminants using the same forage and water remain unaffected (Mostrom MS, veterinary toxicologist, North Dakota State University, personal communication, 2006; and Reagor JC, toxicologist, Texas Veterinary Medical Diagnostic Laboratory, personal communication, 2006).[282] With the exception of 1 study in antelope, there is insufficient dose-response data on which to base safety recommendations in large mammalian wildlife. However, there are reports of elk and deer sharing pastures with horses, sheep, and cattle, where the horses developed alkali disease, without any measurable ill effects in the elk and deer.[353] Thus, water that is, safe for horses should be safe for ruminants under the same conditions.

The effects of waterborne Se are, like many other elements, additive with feed content. The chemical form of Se in surface waters is predominately SeO_3^{2-} or SeO_4^{2-}. In theory, small concentrations of Se in water may be sufficient to push animals on moderately high-Se forages over the edge of toxicity. However, the Se content of forage and hay in the high plains varies from marginally deficient to downright toxic, and other dietary factors may modify the effects of a given concentration of dietary Se. For the purposes of this article, the author assumed a typical forage containing 1 ppm Se (mostly as selenomethionine), and normal protein, vitamin E, and other trace nutrient concentrations. The threshold for chronic poisoning in horses from the literature is 0.05 to 0.1 mg/kg BW/d, which agrees with unpublished observations from my laboratory. Thus, water that contains 0.25 mg Se/L, consumed at a rate of 10% BW, combined with average-Se forage, would constitute a potentially hazardous dose. In extremely hot weather, working horses drinking 20% BW of 0.125 mg Se/L water (a very conservative assumption) would receive a hazardous dose.

In areas where forage Se concentrations are higher, or if animals are receiving dietary supplements that contain Se, safe water concentrations have to be adjusted downward, but, under normal conditions, 0.1 mg/L should not cause problems. This recommendation is very conservative for ruminant livestock.

DISCLOSURE

This is a compilation of 30 years of clinical experience and research funded by many different agencies, including the Wyoming Dept of Environmental Quality, the US Office of Surface Mining, and smaller in kind contributions by various liproducers.

REFERENCES

1. Casteel SW, Bailey EM, Murphy MJ, et al. Arsenic poisoning in Texas cattle: The implications for your practice. Vet Med 1986;81:1045–9.

2. Eisler R. Arsenic hazards to humans, plants, and animals from gold mining. Rev Environ Contam Toxicol 2004;180:133–65.
3. Franke KW, Moxon AL. A comparison of the minimum fatal doses of selenium, tellurium, arsenic and vanadium. J Pharmacol Exp Ther 1936;58:454–9.
4. Hughes MF. Arsenic toxicity and potential mechanisms of action. Toxicol Lett 2002;133:1–16.
5. Moxham JW, Coup MR. Arsenic poisoning of cattle and other domestic animals. N Z Vet J 1968;16:161–5.
6. Wang S, Mulligan CN. Occurrence of arsenic contamination in Canada: Sources, behavior and distribution. Sci Total Environ 2006;366:701–21.
7. Hindmarsh JT, McCurdy RF. Clinical and environmental aspects of arsenic toxicity. Crit Rev Clin Lab Sci 1986;23:315–47.
8. Sasaki A, Oshima Y, Fujimura A. An approach to elucidate potential mechanism of renal toxicity of arsenic trioxide. Exp Hematol 2007;35:252–62.
9. Frost DV. The arsenic problem. Adv Exp Med Biol 1977;91:259–79.
10. Gupta R, Dubey DK, Kannan GM, et al. Concomitant administration of Moringa oleifera seed powder in the remediation of arsenic-induced oxidative stress in mouse. Cell Biol Int 2006;31:44–56.
11. Hirano S, Kobayashi Y. Cytotoxic effects of S-(dimethylarsino)-glutathione: A putative intermediate metabolite of inorganic arsenicals. Toxicology 2006;227: 45–52.
12. Wang A, Holladay SD, Wolf DC, et al. Reproductive and developmental toxicity of arsenic in rodents: A review. Int J Toxicol 2006;25:319–31.
13. Calabrese EJ, Baldwin LA. Inorganics and hormesis. Crit Rev Toxicol 2003;33: 215–304.
14. Snow ET, Sykora P, Durham TD, et al. Arsenic, mode of action at biologically plausible low doses: What are the implications for low dose cancer risk? Toxicol Appl Pharmacol 2005;207:S557–64.
15. National Research Council. Arsenic. In: Mineral tolerance of animals. Washington, DC: National Academies Press; 2005. p. 31–45.
16. Nielsen FH, Givand SH, Myron DR. Evidence of a possible requirement for arsenic by the rat. Fed Proc 1975;34:923.
17. Anke M. Arsenic. In: Mertz W, editor. Trace elements in human and animal nutrition. Orlando (FL): Academic Press; 1986. p. 347–72.
18. Jain CK, Ali I. Arsenic: Occurrence, toxicity and speciation techniques. Water Res 2000;34:4304–12.
19. Tseng CH. Arsenic methylation, urinary arsenic metabolites and human diseases: Current perspective. J Environ Sci Health 2007;25:1–22.
20. Upreti RK, Kannan A, Pant AB. Experimental exposure of arsenic in cultured rat intestinal epithelial cells and cell line: Toxicological consequences. Toxicol In Vitro 2007;21:32–40.
21. Mitchell RD, Ayala-Fierro F, Carter DE. Systemic indicators of inorganic arsenic toxicity in four animal species. J Toxicol Environ Health 2000;59:119–34.
22. Vahter M, Concha G. Role of metabolism in arsenic toxicity. Pharmacol Toxicol 2001;89:1–5.
23. Vahter M. Methylation of inorganic arsenic in different mammalian species and population groups. Sci Prog 1999;82:69–88.
24. Gregus Z, Gyurasics A, Csanaky I. Effects of arsenic, platinum and gold-containing drugs on the disposition of exogenous selenium in rats. Toxicol Sci 2000;57:22–31.

25. Hill CH. Interrelationships of selenium with other trace elements. Fed Proc 1975; 34:2096–100.
26. Minyard JA, Dinkel CA, Olson OE. Effect of arsanilic acid in counteracting selenium poisoning in beef cattle. J Anim Sci 1960;19:260–4.
27. Rhian M, Moxon AL. Chronic selenium poisoning in dogs and its prevention by arsenic. J Pharmacol Exp Ther 1943;78:249–64.
28. Modi M, Kaul RK, Kannan GM, et al. Co-administration of zinc and n-acetylcysteine prevents arsenic-induced tissue oxidative stress in male rats. J Trace Elem Med Biol 2006;20:197–204.
29. Mukherjee S, Das D, Mukherjee M, et al. Synergistic effect of folic acid and vitamin B12 in ameliorating arsenic-induced oxidative damage in pancreatic tissue of rat. J Nutr Biochem 2006;17:319–27.
30. Yokel RA, Lasley SM, Dorman DC. The speciation of metals in mammals influences their toxicokinetics and toxicodynamics and therefore human health risk assessment. J Toxicol Environ Health B Crit Rev 2006;9:63–85.
31. Hornfeldt CS, Borys DJ. Inorganic arsenic poisoning in cats. Feline Pract 1986; 16:20–4.
32. Thomas DJ, Styblo M, Lin S. The cellular metabolism and systemic toxicity of arsenic. Toxicol Appl Pharmacol 2001;176:127–44.
33. el Bahri L, Ben Romdane S. Arsenic poisoning in livestock. Vet Hum Toxicol 1991;33:259–64.
34. Weaver AD. Arsenic poisoning in cattle following pasture contamination by drift of spray. Vet Rec 1962;74:249–51.
35. McLennan MW, Dodson ME. Arsenic poisoning in cattle. Aust Vet J 1972; 48:367.
36. Selby LA, Case AA, Dorn CR, et al. Public health hazards associated with arsenic poisoning in cattle. J Am Vet Med Assoc 1974;165:1010–4.
37. Bergeland ME, Ruth GR, Stack RL, et al. Arsenic toxicosis in cattle associated with soil and water contamination from mining operations. Proc Am Assoc Vet Lab Diagn 1976;19:311–6.
38. Riviere JE, Boosinger TR, Everson RJ. Inorganic arsenic toxicosis in cattle: A review of selected cases. Mod Vet Pract 1981;62:209–11.
39. Morgan SE, Morgan GL, Edwards WC. Pinpointing the source of arsenic poisoning in a herd of cattle. Vet Med 1984;79:1525–8.
40. Valentine BA, Rumbeiha WK, Hensley TS, et al. Arsenic and metaldehyde toxicosis in a beef herd. J Vet Diagn Invest 2007;19:212–5.
41. Bennett J, Schwartz TE. Cumulative toxicity of lead arsenate in phenothiazine given to sheep. Am J Vet Res 1971;32:727–30.
42. Kahrs RF, Braun RK, Edds GT, et al. Fatal lead arsenate toxicosis resembling acute bovine diarrhea-mucosal disease (a case report). Proc Am Assoc Vet Lab Diagn 1979;22:321–32.
43. Pace LW, Turnquist SE, Casteel SW, et al. Acute arsenic toxicosis in five horses. Vet Pathol 1997;34:160–4.
44. McParland PJ, Thompson RJ. Deaths in cattle following ingestion of lead arsenate. Vet Rec 1971;89:450–1.
45. Faires MC. Inorganic arsenic toxicosis in a beef herd. Can Vet J 2004;45: 329–31.
46. Robertson ID, Harms WE, Ketterer PJ. Accidental arsenical toxicity of cattle. Aust Vet J 1984;61:366–7.
47. Thatcher CD, Meldrum JB, Wikse SE, et al. Arsenic toxicosis and suspected chromium toxicosis in a herd of cattle. J Am Vet Med Assoc 1985;187:179–82.

48. Maitai CK, Kamau JA, Gacuhi DM, et al. An outbreak of arsenic and toxaphene poisoning in Kenyan cattle. Vet Rec 1975;96:151–2.

49. Dickinson JO. Toxicity of the arsenical herbicide monosodium acid methanarsonate in cattle. Am J Vet Res 1972;33:1889–93.

50. McCulloch EC, St. John JL. Lead-arsenate poisoning of sheep and cattle. J Am Vet Med Assoc 1940;96:321–6.

51. Nelson HA, Crane MR, Tomson K. Inorganic arsenic poisoning in pastured feeder lambs. J Am Vet Med Assoc 1971;158:1943–5.

52. Swiggart RC, Whitehead CJ, Curley A, et al. Wildlife kill resulting from the misuse of arsenic acid herbicide. Bull Environ Contam Toxicol 1972;8:122–8.

53. Sutherland GN, Fawell EV, Brown JK. Arsenical poisoning of racehorses. Vet Rec 1964;76:275–8.

54. Vantroyen B, Heilier JF, Meulemans A, et al. Survival after a lethal dose of arsenic trioxide. J Toxicol Clin Toxicol 2004;42:889–95.

55. Furr AA, Buck WB. Sodium arsenate toxicity in the domestic cat induced by a commercial ant bait. Vet Hum Toxicol 1974;16:41–2.

56. USFDA: Arsenic-based Animal Drugs and Poultry. Available at: https://www.fda.gov/animal-veterinary/product-safety-information/arsenic-based-animal-drugs-and-poultry. Accessed December 1, 2019.

57. Harding JD, Lewis G, Done JT. Experimental arsanilic acid poisoning in pigs. Vet Rec 1968;83:560–4.

58. Keenan DM, Oe RD. Acute arsanilic acid intoxication in pigs. Aust Vet J 1973;49: 229–31.

59. Ledet AE, Duncan JR, Buck WB, et al. Clinical, toxicological and pathological aspects of arsanilic acid poisoning in swine. Clin Toxicol 1973;6:439–57.

60. Menges RW, Kintner LD, Selby LA, et al. Arsanilic acid blindness in pigs. Vet Med Small Anim Clin 1970;65:565–8.

61. Oliver WT, Roe CK. Arsanilic acid poisoning in swine. J Am Vet Med Assoc 1957; 130:177–8.

62. Vorhies MW, Sleight SD, Whitehair CK. Toxicity of arsanilic acid in swine as influenced by water intake. Cornell Vet 1969;59:3–9.

63. Witzel DA, Smith EL, Beerwinkle KR, et al. Arsanilic acid-induced blindness in swine: Electroretinographic and visually evoked responses. Am J Vet Res 1976;37:521–4.

64. Baird AC. Salt poisoning in the dog. Vet Rec 1969;85:756.

65. Shen J, Wanibuchi H, Waalkes MP, et al. A comparative study of the sub-chronic toxic effects of three organic arsenical compounds on the urothelium in F344 rats; gender-based differences in response. Toxicol Appl Pharmacol 2006; 210:171–80.

66. Irvine L, Boyer IJ, DeSesso JM. Monomethylarsonic acid and dimethylarsinic acid: Developmental toxicity studies with risk assessment. Birth Defects Res B Dev Reprod Toxicol 2006;77:53–68.

67. Tucker WB, Hogue JF. Influence of sodium chloride or potassium chloride on systemic acid- base status, milk yield and mineral metabolism in lactating dairy cows. J Dairy Sci 1990;73:3485–93.

68. Domingo JL. Metal-induced developmental toxicity in mammals: A review. J Toxicol Environ Health 1994;42:123–41.

69. Peoples SA. Arsenic toxicity in cattle. Ann N Y Acad Sci 1964;111:644–9.

70. Neiger RD, Osweiler GD. Effect of subacute low level dietary sodium arsenite on dogs. Fund Appl Toxicol 1989;13:439–51.

71. Byron WR, Bierbower GW, Brouwer JB, et al. Pathologic changes in rats and dogs from two year feeding of sodium arsenite and sodium arsenate. Toxicol Appl Pharmacol 1967;10:132–47.

72. Lancaster RJ, Coup MR, Hughes JW. Toxicity of arsenic present in lakeweed. N Z Vet J 1971;19:141–5.

73. Bucy LL, Garrigus US, Forbes RM, et al. Arsenical supplements in lamb fattening rations. J Anim Sci 1954;13:668–76.

74. Bucy LL, Garrigus US, Forbes RM, et al. Toxicity of some arsenicals fed to growing- fattening lambs. J Anim Sci 1955;14:435–45.

75. Kocar BD, Garrot RA, Inskeep WP. Elk exposure to arsenic in geothermal watersheds of Yellowstone National Park. Environ Toxicol Chem 2004;23:982–9.

76. Forsberg CW. Some effects of arsenic on the rumen microflora; an in vitro study. Can J Microbiol 1978;24:36–44.

77. Langner HW, Jackson CR, McDermott TR, et al. Rapid oxidation of arsenite in a hotspring ecosystem, Yellowstone National Park. Environ Sci Technol 2001;35: 3302–9.

78. Roth TR, Reddy KJ. Arsenic in the environment and its remediation by a novel filtration method. In: Bundschuh, et al, editors. Natural Arsenic in Groundwaters of Latin America. 2008. p. 602–23.

79. National Research Council. Arsenic. In: Armienta MA, Birkle P, editors. Mineral tolerance of domestic animals. Washington, DC: National Academies Press; 1980. p. 40–53.

80. Tolgyesi G, Elmoty IA. Elimination of excess molybdenum by cattle. Acta Vet Acad Sci Hung 1967;17:39–44.

81. Garner RJ. Mineral or inorganic substances. In: Clarke EG, Clarke ML, editors. Veterinary Toxicology. London: Bailliere, Tindal & Cassell; 1967. p. 44–59.

82. Monies B. Arsenic poisoning in cattle. In Pract 1999;21:602–7.

83. Selby LA, Case AA, Osweiler GD, et al. Epidemiology and toxicology of arsenic poisoning in domestic animals. Environ Health Perspect 1977;19:183–9.

84. Stumm W, Morgan JJ. Aquatic Chemistry; chemical Equilibria and rates in natural waters. 3rd edition. New York: John Wiley & Sons Inc.; 1996.

85. Ng A, Patterson CC. Changes of lead and barium with time in California offshore basin sediments. Geochim Cosmochim Acta 1996;46:2307–21.

86. Chernick WS. Drill's Pharmacology in medicine. 4th edition. New York: McGraw-Hill; 1971.

87. Reeves AL. Barium. In: Friberg L, Nordberg GF, Vouk VB, editors. Handbook on the toxicology of metals. Amsterdam (the Netherlands): Elsevier Science Publishers B.V.; 1986. p. 84–94.

88. Cuddihy RG, Griffith WC. A biological model describing tissue distribution and whole-body retention of barium and lanthanum in beagle dogs after inhalation and gavage. Health Phys 1972;23:621–33.

89. Dhillon KS, Sandhu HS, Singh TJ. Chronic molybdenosis in buffaloes. Indian J Anim Sci 1993;63:1072–4.

90. Choudhury H, Cary R. Barium and barium compounds. In: Concise International chemical Assessment. Geneva (Switzerland): World Health Organization; 2001. p. 1–57.

91. National Research Council. Barium. In: Mineral tolerance of animals. Washington, DC: National Academies Press; 2005. p. 46–53.

92. Stevens Y, Moffett D, Ingerman L, et al. Draft toxicological profile for barium and barium compounds. Washington, DC: ATSDR: Agency for Toxic Substances and Disease Registry; 2005. p. 1–77.

93. Garner RJ, Jones HG, Sansom BF. Fission products and the dairy cow. Biochem J 1960;76:572–9.
94. Newton D, Ancill AK, Naylor KE, et al. Long term retention of injected barium-133 in man. Radiat Prot Dosimetry 2001;97:231–40.
95. Shanbaky IO, Borowitz JL, Kessler WV. Mechanisms of cadmium- and barium-induced adrenal catecholamine release. Toxicol Appl Pharmacol 1978;44: 99–105.
96. Smith RP, Gosselin RE. Current concept about the treatment of selected poisons: Nitrite, cyanide, sulfide, barium, and quinidine. Annu Rev Pharmacol Toxicol 1976;16:189–99.
97. Gosselin RE, Smith RP, Hodge HC, et al. Clinical Toxicology of Commercial Products. 5th edition. London: Williams and Wilkins; 1984.
98. Kojola WH, Brenniman GR, Carnow B, et al. A review of environmental characteristics and health effects of barium in public water supplies. Rev Environ Health 1979;3:79–95.
99. Roza O, Berman LB. The pathophysiology of barium: Hypokalemic and cardiovascular effects. J Pharmacol Exp Ther 1971;177:433–9.
100. National Research Council. Barium. In: Mineral tolerance of domestic animals. Washington, DC: National Academies Press; 1980. p. 54–9.
101. Johnson CH, VanTassell VJ. Acute barium poisoning with respiratory failure and rhabdomyolysis. Ann Emerg Med 1991;20:1138–42.
102. Ram L, Schonewille JT, van't Klooster AT, et al. Lethal effect of intraruminal barium chloride administration in goats. N Z Vet J 1999;47:150.
103. Richards T, Erickson DL, Talcott PA, et al. Two cases of barium poisoning in cattle. Proc Am Assoc Vet Lab Diagn 2006;49:155.
104. Malhi CS, Parshad VR, Ahmad N. Determination of potential of barium carbonate for the control of house rat (Rattus rattus). Z Angewandte Zool 1993;80:42–9.
105. Mattila MJ, Anyos K, Puisto EL. Cardiotoxic actions of doxepin and barium chloride in conscious rabbits. Arch Toxicol 1986;9:205–8.
106. Gould DB, Sorrell MR, Lupariello AD. Barium sulfide poisoning: Some factors contributing to survival. Arch Intern Med 1973;132:891–4.
107. Wones RG, Stadler BL, Frohman LA. Lack of effect of drinking water barium on cardiovascular risk factors. Environ Health Perspect 1990;35:355–9.
108. Brenniman GR, Levy PS. Epidemiological study of barium in Illinois drinking water supplies. In: Calabrese EJ, editor. Advances in modern Toxicology. Princeton (NJ): Princeton Scientific; 1984. p. 231–49.
109. Borzelleca JF, Condie LW, Egle JL. Short-term toxicity (one- and ten-day gavage) of barium chloride in male and female rats. J Am Coll Toxicol 1988;7: 675–85.
110. Schroeder HA, Mitchener M. Life-term studies in rats: Effects of aluminum, barium, beryllium, and tungsten. J Nutr 1974;105:421–7.
111. Kopp SJ, Perry JHM, Feliksik JM, et al. Cardiovascular dysfunction and hypersensitivity to sodium pentobarbital induced by chronic barium chloride ingestion. Toxicol Appl Pharmacol 1985;77:303–14.
112. Perry HM, Kopp SJ, Perry EF, et al. Hypertension and associated cardiovascular abnormalities induced by chronic barium feeding. J Toxicol Environ Health 1989;28:373–88.
113. Perry J HM, Kopp SJ, Erlanger MW, et al.: Cardiovascular effects of chronic barium ingestion. Trace Substances in Environmental Health; Proceedings of the University of Missouri's Annual Conference on Trace Substances in Environmental Health 17, June 13-16, 1983 Columbia, MO. pp. 155–64.

114. Dietz DD, Elwell MR, Davis JWE, et al. Subchronic toxicity of barium chloride dihydrate administered to rats and mice in the drinking water. Fund Appl Toxicol 1992;19:527–37.

115. Tardiff RG, Robinson M, Ulmer NS. Subchronic oral toxicity of BaCl2 in rats. J Environ Pathol Toxicol 1980;4:267–75.

116. McCauley PT, Douglas BH, Laurie RD, et al. Investigations into the effect of drinking water barium on rats. In: Condie L, editor. Inorganics in drinking water and cardiovascular disease (Advances in modern environmental toxicology). Princeton (NJ): Princeton Scientific Pub.; 1985. p. 197–211.

117. National Toxicology Program. Toxicology and carcinogenesis studies of barium chloride dihydrate in F344/N rats and B6C3F1 mice: Technical report series 432. Washington, DC: U.S. Department of Health and Human Services; 1994.

118. Tarasenko NY, Pronin OA, Silasev AA. Barium compounds as industrial poisons (an experimental study). J Hyg Epidemiol Microbiol Immunol 1977;21:361–73.

119. Ahmed KE, Adam SE, Idrill OF, et al. Experimental selenium poisoning in nubian goats. Vet Hum Toxicol 1990;32:249–51.

120. Kubota J, Naphan EA, Oberly GH. Fluoride in thermal spring water and in plants of Nevada and its relationship to fluorosis in animals. J Range Manage 1982;35: 188–92.

121. National Research Council. Fluorine. In: Mineral tolerance of animals. Washington, DC: National Academies Press; 2005. p. 154–81.

122. Shupe JL, Alther EW. The effects of fluorides on livestock, with particular reference to cattle. In: Eichler O, Farah A, Herken H, et al, editors. Handbook of experimental Pharmacology. Berlin: Springe-Verlag; 1966. p. 307–54.

123. Cerklewski FL. Fluoride bioavailability. Nutr Res 1997;17:907–27.

124. Carlson CH, Armstrong WD, Singer L. Distribution, migration and binding of whole blood fluoride evaluated with radiofluoride. Am J Physiol 1960;199:187–9.

125. Davis RK. Fluorides: A critical review. V. Fluoride intoxication in laboratory animals. J Occup Med 1961;3:593–601.

126. Whitford GM. Intake and metabolism of fluoride. Adv Dent Res 1994;8:5–14.

127. Reed OE, Huffman CF. The results of a five year mineral feeding investigation with dairy cattle. Michigan State College Agricultural Experiment Station Bulletin 1930;105:1–63.

128. Slagsvold L. Fluoride poisoning in animals. Vet Med 1934;30:375.

129. Suttie W. Nutritional aspects of fluoride toxicosis. J Anim Sci 1980;51:759–66.

130. Agency for Toxic Substances and Disease Registry. Toxicological profile for fluorides, hydrogen fluoride, and fluorine. Atlanta (GA): U.S. Department of Health and Human Services; 2003.

131. Boink AB, Wemer J, Meulenbelt J, et al. The mechanism of fluoride-induced hypocalcaemia. Hum Exp Toxicol 1994;13:149–55.

132. Guan Z, Xiao K, Zeng X, et al. Changed cellular membrane lipid composition and lipid peroxidation of kidney in rats with chronic fluorosis. Mol Toxicol 2000;74:602–8.

133. Kessabi M, Hamliri A, Braun JP, et al. Experimental acute sodium fluoride poisoning in sheep: Renal, hepatic, and metabolic effects. Fund Appl Toxicol 1985;5:1025–33.

134. Chinoy NJ, Pradeep PK, Sequeira E. Effect of fluoride ingestion on the physiology of reproductive organs of male rat. J Environ Biol 1992;13:55–61.

135. Pillai KS, Mathai AT, Deshmukh PB. Effect of fluoride on reproduction in mice. Fluoride 1989;22:165–8.

136. Susheela S, Kumar A. A study of the effect of high concentrations of fluoride on the reproductive organs of male rabbits, using light and scanning electron microscopy. J Reprod Fertil 1991;92:353–60.

137. Bawden JW, Crenshaw MA, Wright JT, et al. Consideration of possible biologic mechanisms of fluorosis. J Dent Res 1995;74:1349–52.

138. Cass JS. Fluorides: A critical review. IV. Response of livestock and poultry to absorption of inorganic fluorides. J Occup Med 1961;3:471–7.

139. Choubisa SL. Some observations on endemic fluorosis in domestic animals in southern Rajasthan (India). Vet Res Commun 1999;23:457–65.

140. Clarke EGC. Clinical toxicology XII. Poisoning in domestic animals. Practitioner 1973;211:818–22.

141. Kierdorf U, Kierdorf H. Dental fluorosis in wild deer: Its use as a biomarker of increased fluoride exposure. Environ Monit Assess 1999;57:265–75.

142. Peirce AW. Chronic fluorine intoxication in domestic animals. Nutr Abstr Rev 1939;9:253–61.

143. Suttie JW. The influence of nutrition and other factors on fluoride tolerance. In: Shupe JL, Peterson HB, Leone NC, editors. Fluorides: effects on vegetation, animals, and humans. Salt Lake City (UT): Paragon Press; 1983. p. 291–302.

144. Mullenix PJ, Denbesten PK, Schunior A, et al. Neurotoxicity of sodium fluoride in rats. Neurotoxicology 1995;17:169–77.

145. Shan K, Qi X, Long Y, et al. Decreased nicotinic receptors in PC12 cells and rat brains influenced by fluoride toxicity- A mechanism relating to a damage at the level in post-transcription of the receptor genes. Toxicology 2004;200:169–77.

146. Paul V, Ekambaram P, Jayakumar AR. Effects of sodium fluoride on locomotor behavior and a few biochemical parameters in rats. Environ Toxicol Pharmacol 1998;6:187–91.

147. Wang Y, Xiao K, Liu J, et al. Effect of long term exposure on lipid composition in rat liver. Toxicology 2000;146:161–9.

148. Ekambaram P, Paul V. Modulation of fluoride toxicity in rats by calcium carbonate and by withdrawal of fluoride exposure. Pharmacol Toxicol 2002;90:53–8.

149. Grucka-Mamczar E, Machoy Z, Tarnawski R, et al. Influence of long- term sodium fluoride administration on selected parameters of rat blood serum and liver function. Fluoride 1997;30:157–64.

150. Heindel JJ, Bates HK, Price CJ, et al. Developmental toxicity evaluation of sodium fluoride administered to rats and rabbits in drinking water. Fund Appl Toxicol 1996;30:162–77.

151. Varner JA, Jensen KF, Horvath W, et al. Chronic administration of aluminum- fluoride or sodium-fluoride to rats in drinking water: Alterations in neuronal and cerebrovascular integrity. Brain Res 1998;784:284–98.

152. Ahn H, Fulton B, Moxon D, et al. Interactive effects of fluoride and aluminum uptake and accumulation in bones of rabbits administered both agents in their drinking water. J Toxicol Environ Health 1995;44:337–50.

153. Kessabi M, Hamliri A, Braun JP. Experimental fluorosis in sheep: Alleviating effects of aluminum. Vet Hum Toxicol 1986;28:300–4.

154. National Toxicology Program TR-393. Toxicology and carcinogenesis studies of sodium fluoride (CAS No. 7681-49-4) in F344/N rats and B6C3F1 mice (drinking water studies). Washington, DC: Department of Health and Human Services, National Toxicology Program; 1990.

155. Newman JR, Markey D. Effects of elevated levels of fluoride on deer mice (Peromyscus maniculatus). Fluoride 1976;9:47–53.

156. Patra RC, Dwivedi SK, Bhardwaj B, et al. Industrial fluorosis in cattle and buffalo around Udaipur, India. Sci Total Environ 2000;253:145–50.
157. Lopez TA, Busetti MR, Fort MC, et al. Fluoride-induced early teeth wearing in Argentinian cattle. Biomed Environ Sci 1994;7:205–15.
158. Neeley KL, Harbaugh FG. Effects of fluoride ingestion on a herd of dairy cattle in the Lubbock, Texas area. J Am Vet Med Assoc 1954;124:344–50.
159. Rand WE, Schmidt HJ. The effect upon cattle of Arizona waters of high fluoride content. Am J Vet Res 1952;13:50–61.
160. Araya O, Wittwer F, Villa A. Evolution of fluoride concentrations in cattle and grass following a volcanic eruption. Vet Hum Toxicol 1993;35:437–40.
161. Schultheiss WA, Godley GA. Chronic fluorosis in cattle due to the ingestion of a commercial lick. J S Afr Vet Assoc 1995;66:83–4.
162. Merriman GM, Hobbs CS. Bovine fluorosis from soil and water sources. Univ Tenn Agr Exper Sta Bull 1962;347:1–47.
163. Suttie JW, Carlson JR, Faltin EC. Effects of alternating periods of high- and low-fluoride ingestion on dairy cattle. J Dairy Sci 1972;55:790–804.
164. Hobbs CS, Merriman GM. Fluorosis in beef cattle. Tenn Agr Exper Sta Bull 1962; 351:1–181.
165. Ammerman CB, Arrington LR, Shirley RL, et al. Comparative effects of fluorine from soft phosphate, calcium fluoride, and sodium fluoride on steers. J Anim Sci 1964;23:409–13.
166. Shupe JL, Christofferson PV, Olson AE, et al. Relationship of cheek tooth abrasion to fluoride-induced permanent incisor lesions in livestock. Am J Vet Res 1987;48:1498–503.
167. Heller VG, Larwood CH. Saline drinking water. Science 1930;71:223–4.
168. Eckerlin HR, Maylin GA, Krook L. Milk production of cows fed fluoride contaminated commercial feed. Cornell Vet 1986;76:403–14.
169. Maylin GA, Eckerlin RH, Krook L. Fluoride intoxication in dairy calves. Cornell Vet 1987;77:84–98.
170. Harris LE, Raleigh RJ, Stoddard GE, et al. Effects of fluorine on dairy cattle. III. Digestion and metabolism trials. J Anim Sci 1964;23:537–46.
171. McLaren JB, Merriman GM. Effects of fluorine on productivity and longevity in beef cows. Tenn Agr Exper Sta Bull 1975;549:1.
172. Shupe JL, Miner ML, Harris LE, et al. Relative effects of feeding hay atmospherically contaminated by fluoride residue, normal hay plus calcium fluoride, and normal hay plus sodium fluoride to dairy heifers. Am J Vet Res 1962;23:777–87.
173. van Rensburg SW, de Vos WH. The influence of excess fluorine intake in the drinking water on reproductive efficiency in bovines. Onderstepoort J Vet Res 1966;33:185–94.
174. Harvey JM. Chronic endemic fluorosis of Merino sheep in Queensland. Queensland Journal of Agricultural Science 1952;9:47–138.
175. Schultheiss WA, Van Niekerk JC. Suspected chronic fluorosis in a sheep flock. J S Afr Vet Assoc 1994;65:84–5.
176. Botha CJ, Naude TW, Minnaar PP, et al. Two outbreaks of fluorosis in cattle and sheep. J S Afr Vet Assoc 1995;64:165–8.
177. Hibbs CM, Thilsted JP. Toxicosis in cattle from contaminated well water. Vet Hum Toxicol 1983;25:253–4.
178. Shupe JL, Olson AE. Clinical aspects of fluorosis in horses. J Am Vet Med Assoc 1971;158:167–74.
179. Comar CL, Visek WJ, Lotz WE, et al. Effects of fluorine on calcium metabolism and bone growth in pigs. Am J Anat 1953;92:361–89.

180. Shupe JL, Olson AE, Peterson HB, et al. Fluoride toxicosis in wild ungulates. J Am Vet Med Assoc 1984;185:1295–300.
181. Suttie JW, Dickie R, Clay AB, et al. Effects of fluoride emissions from a modern primary aluminum smelter on a local population of white-tailed deer (Odocoileus virginianus). J Wildl Dis 1987;23:135–43.
182. Newman JR, Yu MH. Fluorosis in black-tailed deer. J Wildl Dis 1976;12:39–41.
183. Suttie JW, Hamilton RJ, Clay AC, et al. Effects of fluoride ingestion on white-tailed deer (Odocoileus virginianus). J Wildl Dis 1985;21:283–8.
184. Vikoren T, Stuve G, Froslie A. Fluoride exposure in cervids inhabiting areas adjacent to aluminum smelters in Norway. I. Residue levels. J Wildl Dis 1996;32:169–80.
185. National Research Council. Molybdenum. In: Mineral tolerance of animals. Washington, DC: National Academies Press; 2005. p. 262–70.
186. Thomson I, Thornton I, Webb JS. Molybdenum in black shales and the incidence of bovine hypocuprosis. J Sci Food Agric 1972;23:879–91.
187. Alary J, Bourbon P, Esclassan J, et al. Environmental molybdenum levels in industrial molybdenosis of grazing cattle. Sci Total Environ 1981;19:111–9.
188. Buxton JC, Allcroft R. Industrial molybdenosis of grazing cattle. Vet Rec 1955;67:273–6.
189. Erdman JA, Ebens RJ, Case AA. Molybdenosis: A potential problem in ruminants grazing on coal mine spoils. J Range Manage 1978;31:34–6.
190. Gardner AW, Hall-Patch PK. An outbreak of industrial molybdenosis. Vet Rec 1962;74:113–6.
191. Gardner WC, Broersma K, Popp JD, et al. Copper and health status of cattle grazing high-molybdenum forage from a reclaimed mine tailing site. Can J Anim Sci 2003;83:479–85.
192. Parker WM, Rose TH. Molybdenum poisoning (Teart) due to aerial contamination of pastures. Vet Rec 1955;67:276–9.
193. Barceloux DG. Molybdenum. Clin Toxicol 1999;37:231–7.
194. Reddy KJ, Munn LC, Wang L. Chemistry and mineralogy of molybdenum in soils. In: Gupta UC, editor. Molybdenum in Agriculture. New York: Cambridge University Press; 1997. p. 6–9.
195. Ward GM. Acceptable limits of molybdenum for ruminants exist. Feedstuffs 1991;14:15–22.
196. Pitt M, Fraser J, Thurley DC. Molybdenum toxicity in sheep: Epiphysiolysis, exotoses and biochemical changes. J Comp Pathol 1980;90:567–76.
197. Kubota J. Areas of molybdenum toxicity to grazing animals in the Western States. J Range Manage 1975;28:252–6.
198. Ward GM. Molybdenum requirements, toxicity, and nutritional limits for man and animals. In: Braithwaite ER, Haber J, editors. Molybdenum: an outline of its Chemistry and Uses. Amsterdam (the Netherlands): Elsevier; 1994. p. 452–76.
199. Mason J. The relationship between copper, molybdenum and sulphur in ruminant and non- ruminant animals: A preview. Vet Sci Commun 1978;2:85–94.
200. Dale JE, Ewan RC, Speer VC, et al. Copper, molybdenum and sulfate interaction in young swine. J Anim Sci 1973;37:913–7.
201. Gray LF, Daniel LJ. Some effects of excess molybdenum on the nutrition of the rat. J Nutr 1954;53:43–51.
202. Mills CF, Monty KJ, Ichihara A, et al. Metabolic effects of molybdenum toxicity in the rat. J Nutr 1958;65:129–42.
203. Van Reen R, Williams MA. Studies on the influence of sulfur compounds on molybdenum toxicity in rats. Arch Biochem Biophys 1956;63:1–81.

204. Bell MC, Diggs BG, Lowrey RS, et al. Comparison of Mo-99 metabolism in swine and cattle as affected by stable molybdenum. J Nutr 1964;84:367–72.
205. Hogan KG, Hutchinson AJ. Molybdenum and sulphate in the diet and the effect on the molybdenum content of the milk of grazing sheep. N Z J Agric Res 1965; 8:625–9.
206. Scaife JF. Molybdenum excretion and retention in the sheep. N Z J Sci Technol 1956;38a:293–8.
207. Norheim G, Soli NE, Froslie A, et al. Fractionation of soluble molybdenum- binding proteins from liver, kidney, plasma and erythrocytes from sheep supplemented with molybdenum. Acta Vet Scand 1980;21:428–37.
208. Suttle NF. Recent studies of the copper-molybdenum antagonism. Proc Nutr Soc 1974;33:299–305.
209. Allen JD, Gawthorne JM. Involvement of the solid phase of rumen digesta in the interaction between copper, molybdenum and sulphur in sheep. Br J Nutr 1987; 58:265–76.
210. Gooneratne SR, Buckley WT, Christensen DA. Review of copper deficiency and metabolism in ruminants. Can J Anim Sci 1989;69:819–45.
211. Ivan M, Veira DM. Effects of copper sulfate supplement on growth, tissue concentration, and ruminal solubilities of molybdenum and copper in sheep fed low and high molybdenum diets. J Dairy Sci 1985;68:891–6.
212. Spears JW. Trace mineral bioavailability in ruminants. J Nutr 2003;133: 1506S–9S.
213. Suttle NF. The interactions between copper, molybdenum, and sulphur in ruminant nutrition. Annu Rev Nutr 1991;11:121–40.
214. Hynes M, Woods M, Poole D, et al. Some studies on the metabolism of labeled molybdenum compounds in cattle. J Inorg Biochem 1985;24:279–88.
215. Hynes M, Lamand M, Montel G, et al. Some studies on the metabolism and the effects of 99-Mo and 35-S labelled thiomolybdates after intravenous infusion in sheep. Br J Nutr 1984;52:149–58.
216. Mason J, Woods M, Poole DBR. Accumulation of copper on albumin in bovine plasma in vivo after intravenous trithiomolybdate administration. Res Vet Sci 1986;41:108–13.
217. Mason J. The putative role of thiomolybdates in the pathogenesis of Mo-induced hypocupraemia and molybdenosis: Some recent developments. Irish Vet J 1982;36:164–8.
218. Arthington JD, Corah LR, Blecha F. The effect of molybdenum-induced copper deficiency on acute-phase protein concentrations, superoxide dismutase activity, leukocyte numbers and lymphocyte proliferation in beef heifers inoculated with bovine herpesvirus-1. J Anim Sci 1996;74:211–7.
219. Auza N, Braun JP, Benard P, et al. Hematological and plasma biochemical disturbances in experimental molybdenum toxicosis in sheep. Vet Hum Toxicol 1989;31:535–7.
220. Boyne R, Arthur JR. Effects of molybdenum or iron induced copper deficiency on the viability and function of neutrophils from cattle. Res Vet Sci 1986;41: 417–9.
221. Cerone S, Sansinanea A, Streitenberger S, et al. Bovine neutrophil functionality in molybdenum-induced copper deficiency. Nutr Res 1998;18:557–66.
222. Dowdy RP, Matrone G. A copper-molybdenum complex: Its effects and movement in the piglet and sheep. J Nutr 1968;95:197–201.
223. Gengelbach GP, Ward JD, Spears JW, et al. Effects of copper deficiency and copper deficiency coupled with high dietary iron or molybdenum on phagocytic

cell function and response of calves to a respiratory disease challenge. J Anim Sci 1997;75:1112–8.

224. Jones DG, Suttle NF. Some effects of copper deficiency on leukocyte function in sheep and cattle. Res Vet Sci 1981;31:151–6.

225. Kincaid RL, White CL. The effects of ammonium tetrathiomolybdate intake of tissue copper and molybdenum in pregnant ewes and lambs. J Anim Sci 1988;66: 3252–8.

226. Lannon B, Mason J. The inhibition of bovine ceruloplasmin oxidase activity by thiomolybdates in vivo and in vitro: A reversible reaction. J Inorg Biochem 1986;26:107–15.

227. Mason J, Lamand M, Kelleher CA. The fate of 99-Mo-labelled sodium tetrathiomolybdate after duodenal administration in sheep: The effect on caeruloplasmin (EC 1.16.3.1) diamine oxidase activity and plasma copper. Br J Nutr 1980;43: 515–23.

228. Vyskocil A, Viau C. Assessment of molybdenum toxicity in humans. J Appl Toxicol 1999;19:185–92.

229. Woods, Mason J. Spectral and kinetic studies on the binding of trithiomolybdate to bovine and canine serum albumin in vitro: The interaction with copper. J Inorg Biochem 1987;30:261–72.

230. Haywood S, Dincer Z, Holding J, et al. Metal (molybdenum, copper) accumulation and retention in brain, pituitary and other organs of ammonium tetrathiomolybdate-treated sheep. Br J Nutr 1998;79:329–31.

231. Phillippo M, Humphries WR, Garthwaite PH. The effect of dietary molybdenum and iron on copper status and growth in cattle. J Agric Sci Camb 1987;109: 315–20.

232. Phillippo M, Humphries WR, Atkinson T, et al. The effect of dietary molybdenum and iron on copper status, puberty, fertility and oestrus cycles in cattle. J Agric Sci Camb 1987;109:321–36.

233. Miltimore JE, Mason JL. Copper to molybdenum ratio and molybdenum and copper concentrations in ruminant feeds. Can J Anim Sci 1971;51:193–200.

234. Thomas JW, Moss S. The effect of orally administered molybdenum on growth, spermatogenesis and testes histology of young dairy bulls. J Dairy Sci 1951;34: 929–34.

235. Ward GM. Molybdenum toxicity and hypocuprosis in ruminants: A review. J Anim Sci 1978;46:1078–85.

236. ANZECC. Australian and New Zealand Guidelines for fresh and marine water quality. Canberra, ACT, Australia: Livestock drinking water guidelines; 2000.

237. Swan DA, Creeper JH, White CL, et al. Molybdenum poisoning in feedlot cattle. Aust Vet J 1998;76:345–9.

238. Arrington LR, Davis GK. Molybdenum toxicity in the rabbit. J Nutr 1953;51: 295–304.

239. Singh J, Randhawa CS, Randhawa SS, et al. Role of dietary molybdenum in production of hypophosphatemia in crossbred calves. Ind J Dairy Sci 1994;47:926.

240. Smith BP, Fisher GL, Poulos PW, et al. Abnormal bone development and lameness associated with secondary copper deficiency in young cattle. J Am Vet Med Assoc 1975;166:682–8.

241. Fungwe TV, Buddingh F, Demick DS. The role of dietary molybdenum on estrous activity, fertility, reproduction and molybdenum and copper enzyme activities of female rats. Nutr Res 1990;10:515–24.

242. Jeter MA, Davis GK. The effect of dietary molybdenum upon growth, hemoglobin, reproduction and lactation of rats. J Nutr 1954;54:215–20.

243. Van Niekerk FE, Van Niekerk CH. The influence of experimentally induced copper deficiency on the fertility of rams. I. Semen parameters and peripheral plasma androgen concentration. J S Afr Vet Assoc 1989;60:28–31.

244. Van Niekerk FE, Van Niekerk CH. The influence of experimentally induced copper deficiency on the fertility of rams. II. Macro- and microscopic changes in the testes. J S Afr Vet Assoc 1989;60:32–5.

245. Ferguson WS, Lewis AH, Watson SJ. Action of molybdenum in nutrition of milking cattle. Nature 1938;141:553.

246. Lloyd WE, Hill HT, Meerdink GL. Observations of a case of molybdenosis-copper deficiency in a South Dakota dairy herd. In: Chappell W, Peterson KK, editors. Molybdenum in the environment. New York: Marcel Dekker; 1976. p. 85–95.

247. Tolgyesi G, Elmoty I. Excretion of molybdenum given to cattle in large doses. Vet Bull 1968;1071:167.

248. Sas B. Secondary copper deficiency in cattle caused by molybdenum contamination of fodder: A case history. Vet Hum Toxicol 1989;31:29–33.

249. Cunningham HM, Brown JM, Edie AE. Molybdenum poisoning of cattle in the Swan River Valley of Manitoba. Can J Agric Sci 1953;33:254–60.

250. Cook GA, Lesperance AL, Bohman VR, et al. Interrelationship of molybdenum and certain factors to the development of the molybdenum toxicity syndrome. J Anim Sci 1966;25:96–101.

251. Majak W, Steinke D, McGillivray J, et al. Clinical signs in cattle grazing high molybdenum forage. J Range Manage 2004;57:269–74.

252. Barshad I. Molybdenum content of pasture plants in relation to toxicity to cattle. Soil Sci 1948;66:187–95.

253. Dollahite JW, Rowe LD, Cook LM, et al. Copper deficiency and molybdenosis intoxication associated with grazing near a uranium mine. Southwest Vet 1972;9:47–50.

254. Lesperance AL, Bohman VR, Oldfield JE. Interaction of molybdenum, sulfate and alfalfa in the bovine. J Anim Sci 1985;60:791–802.

255. Vanderveen JE, Keener HA. Effects of molybdenum and sulfate sulfur on metabolism of copper in dairy cattle. J Dairy Sci 1984;47:1224–8.

256. Huber JT, Price NO, Engel RW. Response of lactating dairy cows to high levels of dietary molybdenum. J Anim Sci 1971;32:364–7.

257. Britton JW, Goss H. Chronic molybdenum poisoning in cattle. J Am Vet Med Assoc 1946;108:176–8.

258. Kincaid RL. Toxicity of ammonium molybdate added to drinking water of calves. J Dairy Sci 1980;63:608–10.

259. Mills CF, Fell BF. Demyelination in lambs born of ewes maintained on high intakes of sulphate and molybdate. Nature 1960;185:20–2.

260. Hogan KG, Money DFL, White DA, et al. Weight responses of young sheep to copper, and connective tissue lesions associated with the grazing of pastures of high molybdenum content. N Z J Agric Res 1971;14:687–701.

261. Sharma AK, Parihar NS. Pathology of experimental molybdenosis in goats. Indian J Anim Sci 1994;64:114–9.

262. Raisbeck MF, Siemion RS, Smith MS. Modest copper supplementation blocks molybdenosis in cattle. J Vet Diagn Invest 2006;18:566–72.

263. Gardner W and Broersma K. Cattle grazing high molybdenum pasture on reclaimed mine tailings. In: Molybdenum Issues in Reclamation: Proceedings of the 1999 Workshop, Kamloops, BC, September 24, 1999. pp 66–75.

264. Gardner WG, Quinton DA, Popp JD, et al. The use of copper boli for cattle grazing high-molybdenum forage. In: Garland T, Barr AC, editors. Toxic plants and other natural Toxicants. London: CAB Intl; 1998. p. 115–9.

265. Quinton DA, Mir Z, Mir P, et al. Effects of feeding high molybdenum hay to mature beef steers. Proceedings of the BC Mine Reclamation Symposium 17. Port Hardy, BC, 1993. p. 75–85.

266. National Research Council. Selenium. In: Mineral tolerance of domestic animals. Washington, DC: National Academies Press; 1980. p. 392–420.

267. Girling CA. Selenium in agriculture and the environment. Agric Ecosyst Environ 1984;11:37–65.

268. Boon DY. Potential selenium problems in great plains soils. In: Jacobs LW, editor. Selenium in Agriculture and the environment. Madison (WI): Soil Science Society of America; 1989. p. 107–21.

269. Ohlendorf HM. Bioaccumulation and effects of selenium in wildlife. In: Jacobs LW, editor. Selenium in Agriculture and the environment. Madison (WI): Soil Science Society of America; 1989. p. 133–77.

270. Fessler AJ, Moller G, Talcott PA, et al. Selenium toxicity in sheep grazing reclaimed phosphate mining sites. Vet Hum Toxicol 2003;45:294–8.

271. Talcott PA. Diagnostic report. Pulolman, Washington: Washington animal disease diagnostic Lab; 1999. #99-110127.

272. Ohlendorf HM, Skorupa JP. Selenium in relation to wildlife and agricultural drainage water. In: Carapella SC, editor. Fourth International Symposium on Uses of selenium and Tellurium. Darien (CT): Selenium-Tellurium Development Association; 1989. p. 314–34.

273. Saiki MK. A field example of selenium contamination in an aquatic food chain. Proc Annu Symp Selenium Environ. Fresno, CA, June 10–2, 1986, 1. pp. 67–76.

274. Presser TS, Sylvester MA, Low WH. Bioaccumulation of selenium from natural geologic sources in western states and its potential consequences. Environ Manag 1994;18:423–36.

275. Barceloux DG. Selenium. Clin Toxicol 1999;37:145–72.

276. Tapiero H, Townsend DM, Tew KD. The antioxidant role of selenium and selenocompounds. Biomed Pharmacother 2003;57:134–44.

277. National Research Council. Selenium. In: Mineral tolerance of animals. Washington, DC: National Academies Press; 2005. p. 321–47.

278. Muth OH, Oldfield JE, Remmert LF, et al. Effects of selenium and vitamin E on white muscle disease. Science 1958;128:1090.

279. Oldfield JE, Schubert JR, Muth OH. Implications of selenium in large animal nutrition. Agric Food Chem 1963;11:388–90.

280. FDA. Food additives permitted in feed and drinking water of animals; Selenium. Fed Regist 1987;52:10887–8.

281. Edmondson AJ, Norman BB, Suther D. Survey of state veterinarians and state veterinary diagnostic laboratories for selenium deficiency and toxicosis in animals. J Am Vet Med Assoc 1993;202:865–72.

282. Raisbeck MF, Dahl ER, Sanchez DA. Naturally occurring selenosis in Wyoming. J Vet Diagn Invest 1993;5:84–7.

283. Neuhierl B, Bock A. On the mechanism of selenium tolerance in selenium-accumulating plants: Purification and characterization of a specific selenocysteine methyltransferase from cultured cells of Astragalus bisculatus. Eur J Biochem 1996;239:235–8.

284. Olson OE, Novacek EJ, Whitehead EI, et al. Investigations on selenium in wheat. Phytochemistry 1970;9:1181–8.

285. Wang Y, Bock A, Neuhierl B. Acquisition of selenium tolerance by a selenium non- accumulating Astragalus species via selection. Biofactors 1999;9:3–10.
286. Raisbeck MF. Selenosis. Vet Clin North Am Food Anim Pract 2000;16:465–80.
287. Naftz DL, Rice JA. Geochemical processes controlling selenium in ground-water after mining, Powder River Basin, Wyoming, USA. Appl Geochem 1989; 4:565–676.
288. United States Geological Survey. Detailed study of selenium in soil, representa-tive plants, water bottom sediment, and biota in the Kendrick Reclamation Proj-ect area, Wyoming, 1988-1990. 1st edition. Denver (CO): United States Geological Survey; 1990.
289. Whanger P, Vendeland S, Park YC, et al. Metabolism of subtoxic levels of sele-nium in animals and humans. Ann Clin Lab Sci 1996;26:99–113.
290. Goede AA, Wolterbeek HT. Have high selenium concentrations in wading birds their origins in mercury? Sci Total Environ 1994;144:247–53.
291. Turner JC, Osborn PJ, McVeagh SM. Studies on selenate and selenite absorp-tion by sheep ileum using an everted sac method and an isolated, vascularly perfused system. Comp Biochem Physiol A 1990;95:297–301.
292. Vendeland SC, Butler JA, Whanger PD. Intestinal absorption of selenite, sele-nate and selenomethionine in the rat. J Nutr Biochem 1996;3:359–65.
293. Windisch W, Kirchgessner M. Selenium true absorption and tissue concentration of rats at dietary selenite, seleno cysteine, and seleno methionine. In: Roussel AM, Anderson RA, Favier AE, editors. Trace elements in man and ani-mals. New York: Kluwer Academic/Plenum Publishers; 2000. p. 173–4.
294. Raisbeck MF, O'Toole D, Belden EL. Chronic selenosis in ruminants. In: Garland T, Barr AC, editors. Toxic plants and other natural toxicants. New York: CAB International; 1998. p. 389–96.
295. Wright PL, Bell MC. Comparative metabolism of selenium and tellurium in sheep and swine. Am J Physiol 1996;211:6–10.
296. Hill KE, Zhou J, McMahan WJ, et al. Deletion of selenoprotein P alters distribu-tion of selenium in the mouse. J Biol Chem 2003;278:13640–6.
297. Windisch W, Kirchgessner M. True absorption, excretion, and tissue retention of selenium at widely varying selenium supply to rats. In: Roussel AM, Anderson R, Favier AE, editors. Trace elements in man and animals. New York: Kluwer Aca-demic/Plenum Publishers; 2000. p. 883–6.
298. Hintze KJ, Lardy GP, Marchello MJ, et al. Selenium accumulation in beef: Effect of dietary selenium and geographic area of animal origin. J Agric Food Chem 2002;50:3938–42.
299. Ganther HE, Baumann CA. Selenium metabolism. II. Modifying effects of sulfate. J Nutr 1982;77:408–14.
300. Pope AL, Moir RJ, Somers M, et al. The effect of sulphur on Se absorption and retention in sheep. J Nutr 1979;109:1448–55.
301. Halverson AW, Monty KJ. An effect of dietary sulfate on selenium poisoning in the rat. J Nutr 1960;70:100–2.
302. O'Toole D, Raisbeck MF. Experimentally induced selenosis of adult mallard ducks: Clinical signs, lesions, and toxicology. Vet Pathol 1997;34:330–40.
303. O'Toole D, Raisbeck MF. Magic numbers, elusive lesions: Comparative pathol-ogy and toxicology of selenosis in waterfowl and mammalian species. In: Frankenberger JWT, Engberg RA, editors. Environmental Chemistry of selenium. New York: Marcel Dekker; 1998. p. 355–95.
304. Palmer IS, Olson OE, Halverson AW, et al. Isolation of factors in linseed oil meal protective against chronic selenosis in rats. J Nutr 1980;110:145–50.

305. Mihailovic M, Matic G, Lindberg P, et al. Accidental selenium poisoning of growing pigs. Biol Trace Elem Res 1992;33:63–9.

306. Stowe HD. Effects of copper pretreatment upon the toxicity of selenium in ponies. Am J Vet Res 1980;41:1925–8.

307. Rosenfeld I, Beath OA. The influence of protein diets on selenium poisoning. Am J Vet Res 1946;7:52–6.

308. Van Vleet JF, Meyer KB, Olander HJ. Acute selenium toxicosis induced in baby pigs by parenteral administration of selenium-vitamin E preparations. J Am Vet Med Assoc 1974;165:543–7.

309. Baker DC, James LF, Hartley WJ, et al. Toxicosis in pigs fed selenium-accumulating Astragalus plant species or sodium selenate. Am J Vet Res 1989;50:1396–9.

310. Fitzhugh OG, Nelson AA, Bliss CI. The chronic oral toxicity of selenium. J Pharmacol Exp Ther 1944;80:289–99.

311. Heinz GH, Hoffman DJ, Krynitsky AJ, et al. Reproduction of mallards fed selenium. Environ Toxicol Chem 1987;6:423–33.

312. O'Toole D, Raisbeck MF. Pathology of experimentally induced chronic selenosis (alkali disease) in yearling cattle. J Vet Diagn Invest 1995;7:364–73.

313. Palmer IS, Olson OE. Relative toxicities of selenite and selenate in the drinking water of rats. J Nutr 1974;104:306–14.

314. Glenn MW, Jensen R, Griner LA. Sodium selenate toxicosis: Pathology and pathogenesis of sodium selenate toxicosis in sheep. Am J Vet Res 1964;25:1486–93.

315. Ohlendorf HM, Kilness AW, Simmons JL, et al. Selenium toxicosis in wild aquatic birds. J Toxicol Environ Health 1988;24:67–92.

316. Glenn MW, Jensen R, Griner LA. Sodium selenate toxicosis: The effects of extended oral administration of sodium selenate on mortality, clinical signs, fertility, and early embryonic development in sheep. Am J Vet Res 1964;25:1479–85.

317. Tarantal AF, Willhite CC, Lasley BL, et al. Developmental toxicity of L-selenomethionine in Macaca fascicularis. Fund Appl Toxicol 1991;16:147–60.

318. Willhite CC. Selenium teratogenesis. Species dependent response and influence on reproduction. Ann N Y Acad Sci 1996;678:169–77.

319. Wahlstrom RC, Olson OE. The effect of selenium on reproduction in swine. J Anim Sci 1959;18:141–5.

320. Westfall BB, Stohlman EF, Smith MI. The placental transmission of selenium. J Pharmacol Exp Ther 1938;64:55–7.

321. Raisbeck MF and O'Toole D. Morphologic studies of selenosis in herbivores. In: Garland T, Barr AC, editors. Toxic plants and other natural toxicants. CAB International: New York; 1997. pp. 380–8.

322. Orstadius K. Toxicity of a single subcutaneous dose of sodium selenite in pigs. Nature 1960;188:1117.

323. Shortridge EH, O'Hara PJ, Marshall PM. Acute selenium poisoning in cattle. N Z Vet J 1971;19:47–50.

324. MacDonald DW, Christian RG, Strausz KI. Acute selenium toxicity in neonatal calves. Can Vet J 1981;22:279–81.

325. Blodgett DJ, Bevill RF. Acute selenium toxicosis in sheep. Vet Hum Toxicol 1987;29:233–6.

326. Miller WT, Williams KT. Minimum lethal doses of selenium, as sodium selenite, for horses, mules, cattle, and swine. J Agric Res 1940;60:163–73.

327. Hadjimarkos DM. Effect of selenium on food and water intake in the rat. Experientia 1966;22:117–8.

328. Halverson AW, Palmer IS, Guss PL. Toxicity of selenium to post-weanling rats. Toxicol Appl Pharmacol 1966;9:477–84.

329. Hill J, Allison F, Halpin C. An episode of acute selenium toxicity in a commercial piggery. Aust Vet J 1985;62:207–9.

330. Stowe HD, Eavey AJ, Granger L, et al. Selenium toxicosis in feeder pigs. J Am Vet Med Assoc 1992;201:292–5.

331. Wilson TM, Scholz RW, Drake TR. Selenium toxicity and porcine focal symmetrical poliomyelomalacia: Description of a field outbreak and experimental reproduction. Can J Comp Med 1983;47:412–42.

332. Schoening HW. Production of so-called alkali disease in hogs by feeding corn grown in affected area. North Am Vet 1936;17:22–8.

333. Smyth JBA, Wang JH, Barlow RM, et al. Experimental acute selenium intoxication in lambs. J Comp Pathol 1990;102:197–209.

334. Gabbedy BJ, Dickson J. Acute selenium poisoning in lambs. Aust Vet J 1969;45:470–2.

335. Morrow DA. Acute selenite toxicosis in lambs. J Am Vet Med Assoc 1968;152:1625–9.

336. Maag DD, Orsborn JS, Clopton JR. The effect of sodium selenite on cattle. Am J Vet Res 1960;21:1049–53.

337. Raisbeck MF, Schamber RA, Belden EL. Immunotoxic effects of selenium in mammals. In: Garland T, Barr AC, editors. Toxic plants and other natural toxicants. New York: CAB International; 1998. p. 260–6.

338. Kaur R, Sharma S, Rampal S. Effect of sub-chronic selenium toxicosis on lipid peroxidation, glutathione redox cycle and antioxidant enzymes in calves. Vet Hum Toxicol 2003;45:190–2.

339. Jenkins KJ, Hidiroglou M. Tolerance of the preruminant calf for selenium in milk replacer. J Dairy Sci 1986;69:1865–70.

340. Dewes HF, Lowe MD. Suspected selenium poisoning in a horse. N Z Vet J 1987;35:53–4.

341. Witte ST, Will LA. Investigation of selenium sources associated with chronic selenosis in horses of western Iowa. J Vet Diagn Invest 1993;5:128–31.

342. Witte ST, Will LA, Olsen CR, et al. Chronic selenosis in horses fed locally produced alfalfa hay. J Am Vet Med Assoc 1993;202:406–9.

343. Strange K. Regulation of solute and water balance and cell volume in the central nervous system. J Am Soc Nephrol 1992;3:12–27.

344. Coenen M, Landes E, Assmann G. Selenium toxicosis in the horse - Case report. J Anim Physiol Anim Nutr 1998;80:153–7.

345. Knott SG, McCray CWR. Two naturally occurring outbreaks of selenosis in Queensland. Aust Vet J 1959;35:161–5.

346. Ghosh A, Sarkar S, Pramanik AK, et al. Selenium toxicosis in grazing buffaloes and its relationship with soil and plant of West Bengal. Indian J Anim Sci 1993;63:557–60.

347. Raisbeck MF, O'Toole D, Schamber RA, et al. Toxicologic evaluation of a high-selenium hay diet in captive pronghorn antelope (Antilocapra americana). J Wildl Dis 1996;32:9–16.

348. Lawler TL, Taylor JB, Finley JW, et al. Effect of supranutritional and organically bound selenium on performance, carcass characteristics, and selenium distribution in finishing beef steers. J Anim Sci 2004;82:1488–93.

349. Ellis RG, Herdt TH, Stowe HD. Physical, hematologic, biochemical and immunologic effects of supranutritional supplementation with dietary selenium in Holstein cows. Am J Vet Res 1997;58:760–4.

350. Tucker JO. Preliminary report of selenium toxicity in sheep. Proceedings of the American College of Veterinary Toxicologists, Denver, Colorado, August 14, 1960. p. 41–5.

351. Cristaldi LA, McDowell LR, Buergelt CD, et al. Tolerance of inorganic selenium in wether sheep. Small Rumin Res 2005;56:205–13.

352. Davis PA, McDowell LR, Wilkinson NS, et al. Tolerance of inorganic selenium by range-type ewes during gestation and lactation. J Anim Sci 2006;84:660–8.

353. Kuck L. An evaluation of the effects of selenium on elk, mule deer, and moose in southeastern Idaho. Prepared for the Idaho Mining Association Selenium Committee. Belleview (WA): Montgomery, Watson, Harza; 2003.

Commercial and Industrial Chemical Hazards for Ruminants: An Update

Robert H. Poppenga, DVM, PhD[a],*, Stephen B. Hooser, DVM, PhD[b]

KEYWORDS

- Commercial • Industrial • Ruminant • Poisoning • Industrial chemicals
- Agricultural chemicals • Acute toxicosis • Chronic toxicosis

KEY POINTS

- Cattle can be exposed to many industrial or commercial chemicals.
- Exposures can cause acute or chronic illnesses and deaths or result in asymptomatic animals whose products intended for human consumption are contaminated.
- A diagnosis can be difficult in the absence of a known exposure; therefore, a complete case evaluation is critical.

For the purposes of this article, commercial and industrial chemical hazards will be defined as any chemical hazard associated with nondrug commercial products such as fertilizers, pesticides, feed additives, construction materials, or disinfectants used in or near ruminant livestock environments. Industrial chemical hazards also include those associated with the close proximity of a livestock operation to an industrial activity such as manufacturing, mining, or recycling. Emphasis will be placed on those chemical hazards that are not covered elsewhere in this textbook.

The sources of toxicant exposure and the specific toxicants of concern can change over time. For example, used motor oil is not a common source for livestock exposure to lead, as it was removed from gasoline in the mid-1970s. Also, although lead-containing paint on old farm buildings still poses a risk of intoxication for livestock, the gradual elimination of lead-based paint, along with the repainting or replacement of old farm buildings, has decreased the potential for livestock exposure to lead from this source. The use of certain wood preservatives such as chromated copper arsenate (CCA), creosote, and pentachlorophenol has also been curtailed in recent years

[a] California Animal Health and Food Safety Laboratory, University of California, School of Veterinary Medicine, 620 West Health Sciences Drive, Davis, CA 95616, USA; [b] Toxicology Section, Animal Disease Diagnostic Laboratory, Purdue University, College of Veterinary Medicine, 406 South University Street, West Lafayette, IN 47907, USA
* Corresponding author.
E-mail address: rhpoppenga@ucdavis.edu

Vet Clin Food Anim 36 (2020) 621–639
https://doi.org/10.1016/j.cvfa.2020.08.012
0749-0720/20/© 2020 Elsevier Inc. All rights reserved.
vetfood.theclinics.com

due to concern about potential adverse human health and environmental effects, although exposure of ruminants can still occur if precautions are not taken to properly dispose of older treated materials.

Possible exposure pathways include inhalation, ingestion from various media (water and feed), and dermal contact. Some hazardous materials are actively ingested by livestock. For example, some minerals, such as lead and arsenic, are reportedly attractive due to a saltlike taste; this might be especially problematic in salt-deprived animals. The ingestion of potentially hazardous materials can result from pica induced either by nutritional deficiencies or by boredom.[1]

Veterinarians might be asked to investigate producer claims of decreased livestock productivity, illness, and death following alleged exposure to commercial and industrial toxicants. In most cases, losses can be attributed to other disease conditions or management deficiencies, although it is sometimes difficult to convince the producer that they themselves might be primarily responsible for the situation. Investigation of such cases requires an open mind, thoroughness, and early consultation with outside sources of expertise. Patience in such cases is also a virtue, because their resolution can take years and might involve litigation.

It is important to point out that for most chemicals, no withdrawal periods or tolerances have been established for meat or milk products should exposure occur. The detection of any concentration could result in the product being adulterated. In cases of known exposure, it is important to consult with veterinary toxicologists or the Food Animal Residue Avoidance Databank (FARAD; www.farad.org) for advice on recommended withdrawal times or appropriate disposal of contaminated products. Alternatively, State Department of Agricultures or Boards of Animal Health should be contacted for assistance.

The following discussion focuses on several of the more important commercial or industrial toxicants of concern. It is not possible to cover all potential hazards because numerous products or chemicals are used around livestock. However, it is important to keep in mind that documented cases of intoxication can occur from unexpected sources. For example, in one case, 10 of approximately 340 lactating dairy cows suddenly developed depression, diarrhea, and incoordination.[2] A total of 18 cows were noted to have a reddish brown stain on their dorsal hair coats with welts noted below the stains. The welts were believed to have resulted from full-thickness burns of the skin; no other significant lesions were noted in one animal that died and was examined by necropsy. Routine toxicologic testing revealed high liver and kidney concentrations of chromium. Subsequent investigation revealed that a leaking container of 99.7% chromic acid had been stored above the area through which the cows walked to enter the milking parlor. This case is a good illustration of the need for thorough examination of the premises in disease outbreaks of unknown cause.

ENERGY PRODUCTION
Petroleum Exploration and Production

In certain regions of the country, oil exploration and production occur in close proximity to animal agriculture. Oil- and petroleum-related compounds can be introduced into the environment of livestock in several ways including via oil drilling and refining activities, oil or oil product spills, and from many petroleum product uses. Crude oil is a complex mixture of hundreds of different chemical compounds or petroleum hydrocarbons, and there is considerable variation in the specific chemical composition of oils from different sources.[3,4] In addition, livestock are potentially exposed to a variety of chemicals in drilling muds and additives used in oil exploration.[3,4]

Livestock intoxications from crude oil–related activity are well documented. Ruminants will ingest crude oil or petroleum products when thirsty and water is unavailable, when food or water is contaminated, or when adequate feed and salt are not provided.[3,4] The toxicity of crude oil and clinical signs associated with its ingestion can vary depending on its chemical composition. However, the toxicity of crude oil seems to correlate with its content of volatile components such as kerosene, naphtha, and gasoline. Thus, "sweet" crude oil, which is relatively high in volatiles, is more toxic than "sour" crude oil, which is higher in less volatile components such as gas oil, lubricating distillates, residue, and sulfur.[5] The process of "weathering" decreases the volatile and water soluble components in crude oil, which can further alter its toxicity and clinical effects. Acute clinical signs are attributed to the more volatile components of crude oil.

The major components of crude oil have different mechanisms of toxic action. The volatile components of crude oil have anesthetic properties, are more irritating, and are more likely to be aspirated into the lungs.[3] Volatile components may also sensitize the heart to catecholamines. Crude oil destroys rumen microflora and enzymatic activity, which perhaps contributes to the onset of bloat.

The effect of ingesting crude oil ranges from no clinical signs to sudden death. Reported signs include a petroleum smell on the breath, hypo- or hyperesthesia, depression, mydriasis, ptyalism, epiphora, muscle and head tremors, ataxia, tonic-clonic seizures, hypo- or hyperthermia, and gastrointestinal signs such as emesis, bloat, rumen atony, abomasal displacement, and loose to hard feces with a petroleum smell or visible oil present. Aspiration pneumonia is a commonly reported sequel, and hyperpnea, dyspnea, and moist rales can occur.

Necropsy findings include detection of crude oil in the gastrointestinal tract contents and lung lesions consistent with aspiration pneumonia. The portions of the lungs lowermost at the time of aspiration are most severely affected; following petroleum hydrocarbon ingestion this often involves the caudoventral apical and cardiac and cranioventral diaphragmatic and intermediate lobes.

Diagnosis of intoxication is based on a history of possible access to a source, evidence of consumption, and analysis of gastrointestinal contents and tissues. Mixing rumen or stomach contents with warm water will allow oil or petroleum products such as kerosene to rise the surface, making identification easier.[5] Because of the unique chemical nature of each crude oil source, chromatograms or "fingerprints" from gastrointestinal content and tissue analyses can be matched with those from different potential sources of exposure to assist in confirming the origin of exposure.[3]

Drilling fluids are used to facilitate the drilling of oil wells and serve several purposes including clearing the bore hole of debris, lubrication, and maintenance of the drill hole wall.[3,4] Drilling fluids are liquids that contain suspended solids. The liquids used include fresh or salt water, a water-oil emulsion, or oil. The suspended solids are mixtures of clays and barite (barium sulfate). Various chemicals are added to drilling fluids to change their physical and chemical properties depending on specific needs. Additives are numerous and range from pulverized hard nut shells to organophosphate radicals. In addition to containing various chemical components, drilling fluids can be highly acidic or alkaline.[3,4]

Livestock exposure to drilling fluids can result in acid or alkaline burns. The toxicity of drilling fluids and the clinical sequelae following their ingestion can vary due to their chemical complexity. Intoxications have been attributed to caustic soda, arsenic, zinc chromate, and organic acids.[3] The potential for residues will vary depending on the specific chemical composition of the fluids; there is likely to be an increased chance of harmful residues if certain metals are ingested.

Although proximity of livestock to oil or other petroleum hydrocarbon production facilities is a well-recognized hazard, exposure to petroleum products stored on farms can also present hazards. In one case, a herd of 1600 Angus beef cattle were placed in a new paddock that contained diesel fuel tanks surrounded by a low concrete barrier filled with rainwater.[6] Animals reaching for the water broke a fuel line allowing diesel fuel to contaminate the water source. Eighteen animals were found dead with a strong diesel odor; froth exuding from the nose and mouth; and severe, diffuse pulmonary hemorrhage noted on postmortem examination. Affected animals had histologic lesions consistent with inhalation or aspiration pneumonia. The diesel fuel separated into an upper layer within the water source, which was apparently readily consumed by some individuals. In another case, kerosene intoxication of grazing dairy heifers occurred as a result of contamination of a stream serving as a water source for the animals.[7] The contamination was believed to have originated from an upstream airfield. These cases provide good evidence that ruminants (eg, cattle, sheep, and goats) will voluntarily ingest petroleum hydrocarbons such as diesel fuel or kerosene.

Since crude oil and petroleum products contain compounds suspected of being human carcinogens, meat or milk from exposed animals should not be used for human consumption. Also, the possibility exists that rumen microflora metabolize chemicals found in crude oil or petroleum products to form carcinogenic metabolites. A concentration of total petroleum hydrocarbons as crude oil in drinking water for cattle that will not result in a meat concentration exceeding a human health-based safe consumption level has been determined to be 1120 mg/L (1120 ppm),[8] which is greater than a concentration of total petroleum hydrocarbons in water for cattle that would not cause an adverse health effect (355 mg/L, or 355 ppm). Thus, meat concentrations of concern would most likely be associated with clinically affected cattle. Any petroleum hydrocarbon concentration detected in milk would likely result in the milk being considered adulterated.

The tremendous increase in unconventional oil and gas recovery through hydraulic fracking in recent years has generated concern regarding environmental, human, and animal adverse impacts.[9] The large volumes of hydraulic fracturing fluids used contain many chemical additives that are potentially toxic or are degraded to potentially toxic compounds.[10] In one study, 517 different organic and inorganic chemicals were identified with many of the organic chemicals being carcinogens or endocrine disrupters. Although there are regulations in place to mitigate environmental impacts of "fracking," the long-term effects on water quality and public and animal health require additional study.

MINING AND SMELTING
Lead

Lead is a nonessential, highly toxic heavy metal that is ubiquitous in the environment. It is widely used in batteries, solder, pigments, piping, ammunition, paints, ceramics, and caulking.[11] Lead is one of the easiest metals to mine, and smelting requires only moderate temperatures. Most anthropogenic emissions of lead occur as a result of mining, smelting, and refining of lead and other metal ores, vehicle emissions, and industrial emissions resulting from the production, use, recycling, and disposal of lead-containing products.

Currently, the most common sources of exposure of livestock to lead are from ingestion of lead plates found in storage batteries and lead-based paint or grazing of pastures contaminated by lead mine tailings. In some parts of the country, cattle can be exposed to lead from storage batteries through ingestion of soil containing lead melted while burning junk piles. They can also ingest pieces of lead after batteries left in fields are hit by the blades of lawn mowers. The ingestion of lead-contaminated motor oil is much less likely to occur now than in the past, as lead has been removed from gasoline. Accidental releases of lead from industrial and other point sources can result in significant water contamination, and local soil contamination can occur around storage battery reclamation plants, near mines, and around older buildings where leaded paint has been used and is flaking or has been sanded or scraped. One interesting source of exposure of cattle to lead occurred when rice bran became contaminated with zinc ore during its shipment; one sample of finished feed incorporating the contaminated rice bran contained almost 2200 ppm lead (expressed on a dry weight basis).[12] More than 1800 farms and 50,000 dairy cows were exposed.

Clinical signs associated with the diagnosis of lead intoxication are well described and are not discussed here. However, once a diagnosis of lead intoxication is made, it is extremely important to determine the source of exposure and, if people are likely to be exposed, to suggest that they be examined and tested by their physician.

Because of the toxicity of very low levels of lead to people, especially children, there is justifiable concern about residues of lead in animal products intended for human consumption. Some states quarantine animals exposed to lead until tissue concentrations fall below levels of concern as determined by testing of whole blood samples. Lead accumulates in tissues such as liver, kidney, and bone but muscle and milk accumulate little. Thus, in reality, there is little reason to be concerned about significant lead exposure to humans from lead-intoxicated animals as long as their blood lead levels are normal. In addition, although blood lead concentrations increase in periparturient animals previously exposed to lead due to mobilization of lead from bone storage, there is no detectable increase in milk lead concentrations.[13]

Fluoride

Fluorine in a free form is uncommon in nature; it is most commonly found combined with another element such as aluminum, calcium, and potassium, among others, to form a salt or fluoride. Fluorides are widely distributed in the environment. Although the essentiality of fluorine is unclear, it seems to be necessary for normal tooth development, and fluorides are added to most human drinking water to prevent dental caries.[14] Fluorides are emitted from industrial plants processing fluoride-containing raw materials such as bauxite or phosphate rock, are found in rock phosphate used for livestock mineral supplementation or as fertilizer, and can be found in high concentrations in water obtained from deep wells and geothermal springs in certain geographic regions of the United States.[15,16] Fluoride exposure is most often from a localized source, and most intoxications have been associated with ingestion of contaminated forages due to airborne emissions from industrial facilities. Current limits on industrial emissions of fluorides and removal of fluorine during the processing of rock phosphate intended for livestock mineral supplementation minimize exposure from these sources. Although fluorosis is not common, cases or alleged cases involving various animal species still occur occasionally.[17,18] One of us was recently involved in a series of equine and bovine fluorosis cases in Southern California as a result of naturally contaminated well water (Poppenga, personal communication, 2019).

Fluoride toxicosis can be either acute or chronic.[15,19] Acute toxicosis is uncommon and is generally associated with ingestion of sodium fluoroacetate or sodium fluorosilicate (rodenticides), sodium fluoride, or feeds with very high fluoride concentrations.[15] Chronic fluorosis is more common and is a slowly progressive, debilitating disease, primarily of herbivores, that involves teeth and bones. The toxicity of fluoride depends on several factors including amount, duration, and timing of ingestion, form ingested, species, age, nutritional, and health status of the animal exposed, and normal biological variation within a group of animals.[19]

In chronic fluorosis, fluoride damages ameloblasts and odontoblasts necessary for normal tooth development. Matrix laid down by the damaged cells does not mineralize normally. In bone, fluoride disrupts osteoblastic activity, resulting in defective matrix formation and subsequent mineralization.

Acute fluorosis, resulting from the accidental ingestion of very high concentrations of fluoride-containing compounds, is generally manifested as excitement, clonic convulsions, urine and fecal incontinence, stiffness, weakness, salivation, emesis, depression, cardiovascular collapse, and death.[15,19] Chronic fluorosis is insidious and can be confused with other chronic debilitating diseases such as osteoarthritis and degenerative joint disease. In chronic fluorosis, months to years may pass between the beginning of exposure to excessive fluoride and clinical manifestations of toxicosis.

Animals ingesting sufficient fluoride at the time of permanent tooth development exhibit tooth mottling, brown staining or discoloration (chalky white or creamy yellow to brownish black), hypoplasia, pitting and loss of enamel with exposure of dentine, and increased and uneven wear.[15,19] Excessive tooth involvement secondarily results in difficult mastication, decreased feed intake, slow growth or poor performance, and signs associated with dental pain such as lapping of water. Once teeth have calcified and erupted, fluoride ingestion has little to no effect on them. Bone lesions of chronic fluorosis are manifested grossly as hyperostotic, chalky-white lesions. Lesions can occur at any age. Therefore, depending on the age at which exposure occurs, an animal may have both dental and bone lesions or only bone lesions. Bone lesions are generally bilateral and symmetric and appear first on the medial surfaces of the proximal one-third of the metatarsal bones. As the condition progresses, the mandible, metacarpals, and ribs become involved. Bone involvement results in characteristic, intermittent lameness.

Long-term dietary fluoride tolerances have been established for various livestock species based primarily on controlled feeding trials. Dairy or beef heifers are the most sensitive category of livestock and have the lowest tolerance, whereas poultry are the least sensitive.[19] There is controversy with regard to established tolerances. Some investigators believe that current tolerances are too high to protect animal health.[20]

Most soft tissues do not accumulate fluoride, even during high intakes. However, kidney will usually exhibit elevated fluoride concentrations during high intakes due to excretion of fluoride in urine. Milk fluoride concentrations are affected only minimally by dietary intake. Thus, there is unlikely to be significant human health concern about ingestion of meat or milk from affected animals.

Barium

Barium intoxication has been documented in range cattle driven through an old lead, silver, and zinc mine.[21] Clinical signs included protruding tongues, hypersalivation, mild muscle tremors, hypermotility of the rumen, watery mucoid diarrhea, tachycardia, and tachypnea. High concentrations of barium were found in serum, liver, and kidney samples from affected animals; all other metal concentrations were within acceptable ranges. The source of barium was determined to be a claylike material found in the abomasums of dead animals and also in a tailings pond to which the animals had access. The material contained high concentrations of barium. There are several barium salts (eg, acetate, carbonate, chloride, nitrate, and sulfide), all of which are considered to be highly toxic. Only barium sulfate is relatively nontoxic. Barium causes direct stimulation of smooth, striated, and cardiac muscle, and blockage of potassium channels leads to severe hypokalemia. There are no characteristic gross or microscopic lesions noted on postmortem examination and a diagnosis of intoxication relies on tissue and environmental (eg, feed, water, or other potential sources) testing.

Chromium

Chromium is a metallic element that occurs in several oxidation states, with hexavalent chromium being a strong oxidant and carcinogenic. Both trivalent and hexavalent chromium are used for chrome plating, leather tanning, and manufacturing of pigments and wood preservatives. Hexavalent chromium is present in drinking water and public water systems. Drinking water standards for hexavalent chromium, based on human health concerns, have been established at 10 ppb. Chromium is considered to be an essential element, and chromium supplementation has been shown to have beneficial effects on productivity and disease resistance.[22]

In 2004, the Food and Drug Administration (FDA) investigated an outbreak of disease at a dairy farm in Washington State that was characterized by a reddish black substance and blisters on the backs of approximately 20 cattle. Ten cows were sick, with 2 cows dying (http://www.cidrap.umn.edu/news-perspective/2004/06/fda-says-chromium-compound-poisoned-dairy-cows). The reddish brown substance was identified as a hexavalent chromium compound. During the incident investigation, the dairy farmer had to discard approximately 100,000 pounds of milk although subsequent testing of milk samples by the FDA did not identify a public health risk. Initially, this incident was investigated as a potential malicious or terrorist act.

AGRICULTURE
Pesticides

There are a variety of pesticides in the farm environment to which livestock can be exposed, including herbicides, insecticides, fungicides, and fertilizers. Most herbicides with the exception of atrazine and paraquat, herbicides that can cause acute toxicity under the appropriate circumstances, fungicides, and fertilizers have relatively low toxicity and will not be discussed further. However, many organophosphate (OP) and carbamate insecticides, often collectively referred to as cholinesterase-inhibiting insecticides due to their common mode of action, pose a significant hazard because of their extreme toxicity. Most problems occur when farm chemicals are not stored properly or are accidently incorporated into livestock feed.

Chlorinated insecticides

Chlorinated insecticides include DDT, dieldrin, aldrin, endrin, chlordane, toxaphene, endrin, heptachlor, methoxychlor, and lindane. Most are no longer used in developed countries because of their environmental persistence, devastating effects on certain wildlife species, and development of insect resistance. However, they are still used in many underdeveloped countries and are ubiquitous environmental contaminants. There have been few documented cases of livestock intoxication in recent years due to their unavailability, although there are occasional unpublished cases where livestock have been exposed to old containers of insecticide and intoxicate themselves.

Perhaps of more concern than acute intoxication is the possibility of contamination of meat, milk, and eggs with residue levels above current tolerances. Because of the long half-lives of these insecticides, decontamination following exposure can take a prolonged amount of time and cause considerable economic impact.[23]

Organophosphate and carbamate insecticides

OP and carbamate insecticides are still widely used in the farm environment. They can be applied by the dermal route or orally administered to livestock or applied to soils and crops for pest control. Those that are applied to animals directly are much less toxic than those applied to crops. For example, chlorpyrifos, used by dermal application to cattle, has a rat oral LD_{50} of 96 to 270 mg/kg, whereas fonofos, an insecticide incorporated into soil, has a rat oral LD_{50} of 8 to 17.6 mg/kg.[24] Some OP and carbamate insecticide uses or formulations have been banned due to potential for intoxicating animals. For example, granular diazinon and carbofuran use has been curtailed due to concern about wildlife intoxications. Acute intoxication of livestock still occurs, most often through accidental incorporation of the chemicals into feed or misuse on animals.

As the name implies, these insecticides inhibit cholinesterase enzymes. Specifically, when acetylcholinesterase enzyme is inhibited, the neurotransmitter acetylcholine accumulates within synapses, resulting in continued stimulation of muscarinic and nicotinic postsynaptic receptors. The clinical signs and diagnosis of intoxication have been extensively discussed elsewhere.[25]

Unlike the chlorinated insecticides, OPs and carbamates are rapidly metabolized and generally do not cause persistent residues in meat, milk, or eggs. Those intended for use on livestock will have recommended withdrawal times on product labels. When products are used in an extra-label manner or accidental exposures occur, there are no established withdrawal times. Dermal application of OPs to livestock can result in their persistence for extended periods on hair or in skin and subcutaneous fat depots.[26]

It is likely that with the development of safer insecticides such as pyrethroids or insect growth regulators, availability of genetically engineered, insect-resistant crops, and introduction of integrated pest management techniques, the more toxic OP and carbamate insecticides will be used less frequently in the future and therefore pose less of a hazard to livestock and wildlife.

Herbicides

Although herbicides are widely used, most are considered relatively nontoxic when used according to label directions. However, a select few have been associated with adverse effects on cattle or have received widespread media attention due to public health concerns.

Paraquat

Paraquat is a restricted use pesticide that is used on a wide variety of crops. It is considered extremely hazardous due to its availability and high toxicity.[27] Because of its toxicity it has been banned in many countries. It has a special affinity for the lungs and concentrates in alveolar epithelial cells where it causes damage through production of reactive oxygen species.

Intoxication reportedly occurs in 3 phases. Phase one results from the caustic action of paraquat on the gastrointestinal mucosa. Phase 2 occurs due to acute renal and liver damage.

Assuming that the animal survives early phases, phase 3 is manifested by development of pulmonary damage and resulting fibrosis, recovery from which is unlikely.

Paraquat has been used to maliciously poison animals. Occasionally livestock have been accidently poisoned following direct access to paraquat. One of the authors recently confirmed paraquat intoxication of a group of calves exposed to undiluted product in a combined cotton field—ryegrass pasture. The animals were found dead and necropsy lesions were nonspecific in nature. Without the history of paraquat being present in the animals' environment and subsequent detection of paraquat in lung tissue the diagnosis could have been missed. Exposure of animals to sprayed crops or forage is unlikely to cause intoxication due to dilution of the product before spraying and strong adherence of the herbicide to plants and soil.

Atrazine

Atrazine is a triazine herbicide that is very widely used in the United States to control broadleaf and grassy weeds primarily in corn, sorghum, sugar cane, and to a lesser extent on lawns. It is a restricted use pesticide that can only be purchased and used by certified herbicide users. It has low acute toxicity in mammals, with an oral LD50 in rats of 672 to 2310 mg/kg. Current controversy surrounding its use is related to its widespread use and persistence in the environment and the possibility of chronic reproductive or developmental effects in susceptible species.[28]

There have been several cases of atrazine toxicity reported in cattle. In these cases, cattle became ill after consuming formulations of concentrated atrazine meant for field application. In one case, 8 of 73 cattle became acutely ill within hours of eating a formulation containing 76% atrazine. The cattle broke open four, 5-pound bags of wettable powder most of which was consumed or spilled by an unknown number of the animals (probably more than 8, which exhibited clinical signs of toxicity). One cow became recumbent and died within 6 to 8 hrs. At necropsy, this animal had nonspecific edema of the lungs. Six additional cattle exhibited anorexia, hypersalivation, tenesmus, and died within 3 days. Analysis of rumen contents from the cow that died revealed 12,300 ppm of atrazine.[29] In an additional more recent case, forty 16-month-old cows broke into an old barn containing containers of unused herbicides, broke some of those open and ate an unknown amount. Four cows died within 24 hours. Some of the remaining animals exhibited clinical signs including hypersalivation, agitation, and muscle tremors. An additional 6 died between 24 and 48 hours following ingestion for a total of 10 of 40 fatalities. Autolysis precluded necropsy examination; however, analysis of rumen contents and liver revealed the presence of large amounts of atrazine (Hooser, personal communication).

Glyphosate

Glyphosate is one of the most widely used herbicides as a result of widespread use of glyphosate-tolerant crops. It is a nonselective systemic herbicide that is applied directly to plant foliage. There are several formulations of glyphosate, with the isopropylamine salt found in the most widely used product. It is considered to have low toxicity, with the isopropylamine salt having a rodent oral LD$_{50}$ of greater than 5000 mg/kg. The current controversy surrounding the herbicide relates to its potential as a human carcinogen, although evidence for carcinogenicity is debated. Livestock are most likely to be exposed via residues in their feed. The USEPA has established tolerances for glyphosate for various crops and animal products. Based on several reviews, livestock are not exposed to concentrations of glyphosate in their feed that would adversely affect their health.[30,31]

There are no specific antidotes or therapeutic regimens to treat herbicide intoxications. Appropriate oral decontamination procedures such as administration of activated charcoal and a cathartic might be useful if instituted early after exposure. Otherwise, symptomatic and supportive care is provided as needed.

When using pesticides, it is critical that label directions be followed with regard to product dilutions and use conditions (eg, wind speed). In addition, many labels will have recommended reentry times during which livestock should not be placed on treated areas. Calls to veterinary toxicologists often are made when animals are exposed to pesticide spray drifts either directly or through exposure of their pastures. Although theoretically possible to be exposed to toxic amounts of a pesticide via spray drift, documented cases are rare. This is likely due to use of diluted active ingredient and relatively low exposures.

Grain Fumigants

Currently, only 3 fumigants are labeled for use in stored grain: phosphine, chloropicrin, and methyl bromide. Each of these products has special limitations and restrictions governing its use.

Chloropicrin

Chloropicrin is still registered for grain fumigation as well as empty bin fumigation to combat insect infestations. It is especially useful for the control of insects in the sub-floor aeration area of empty bins. Chloropicrin has also been used as a soil fumigant and as a riot control agent and is classified as a lacrimator.[32] Undiluted chloropicrin is severely and immediately irritating to the upper respiratory tract, eyes, and skin on direct contact. In humans, exposure to airborne concentrations of chloropicrin exceeding 0.15 ppm (1 mg/meters cubed) can cause tearing and eye irritation, which is reversible on termination of exposure.[33] Prolonged inhalation exposures at airborne concentrations greater than 1 ppm may cause symptoms of respiratory system damage including irritation of the airways, shortness of breath and/or tightness in chest, and difficulty in breathing. Inhalation exposure to very high levels, even if brief, can lead to pulmonary edema, unconsciousness, and even death. No documented cases of chloropicrin intoxication of livestock were identified.

Methyl bromide (bromomethane)

Methyl bromide is an effective grain fumigant for the control of stored grain insects at all stages of development. It evolves into a gas at temperatures higher than 39° F and has virtually no odor or irritating qualities to indicate its presence. Because methyl bromide is a gas at ambient temperatures, the most significant route of exposure is via inhalation.[34] Methyl bromide can be highly irritating on contact to the mucous membranes of the eyes and airways and to skin. About 1000 human poisoning incidents caused by methyl bromide exposure have been documented, with effects ranging from skin and eye irritation to death. Most fatalities and injuries occurred when methyl bromide was used as a fumigant. The lowest inhalation level found to cause toxicity in humans is 0.14 mg/L in air. The use of methyl bromide has been or is being phased out in many regions, but in the United States there remain some critical use exceptions. No documented cases of methyl bromide intoxication of livestock were identified. However, in 2006 adverse health effects in cattle from ingesting bromide-contaminated forage were alleged after methyl bromide was used as a soil fumigant to control potato cyst nematode in Idaho (https://www.boisestate.edu/agriculturalhealth/methyl-bromide-pcn-eradication/). Complaints included low birth rates, high calf mortality, and skin lesions. The potential adverse health effects from such use remain to be proved.

Phosphides

Phosphine-producing materials (primarily aluminum phosphide) have become the predominant fumigants used for the treatment of bulk-stored grain throughout the world. Zinc phosphide is used primarily as a rodenticide and is likely to be of less concern to livestock. Fumigant phosphides are available in solid formulations of aluminum phosphide or magnesium phosphide. When exposed to heat and moisture the formulations release phosphine, a highly toxic gas. The time required for release of phosphine will vary with temperature, grain moisture, and formulation. Phosphine gas is heavier than air and has a distinct odor that has been described as similar to rotten fish, garlic, or acetylene. Intoxication can occur via ingestion of solid formulations or via inhalation of phosphine gas. Documented instances of livestock intoxication from phosphides have involved the contamination of feed with aluminum phosphide.[35,36]

Intoxication is believed to be, in part, due to inhibition of oxidative phosphorylation.[37] Peroxidation of cell membranes and other cellular oxidative damage might also occur and contribute to disease pathogenesis. An acute oral LD_{50} of zinc phosphide for ruminants is reportedly 60 mg/kg body weight; presumably toxic dosages of the other phosphides would be similar.[37]

Clinical signs in ruminants can include rumen tympany and bloat followed by ataxia, weakness, recumbence, hypoxia, and struggling. Central nervous system stimulation, characterized by hyperesthesia and seizures, might also be noted. Acidosis, circulatory shock, and liver damage are possible as well. Intoxication by phosphine does not cause any characteristic postmortem lesions on gross examination but has been reported to result in hepatic, renal, or myocardial lesions microscopically. A diagnosis relies on a history of exposure and the detection of phosphine in gastrointestinal (GI) contents or tissues such as liver and kidney. Because of the rapid hydrolysis of aluminum or zinc phosphide, along with rapid dissipation of phosphine gas once formed, it is important to place samples in airtight containers and keep them frozen when shipping to a diagnostic laboratory for testing. It is also important to exercise caution when opening and examining samples that may contain zinc phosphide, as phosphine gas can be liberated and clinic/laboratory personnel can be exposed.[38] Also see AVMA Phosphine Product Precautions at https://www.avma.org/phosphine-product-precautions.

There is no specific antidote or therapeutic regimen to treat intoxication. Appropriate decontamination procedures such as administration of activated charcoal and a cathartic might be useful if instituted early after exposure. Otherwise, symptomatic and supportive care is provided as needed.

Fertilizers

Fertilizers are soil amendments used to promote plant growth. The 3 primary macronutrients in fertilizers are nitrogen, phosphorus, and potassium. Secondary macronutrients in fertilizers are calcium, sulfur, and magnesium. Fertilizers can also contain several micronutrients, including boron, chlorine, manganese, iron, zinc, copper, molybdenum, and selenium. Fertilizers are available in various forms including granular and liquid forms. Fertilizers can be broadly categorized as inorganic or organic. Inorganic fertilizers are composed of synthetic chemicals and minerals, whereas organic fertilizers are composed of plant or animal organic matter. Examples of synthetic agricultural fertilizers are granular triple superphosphate, potassium chloride, urea, and anhydrous ammonia.

Toxicosis from phosphorus is rare in food-producing animals.[39] Phosphates are readily excreted via the urine, and animals tolerate a wide range of phosphorus intakes, particularly if diets are appropriately balanced with calcium. Phosphorus intoxication is associated with metabolic disorders of calcium absorption and function (ie, hypocalcemia).[39] The maximum tolerable level of dietary phosphorus for cattle is 0.7% (dry matter basis). Likewise, potassium toxicosis in healthy animals is rare due to the ability of the body to readily excrete the mineral. Potassium toxicosis is associated with potentially fatal arrhythmias. A conservative safe maximum tolerable level for ruminants is 20,000 mg/kg.[40]

Urea intoxication of ruminants is well described in the veterinary literature and is not discussed here. Another common nitrogen source, anhydrous ammonia, is a clear, colorless gas at standard temperature and pressure conditions and has a very characteristic odor. The odor is the strongest safety feature of the product. At a concentration of only 50 parts per million (ppm), it is readily identified. Normally, the odor at that concentration will drive a person away from the area. Anhydrous ammonia combines with moisture in mucous membranes of the mouth, respiratory tract, and cornea to form ammonium hydroxide, a strong alkaline caustic. At concentrations greater than 5000 ppm, people become incapacitated such that escape is impossible and suffocation results.

Intoxication of cattle unable to escape exposure has been documented. In one case, 72 dairy cows and replacement heifers died acutely after they were exposed to anhydrous ammonia leaking from a nurse tank.[41] Most animals died within several minutes of exposure. Animals surviving the acute exposure developed red and peeling skin on the nose and udder, severe damage to the respiratory tract resulting in dyspnea, and copious nasal discharge and corneal opacity. Several animals died up to 4 weeks after exposure due to bacterial pulmonary infections, which were believed to be secondary to extensive epithelial damage to the respiratory tract.

PIT GASES
Hydrogen Sulfide

Hydrogen sulfide (H_2S) is a highly toxic gas that is produced by the anaerobic decomposition of protein or other sulfur-containing organic matter. It is frequently associated with decomposition of manure collected in pits beneath animal confinement facilities. When the manure is agitated before removal by pumping, H_2S gas can be released and forced up above the slatted floor, thus exposing animals laying on the floor above. High concentrations can have a direct paralyzing effect on the respiratory center, resulting in respiratory paralysis and death within a few minutes. In one case, 26 of 158 cattle in confinement pens in an enclosed barn died a few minutes after pit manure agitators were turned on before pumping. Microscopic examination following necropsy revealed massive, diffuse cerebral laminar necrosis with subcortical white matter vacuolation.[42]

There are no specific antidotes for H_2S poisoning. The rapidity with which H_2S kills precludes successful treatment. If possible to do so remotely and safely, the enclosed area should be opened to outside air as quickly as possible to allow for safe dissipation and dilution of the H_2S with uncontaminated air. This must be done with the utmost caution. Many human deaths have occurred resulting from H_2S exposure in manure pits. Therefore, only emergency personnel wearing fully contained breathing apparatus should ever enter one of these areas.

CONSTRUCTION MATERIALS
Chromated Copper Arsenate

CCA is a chemical wood preservative containing chromium, copper, and arsenic. CCA is used in pressure-treated wood to protect wood from rotting due to insects and microbial agents. The USEPA has classified CCA as a restricted use product, for use only by certified pesticide applicators. CCA has been used to pressure treat lumber since the 1940s. Since the 1970s, most of the wood used in outdoor residential settings has been CCA-treated wood. Pressure-treated wood containing CCA is no longer being produced for use in most residential settings. However, CCA-treated wood can still be used by animal production facilities and is not considered to be hazardous when used in structures to house animals. The greatest risk to ruminants occurs following exposure to ashes from burning treated wood, which serves to concentrate arsenic in the ashes.[43] Cattle, especially if salt-deprived, readily ingest the ashes due to a salty taste.

Arsenic intoxication is typically acute with major effects on the GI and cardiovascular systems.[44] Arsenic has a direct damaging effect on capillaries, which leads to transudation of plasma, hemorrhage, and circulatory shock. Signs include severe watery and hemorrhagic diarrhea, severe colic, dehydration, weakness, depression, and a weak pulse. Postmortem lesions include necrosis of epithelial and subepithelial tissues along the GI tract and diffuse inflammation of the liver, kidneys, and other visceral organs. Fatty degeneration and necrosis can be noted in the liver, and tubular damage is noted in the kidneys. Diagnosis of arsenic intoxication requires analysis of whole blood or urine sample antemortem or liver and kidney samples post mortem. Analysis of potential sources of exposure is recommended as well.

Treatment of affected animals is largely symptomatic and supportive with particular attention paid to fluid replacement and cardiovascular support. Although dimercaprol is used to chelate arsenic, its efficacy in large animals when used alone is questionable. The water soluble analogue of dimercaprol, succimer, is less toxic and more effective, but its use in ruminants is cost prohibitive. ᴅ-penicillamine is also an arsenic chelator that has been used successfully in people.

Pentachlorophenol

The use of pentachlorophenol as a wood preservative was canceled in 1986. Because of its toxicity, agricultural and residential use is prohibited. Pentachlorophenol can be absorbed through the skin and lungs and is quite irritating to skin and mucous membranes. Animals fed in troughs made from lumber treated with pentachlorophenol salivate and have irritated oral mucosa.[45] Inhalation of pentachlorophenol from enclosed animal holding areas has caused illness and death. Acutely toxic doses are reported to range from 27 to 350 mg/kg.[45]

Once absorbed, pentachlorophenol uncouples oxidative phosphorylation. Clinical signs of intoxication include nervousness, tachycardia, tachypnea, weakness, muscle tremors, fever, and convulsions, followed by death. Chronic exposure results in fatty liver, nephrosis, and weight loss. A diagnosis of intoxication relies on a history of exposure, occurrence of compatible clinical signs, and, in some cases, identification of pentachlorophenol in source materials or biological samples.

There is no specific treatment of pentachlorophenol intoxication. Termination of exposure, dermal decontamination, administration of activated charcoal, and symptomatic and supportive care are recommended. Possible violative meat and milk residues can occur with exposure.

Creosote

The distillation of coal tar results in the production of cresols (phenolic compounds), crude creosote (cresols, heavy oils, and anthracene), and pitch. Cresols can be used as disinfectants, whereas creosote has been used as a wood preservative. Exposure of ruminants to creosote is most often due to ingestion of a product or treated material in contrast to exposure via food or water contamination. Phenol is the most toxic chemical in coal tar products with an approximate acute oral LD_{50} for most species of 0.5 g/kg. The lethal dose of creosote in calves is reported to be 4 g/kg.[46]

There is no specific treatment of phenol intoxication. Appropriate decontamination and symptomatic and supportive care are recommended.

Irrigation

In many areas of the western United States, irrigation wastewater can accumulate in confined shallow aquifers. If not drained away, the accumulated wastewater increases to levels that adversely affect crop production. Systems for the drainage and disposal of the wastewater have been constructed and in many areas the water is discharged either directly into surface aquatic systems or to evaporation ponds. Irrigation drainage water can contain several chemicals that are either applied to crops or leached from native soils. The most troublesome leachate in many irrigated areas is selenium. The concentration of selenium in evaporation ponds in the San Joaquin valley in southern California and its subsequent bioaccumulation in aquatic food chains resulted in substantial aquatic bird mortality in the early 1980s.[47] To prevent further wildlife mortality, the ponds were filled and the area converted into grassland habitat.[48] Although there has been no documented livestock morbidity or mortality from ingestion of selenium from irrigation sources, the possibility exists that animals could be chronically exposed to elevated selenium in water or pasture plants resulting in chronic selenosis.

POLYCHLORINATED BIPHENYLS, POLYBROMINATED BIPHENYLS, DIOXINS, AND FURANS

Polychlorinated biphenyls (PCBs), polybrominated biphenyls (PBBs), dioxins, and furans belong to a group of related chemical compounds widely distributed in the environment. They are not single compounds but each group includes several chemically similar compounds or "congeners." For example, there are 209 different congeners of PCBs. Not all of the congeners within each group are toxic; only 30 of the 209 PCBs are considered toxic.

PCBs and PBBs were used in many commercial applications due to their inertness; they resist acids and alkalis, they have low dielectric constants, and are thermally stable. PCBs were used as heat exchange and hydraulic fluids, lubricants, dielectric fluids in transformers and capacitors, and as plasticizers in applications where flame resistance was important. PCBs and PBBs are no longer manufactured in the United States although they continue to be manufactured and used in other countries. Unfortunately, because of their environmental persistence and wide atmospheric distribution, PCBs are now ubiquitous and found throughout the world. PCBs serve as a good example of a class of compound that can still be of concern in the United States due to their widespread distribution even though they are no longer manufactured in this country.

Widespread exposure of food animals to PBBs occurred in the mid-1970s as a result of contamination of feed with a fire retardant when it was confused with a similarly packaged feed supplement, magnesium oxide.[49] Dairy cattle, pigs, sheep, and chickens were exposed. More recently, Belgian livestock were exposed to PCBs and dioxins as a result of contaminated fat being incorporated into livestock feed. In the United States, poultry and catfish were found to be contaminated with dioxins; the ultimate source was determined to be ball clay used as an anticaking agent for soybean meal.[40]

In contrast to PCBs and PBBs, dioxins and furans have no commercial use. The most infamous of these compounds is 2,3,7,8-tetrachlorodibenzodioxin (TCDD). TCDD is one of the most toxic compounds yet encountered.[50] Dioxins and furans have been released into the environment primarily as contaminants of chemical and combustion processes. With the exception of the dioxin-contaminated clay from a site in Mississippi, they are not known to occur naturally.

The mechanisms of toxic action of these compounds have not been clearly established, but clinical affects are multiple. Toxic congeners bind a cytosolic receptor called the Ah receptor, which in turn affects gene regulation.[50] The Ah receptor is found in a variety of species and is expressed in multiple tissues. Ah receptor binding and subsequent induction of aryl hydrocarbon hydroxylase activity and other P450-dependent enzymes affect the metabolism of steroids and other hormones. Toxic effects can be manifested in several organ systems, including the immune, reproductive, and nervous systems. These compounds are also teratogenic and have tumor-promoting effects.

These chemicals are either not considered very toxic (PCBs and PBBs) or are quite toxic but present at extremely low concentrations (TCDD). Thus, acute intoxications are unusual. However, animal and human health effects following chronic exposure are well documented. Dairy cattle exposed to PBBs in Michigan exhibited many nonspecific clinical signs such as unthriftiness, decreased milk production, abscesses, abnormal hoof growth, and decreased appetite.[49] A wasting syndrome is well described in several animal species.[49,50] In Missouri, horses unintentionally exposed to TCDD-contaminated oil exhibited a progressive deterioration in health, including anorexia, listlessness, loss of body weight and emaciation, dermatitis, weakness, an unsteady gait, and chronic cough.[51] There is a case report of dioxin intoxication of horses following chronic exposure to pentachlorophenol-contaminated wood shavings.[52]

Residues are a major concern with these chemicals. They are extremely lipophilic and resistant to metabolic transformation. Once ingested, they have long half-lives; the estimated half-life of PBBs in human serum is 10.8 years.[49] Because of their lipophilicity, they are found in muscle and milk fat and egg yolks. Tolerances have been established for PCBs in foods and feed ranging from 0.2 ppm for finished feed for food-producing animals and human infant and junior foods to 10 ppm for food-packaging paper material.[49] No safe level, tolerance, or action level has been established for dioxins or furans in animal feed, feed components, or food, although an interim level of concern for TCDD of 1 part per trillion was established for catfish, eggs, and poultry exposed to dioxin-contaminated ball clay. The extremely low tolerance set for TCDD compared with that for PCBs reflects its much greater toxicity.

PERFLUORINATED COMPOUNDS (PERFLUOROOCTANOIC ACID AND PERFLUOROOCTANE SULFONATE)

Perfluorooctanoic acid and perfluorooctane sulfonate are part of a larger group of chemicals called per- and polyfluoroalkyl substances (PFAS). These are highly fluorinated aliphatic molecules that have been released into the environment via industrial manufacturing and use and disposal of PFAS-containing products. They are widely distributed in soil, air, and groundwater at sites throughout the United States. The toxicity, mobility, and bioaccumulation potential of these chemicals is an environmental, human, and animal health concern. Human health concerns include developmental, reproductive, immunologic, and carcinogenic effects (https://www.atsdr.cdc. gov/pfas/health-effects.html). As a result, production has been phased out in the United States. However, their environmental persistence and bioaccumulation potential continues to pose risks to health. Although specific health effects have not been reported in cattle, there is the potential for contamination of meat and milk products derived from exposed animals.[53] Fortunately, these compounds have not yet been shown to occur in meat or milk above regulatory exposure limits.[54,55]

MISCELLANEOUS HAZARDS
Ethylene Glycol (or Solvents)

There is one case report of ethylene glycol (EG) intoxication of a calf.[56] Oxalate crystalluria is often found in ruminant urine or kidney tissue due to exposure to soluble oxalate-containing plants such as *Sarcobatus vermiculatus* (greasewood), *Halogeton glomeratus* (halogeton), *Rumex* spp. (dock), *Amaranthus* spp. (pigweed), *Oxalis* spp., among others.[57] Because both EG and soluble oxalate-containing plants might be present in a ruminant environment, they should be considered in cases of acute renal failure. Clinical signs in cattle include dyspnea, incoordination, paraparesis, recumbence, and hypocalcemia. A toxic dose for adult cattle and nonruminating calves is reported to be 5 to 10 mL/kg and 2 mL/kg body weight, respectively.[56]

Tests are readily available for the identification of EG in antemortem or postmortem samples to help differentiate between the 2, although the rapid metabolism of EG might result in failure to detect the toxicant in biological samples. Laboratory indicators of EG poisoning include hypocalcemia, acidosis, elevated EG blood levels, positive urine oxalate crystals, and renal oxalosis detected by histopathology.

If a diagnosis of ethylene glycol exposure or intoxication is made soon after ingestion, ethanol or fomepizole is antidotal, although the use of fomepizole is most likely cost prohibitive in food production animals. Additional treatment involves correction of acid-base imbalances and attempting to maintain urine flow; other therapeutic interventions are symptomatic and supportive.

DISCLOSURE

The authors have nothing to disclose.

REFERENCES

1. Radostits OM, Gay CC, Hinchcliff KW, et al. Disturbances of appetite, food intake and nutritional status. In: Radostits OM, Gay CC, Hinchcliff KW, editors. Veterinary medicine: a textbook of the diseases of cattle, horses, sheep, pigs and goats. 10th edition. Edinburgh (Scotland): Saunders Elsevier; 2007. p. 112–4.
2. Talcott PA, Haldorson GJ, Sathre P. Chromium poisoning in a group of dairy cows. In: 48th Annual Conference Proceedings of the American Association of Veterinary Laboratory Diagnosticians. Hershey; Hershey, PA, November 3-9, 2005, p. 45.
3. Edwards WC, Coppock RW, Zinn LL. Toxicoses related to the petroleum industry. Vet Hum Toxicol 1979;21:328–37.
4. Edwards WC. Toxicology of oil field wastes: hazards to livestock associated with the petroleum industry. Vet Clin North Am Food Anim Pract 1989;5:363–74.
5. Osweiler GD, Carson TL, Buck WB, et al. Crude oils, fuel oils and kerosene. In: Clinical and diagnostic veterinary toxicology. Dubuque (IA): Kendall-Hunt; 1985. p. 177–8.
6. Gailbreath KL, Talcott PA, Baszler TV. Fibrinosuppurative pneumonitis associated with diesel ingestion in a herd of beef cattle. In: 52nd Annual Conference Proceedings of the American Association of Veterinary Laboratory Diagnosticians. San Diego, CA, October 7-14, 2009, p. 60.
7. Barber DML, Cousin DAH, Seawright D. An episode of kerosene poisoning in dairy heifers. Vet Rec 1987;120:462.
8. Ryer-Powder J, Scofield R, Lapierre A, et al. Determination of safe levels of total petroleum hydrocarbons as crude oil in cattle's drinking water and in meat from

cattle. In: Proceedings of the Petroleum Hydrocarbons and Organic Chemicals in Ground Water: Prevention, Detection and Remediation Conference. Houston, TX, November 13-15, 1996, pp. 99–109.

9. Bamberger M, Oswald RE. Long-term impacts of unconventional drilling operations on human and animal health. J Environ Sci Health A 2015;50:447–59.

10. Chen H, Carter KE. Characterization of the chemicals used in hydraulic fracturing fluids for wells located in the Marcellus shale play. J Environ Manage 2000;200: 312–24.

11. Keogh JP, Boyer LV. Lead. In: Sullivan JB, Kreiger GR, editors. Clinical environmental health and toxic exposures. Baltimore (MD): Lppincott, Williams and Wilkins; 2001. p. 879–88.

12. Allen WM. Environmental accidents: the assessment of the significance of an environmental accident due to the feeding of lead-contaminated feedstuffs to several hundred cattle farms. Bov Pract (Stillwater) 1999;33:76–9.

13. Galey FD, Slenning BD, Anderson ML, et al. Lead concentrations in blood and milk from periparturient diary heifers seven months after an episode of acute lead toxicosis. J Vet Diagn Invest 1990;2:222–6.

14. National Academy of Sciences. Fluorine. In: Mineral tolerance of domestic animals. Washington, DC: National Academy of Sciences; 2005. p. 154–81.

15. Osweiler GD, Carson TL, Buck WB, et al. Fluoride. In: Clinical and diagnostic veterinary toxicology. Dubuque (IA): Kendall-Hunt; 1985. p. 183–8.

16. Shupe JL, Olson AE, Peterson HB, et al. Fluoride toxicosis in wild ungulates. J Am Vet Med Assoc 1984;185:1295–300.

17. Botha CJ, Naude TW, Minnaar PP, et al. Two outbreaks of fluorosis in cattle and sheep. J S Afr Vet Assoc 1993;64:165–8.

18. Jubb TF, Annand TE, Main DC, et al. Phosphorus supplements and fluorosis in cattle – a northern Australian experience. Aust Vet 1993;70:379–83.

19. Shupe JL. Clinicopathologic features of fluoride toxicosis in cattle. J Anim Sci 1980;51:746–58.

20. Crissman JW, Maylin GA, Krook L. New York State and U.S. federal fluoride pollution standards do not protect cattle health. Cornell Vet 1980;70:183–92.

21. Richards T, Erickson DL, Talcott PA, et al. Two Cases of Barium Poisoning in Cattle. In: 49th Annual Conference Proceedings of the American Association of Veterinary Laboratory Diagnosticians. Minneapolis, MN, October 12-18, 2006, p. 155.

22. National Academy of Sciences. Chromium. In: Mineral tolerance of domestic animals. Washington, DC: National Academy of Sciences; 2005. p. 115.

23. Raisbeck MF, Kendall JD, Rottinghaus GE. Organochlorine insecticide problems in livestock. Vet Clin North Am Food Anim Pract 1989;5:391–410.

24. Meister RT. Crop protection handbook. Willoughby (OH): Meister Publishing; 2005. p. 85, 204.

25. Meerdink GL. Organophosphorous and carbamate insecticide poisoning in large animals. Vet Clin North Am Food Anim Pract 1989;5:375–89.

26. Henny CJ, Blus LJ, Kolbe EJ, et al. Organophosphate insecticide (famphur) topically applied to cattle kills magpies and hawks. J Wildl Manage 1985;49:648–58.

27. Oehme F, Pickrell JA. Dipyridyl herbicides. In: Plumlee KH, editor. Clinical veterinary toxicology. St Louis (MO): Mosby; 2005. p. 146–8.

28. Agency for Toxic Substances and Disease Registry (ATSDR). Toxicological Profile for atrazine. Atlanta (GA): U.S. Department of Health and Human Services, Public Health Service; 2003.

29. Jowett PLH, Nicholson SS, Gamble GA. Tissue levels of atrazine in a case of bovine poisoning. Vet Hum Toxicol 1986;29:539–40.

30. European Food Safety Authority. Evaluation of the impact of glyphosate and its residues in feed on animal health. 2018. Available at: https://efsa.onlinelibrary.wiley.com/doi/epdf/10.2903/j.efsa.2018.5283. Accessed January 15, 2019.

31. Vicini JL, Reeves WR, Swarthout JT, et al. Glyphosate in livestock feed: feed residues and animal health. J Anim Sci 2019;97:4509–18.

32. Suchard JR. Chemical Weapons. In: Flomenbaum NE, Howland MA, Goldfrank LR, et al, editors. Goldfrank's toxicologic emergencies. 8th edition. New York: McGraw-Hill; 2006. p. 1775–91.

33. EXTOXNET. Available at: http://extoxnet.orst.edu/pips/chloropi.htm. Accessed December 15, 2010.

34. EXTOXNET. Available at: http://extoxnet.orst.edu/pips/methylbr.htm. Accessed December 15, 2010.

35. Easterwood L, Chaffin MK, Marsh PS, et al. Phosphine intoxication following oral exposure of horses to aluminum phosphide-treated feed. J Am Vet Med Assoc 2010;236:446–50.

36. Morgan S, Niles GA, Edwards WC. Case report: phosphine gas detected in the rumen content of dead calves. Bov Pract (Stillwater) 2000;34:127.

37. Albretson JC. Zinc phosphide. In: Plumlee KH, editor. Clinical veterinary toxicology. St Louis (MO): Mosby; 2004. p. 456–8.

38. Occupational Phosphine Gas Poisoning at Veterinary Hospitals from Dogs that Ingested Zinc Phosphide — Michigan, Iowa, and Washington, 2006–2011. MMWR Morb Mortal Wkly Rep 2012;61(16):286–8.

39. National Academy of Sciences. Phosphorus. In: Mineral tolerance of domestic animals. Washington, DC: National Academy of Sciences; 2005. p. 290.

40. National Academy of Sciences. Potassium. In: Mineral tolerance of domestic animals. Washington, DC: National Academy of Sciences; 2005. p. 306.

41. Carson TL, Till DJ, Quinn WJ, et al. Anhydrous ammonia fertilizer poisoning in cattle: peracute death loss and sequelae. In: 39th Annual Conference Proceedings of the American Association of Veterinary Laboratory Diagnosticians. Little Rock, AR, October 12-18, 1996, p. 66.

42. Hooser SB, Van Alstine W, Kiupel M, et al. Acute pit gas (hydrogen sulfide) poisoning in confinement cattle. J Vet Diagn Invest 2000;12:272–5.

43. Hullinger G, Sangster L, Colvin B, et al. Bovine arsenic toxicosis from ingestion of ashed copper-chrome-arsenate treated lumber. Vet Hum Toxicol 1998;40:147–8.

44. Merck Veterinary Manual. Arsenic. In: Kahn CM, editor. Merck veterinary manual. 9th edition. Whitehouse Station (NJ): Merck & Co; 2005. p. 2346–8.

45. Merck Veterinary Manual. Pentachlorophenol poisoning. In: Kahn CM, editor. Merck veterinary manual. 9th edition. Whitehouse Station (NJ): Merck & Co; 2005. p. 2429.

46. Merck Veterinary Manual. Coal-tar poisoning. In: Kahn CM, editor. Merck veterinary manual. 9th edition. Whitehouse Station (NJ): Merck & Co; 2005. p. 2352–3.

47. Ohlendorf HM. Bioaccumulation and effects of selenium in wildlife. In: Selenium in agriculture and the environment. Madison (WI): Soil Science Society Special Publication No. 23; 1989. p. 133–77.

48. Clemings R. Of drainage and baby ducks. In: Mirage: the false promise of desert agriculture. San Francisco: Sierra Club Books; 1996. p. 51.

49. Headrick ML, Hollinger K, Lovell RA, et al. PBBs, PCBs, and dioxins in food animals, their public health implications. Vet Clin North Am Food Anim Pract 1999; 15:109–32.

50. Koss G, Wolfle D. Dioxin and dioxin-like polychlorinated hydrocarbons and biphenyls. In: Marquardt H, Schafer SG, McClellan R, et al, editors. Toxicology. San Diego (CA): Academic Press; 1999. p. 699–728.
51. Case AA, Coffman JR. Waste oil: toxic for horses. Vet Clin North Am 1973;3: 273–7.
52. Kerkvliet NI, Wagner SL, Schmotzer WB, et al. Dioxin intoxication from chronic exposure to pentachlorophenol-contaminated wood shavings. J Am Vet Med Assoc 1992;201:296–302.
53. Fernandes AR, Lake IR, Dowding A, et al. The potential of recycled materials used in agriculture to contaminate food through uptake by livestock. Sci Total Environ 2019;667:359–70.
54. Perez F, Llorca M, Kock-Schulmeyer M, et al. Assessment of perfluoroalkyl substances in food items at global scale. Environ Res 2014;135:181–9.
55. Xing Z, Lu J, Liu Z, et al. Occurrence of perfluorooctanoic acid and perfluorooctane sulfonate in milk and yogurt and their risk assessment. Int J Environ Res Public Health 2016;13:1037.
56. Crowell WA, Whitlock RH, Stout RC, et al. Ethylene glycol toxicosis in cattle. Cornell Vet 1979;69:272–9.
57. Knight AP, Walter RG. Plants causing kidney failure. In: Knight AP, Walter RG, editors. A guide to plant poisoning of animals in North America. Jackson (WY): Teton New Media; 2001. p. 263–77.

Ionophore Use and Toxicosis in Cattle

Steve Ensley, DVM, PhD

KEYWORDS

- Ionophores • Myocardial and skeletal muscle damage • Delayed toxicosis in cattle

KEY POINTS

- Ionophores are a commonly used feed additive used for growth promotion in animals.
- Secondary use of some ionophores is for coccidia control.
- The safety margin for ionophores is narrow for most species.
- There can be a delay of several days from the time a dose that causes toxicosis is consumed and when adverse clinical signs or death will occur.
- Because of the delay from time of ingestion to time of adverse clinical signs it is difficult to have access to the feed that caused the toxicosis. Analyzing the feed present at the time of adverse clinical signs will not provide the concentration of the ionophore that was over-fed several days prior.

The ionophores were first identified in 1951 but not used widely in the cattle industry until 1975.[1] These additives were originally developed to improve feed efficiency in feedlot cattle. A second label was added to the ionophore, Rumensin, for use in feedlot cattle for the prevention of coccidiosis. The ionophores are a commonly used feed additive in many species. Ionophores are produced by various species of Streptomyces.[2] When ionophores are used at the label dose there are usually no adverse effects. Negative impacts on health usually occur when there is a feed mis-mix and a mis-dosing. Ionophores are used in other species so there can be inadvertent use of one or more ionophores intended for other species in the diet that is causing the overdose. When one or more ionophores are used in the same diet, there can be an additive effect of the ionophores and cause a toxicosis. There are also drugs that when used in combination with an ionophore will interfere with metabolism of the ionophore and potentiate a toxicosis. This could cause a toxic concentration of the ionophores in the targeted animal even when the correct concentration of an ionophore is being used in the diet. Cattle are more tolerant to a toxic concentration of an ionophore when compared with other species.[3,4]

Anatomy & Physiology, Kansas State University, 1800 Denison Avenue, Mosier P217, Manhattan, KS 66506, USA
E-mail address: sensley01@ksu.edu

Vet Clin Food Anim 36 (2020) 641–652
https://doi.org/10.1016/j.cvfa.2020.07.001
0749-0720/20/© 2020 Elsevier Inc. All rights reserved.

USEFUL PROPERTIES OF IONOPHORES

The physiologic activity of ionophores is to move monovalent cations such as calcium and sodium across the cell wall in exchange for potassium and hydrogen ions. For this reason, this class of drugs is called ionophores.[5] Ionophores will also cause a shift in the rumen flora to be able to increase feed efficiency in ruminants.[6–8] Gram-positive organisms in the rumen are inhibited allowing gram-negative organisms to predominate.[9] The ionophores can also decrease bloat and ruminal acidosis. Lactic acid production is decreased even when metabolism is increased. The diet composition can be involved with the changes observed in metabolism of ionophores.

The increase in rate of gain and feed efficiency when ionophores are used is due to the changes in volatile fatty acids in the rumen. Propionic acid production is increased over butyric and acetic acids without changing the total volatile fatty acid production.[8–16] Ammonia digestion and rumen protein degradation are affected by ionophores by decreasing the amount of bacterial ammonia fixation. Nitrogen retention and absorption can be increased by ionophores. Ruminal methane production is decreased by ionophores.

Another useful property of ionophores is that they have antimycoplasma activity.[17–19] The ionophores will prevent 3-methylindole toxicosis, which is associated with atypical interstitial pneumonia.[20–22] Monensin and lasalocid have been shown to significantly decrease the rate of conversion of tryptophan to 3-methylindole, thus preventing clinical signs of atypical interstitial pneumonia.

BIOLOGICAL ACTIVITY

Ionophores move ions or compounds across biological membranes and down concentration gradients. Ionophores are known to move cations but they also have been shown to carry biogenic amines.[23] For transport across biological membranes, there must be a concentration gradient so that translocation occurs from higher concentration to a lower concentration. When ions move across a cell wall, this causes a series of events that tries to reestablish the ion gradients. This can result in cell damage and death. The cation translocating capability of the ionophores causes many changes that may influence ruminants as far as growth and feed efficiency. There are many factors that are believed to be involved with improved gain and efficiency. The effects of ionophores in production efficiency are reviewed.[24]

One mechanism by which ionophores alter ruminant metabolism is by altering the ruminal flora. Many studies demonstrate changes in bacterial populations that occur in the rumen.[9,10,12,13] Protozoal numbers are changes by ionophores, and ruminal anaerobic fungi are suppressed by ionophores.[6,14] Ionophores can also change the metabolism of the rumen flora by producing more efficient energy sources for ruminants. These changes in ruminal microbial flora have benefits such as decreasing ruminal acidosis, decreasing bloat, enhancing feed efficiency, and altering microbial metabolism of exogenous compounds. Ionophore effects on systemic metabolism suggest that increased growth and feed efficiency could be influenced by factors in addition to the ruminal effect. Studies have shown that increased weight gain and feed efficiency cannot be completely explained by alterations in ruminal fermentation or site and extent of digestion.[25] Changes in circulating hormones and metabolic products have occasionally been seen but have not been consistently identified.[26,27] Changes in tissue metabolic products have been reported.[7] Some of these changes may be related to induction or inhibition of specific metabolic pathways necessary for the metabolism of the ionophore. Ionophore effects at the cellular level have been associated with changes in primary ion concentrations such as gradient changes across cell membranes and release of intracellular ions. These changes can change the intracellular pH causing damage to the cell or cellular organelles. The systemic toxicity of ionophores is related to change in function of or damage to cellular organelles. Dilation and vacuolization of the golgi apparatus within cardiac muscle, smooth muscle, epithelial cells, and plasma cells also have been reported. Ultrastructural changes consisting of partial or complete swelling and disruption of cellular mitochondria have been reported in several species.[28] Additional cellular effects of ionophores involve inhibition of enzymatic activities.[29]

EFFECTS OF RUMEN METABOLISM AND GROWTH PROMOTION

The ionophores were first introduced as growth promotants for feeder cattle in 1973 in response to evidence of improved weight gain and feed efficiency. Many reviews of ionophore activities in animals have been published.[30] The most prominent effects of ionophores are increased feed efficiency, increased rate of weight gain, and decreased dry matter intake, although some studies have found no increase in weight gain or no increase in feed efficiency.[30] Diet composition has a primary role in the effects observed with ionophore use. Ionophore-induced changes in feed digestibility vary wildly. Monensin in a com silage diet of fistulated steers did not consistently affect dry matter digestibility, fiber digestibility, rate of disappearance of cellulose, rate of ruminal liquid disappearance, or rate of ruminal particulate change.[31] Digesta movement, location of digestion, digestibility, and performance with lasalocid supplementation were found to depend on the type and quality of diets fed to cows and feeders. Adult lactating Holstein cows receiving lasalocid in their concentrate ration had a linear increase in apparent digestibility of dietary crude protein and no change in dietary dry matter digestibility.[32]

VOLATILE FATTY ACIDS

Increased rate of gain and improved feed efficiency is associated with a change in fatty acid production. Laidlomycin, monensin, narasin, salinomycin, and lasalocid change the molar ratio of volatile fatty acids (VFAs) produced by ruminal bacteria so that propionic acid production is increased with a decrease of butyric and acetic acids, without altering total VFA production in cattle or altering fermentation. Studies also show the difference that the time of sample collection postfeeding will have. The time of sampling has a marked difference in the molar ratios of all of the VFAs analyzed. In other studies involving salinomycin, monensin, and lasalocid the ruminal VFA molar ratios are not altered significantly, even though increases in feed efficiency and rate of weight gain were seen in cannulated steers and heifers.[10,16,33,34] In other studies variable results were obtained.[35] The fat content of the diet can increase, decrease, or prevent any VFA molar ratio changes induced by ionophores, and dietary components can alter the degree of response to ionophores.[10]

NITROGEN

Ionophores also affect ruminal protein and ammonia digestion. Ionophores decrease the amount of bacterial ammonia fixation but salinomycin, lasalocid, and a monensin-tylosin combination do not affect rumen ammonia, nitrogen absorption, or nitrogen retention.[26,34] Ruminal ammonia nitrogen increases with increasing salinomycin concentrations in pastured steers and with increasing lasalocid concentration in pastured steers and heifers.[10,36] No change in rumen ammonia was caused by feeding lasalocid or monensin to cannulated cows fed a bloat-inducing alfalfa diet or calves fed milk and starter feeds.[31] No changes were found in steers fed salinomycin or lasalocid with concentrate diets or with laidlomycin propionate in cannulated steers on concentrate diets.[37,38] In cows the effect of lasalocid on protein and diet digestibility depended on the type and quality of the diet.[39] Lasalocid increased feed efficiency in cattle by increasing nitrogen digestibility. Heifers fed lasalocid in a low, undegradable protein diet had increased weight gain and feed efficiency, but when fed in a high, undegradable protein diet, it decreased weight gain and feed efficiency.[40] The effects on nitrogen metabolism vary widely among studies and are likely related to the specific components of the diet.

OTHER BENEFICIAL EFFECTS

Lactic acidosis in feed lot ruminants is at least partially controlled by ionophore effects on the ruminal flora, such that lactic acid production is decreased and its metabolism is increased. Both narasin and salinomycin exhibit an inhibitory effect on rumen lactic acid–producing bacteria and butyric acid–producing bacteria by a bacteriostatic action.[9] Lactic acid–producing bacteria in culture were inhibited by monensin or lasalocid.[12,31,41] Lactic acid–fermenting ruminal bacteria tended to be resistant to narasin, monensin, lasalocid, and salinomycin.[9,12,31,41] Ruminal methane production is decreased by treatment with narasin, monensin, salinomycin, lasalocid, nigericin, and grisorixin.[42,43] In steers medicated with monensin or lasalocid, increased dietary sodium further decreased ruminal methane production. Addition of potassium in the diet decreased methane production with monensin but increased methane production with lasalocid.[44] Steers fed ionophores had a gradual increase in methane production with longer treatment times indicating a possible adaptation of the methanogenic microflora. This also was shown with cultured rumen fluid from naive cattle having decreased gas production but not with cultures from ionophore-adapted cattle.[45] Ionophores also may enhance feed efficiency by decreasing energy loss and bloat. Ionophores have not been approved for use as anticoccidials in cattle, but they have been shown to be effective in coccidia control. Decreased oocyst shedding and clinical signs of coccidiosis were reported in cattle treated with monensin, salinomycin, and lasalocid.[46–49] Coccidial oocyst shedding reoccurs and can increase on discontinuation of the treatment. Calves can have coccidial infection and clinical signs while on ionophore treatment.[50] Decreased clinical and subclinical coccidia, which may occur in feed lot conditions, could account for some of the improvement in weight gain and performance of ruminants. Although better control agents are available, it has been shown that the ionophores have antimycoplasmal activity in vitro and in vivo. Laidlomycin, monensin, and lasalocid were effective at inhibiting the growth of several Mycoplasma sp.[17–19] Ionophores possess antimycoplasmal activity and likely decrease clinical disease. Another benefit of ionophore use is the prevention of 3-methylindole toxicosis. Monensin and lasalocid were shown to significantly decrease the rate of conversion of tryptophan to 3-methylindole or prevent clinical signs.[22,51] Removal of ionophore treatment resulted in rapid return of the faster conversion rate of 3-methylindole. Effects of ionophores on body composition have been evaluated. In heifers fed lasalocid, there were increases in muscle depth and body fat.[40] Carcass fat thickness was lower and cutability was higher in steers fed lasalocid, salinomycin, or monensin.

IONOPHORE TOXICOSIS IN CATTLE

Ionophore toxicosis occurs in all species, including cattle. The ionophores are a common additive in cattle feed because of the many positive changes that ionophores can induce. The inclusion rate in cattle diets is widespread. E. L. Potter published a paper titled "Monensin toxicity in cattle" in 1982 that is a very good review of monensin toxicosis specifically and ionophore toxicity in cattle in general. For monensin, an LD50, LD10, and LD1 were published as 26.4, 11.2, and 5.5 mg/kg of body weight. The LD50 for monensin in cattle is accepted as 26.4 mg/kg bd wt. In the Potter paper they also mention when cattle were gavaged daily for 7 days with monensin that death loss occurred at 7.6 mg/kg bd wt of monensin. The LD50 for lasalocid in cattle is 50 mg/kg bd wt.[52–54]

In general, cattle are not as susceptible to the adverse effects of ionophores as are other species. Several factors could account for this decreased susceptibility to ionophore toxicosis, including ruminal breakdown, decreased absorption, increased first pass effect by the liver, or differences in cell wall structure, resulting in reduced cellular uptake. The toxic effects of polyether ionophores in feed lot cattle and monensin toxicity or safety in cattle, including effects on reproduction, have been reviewed.[55] The acute oral LD50 for monensin in cattle was found to be 26.4 mg/kg, and the LD10 was estimated to be 11.2 mg/kg.[55] These lethal dose findings would indicate a very steep dose-response curve. Lethality with lasalocid has occurred at concentrations of 50 mg/kg. Poultry litter containing maduramicin was toxic to cattle.[56]

CLINICAL SIGNS

The clinical signs of ionophore toxicosis in cattle follow a predictable time line depending on the concentration of the overdose. When cattle consume a toxic concentration of an ionophore the first clinical sign observed within hours after the overdose is anorexia. The typical history in a feedlot is that cattle were fed in the morning normally; when the bunk was checked in the afternoon there was still feed remaining so no additional feed is delivered. The next morning after the previous day's overdose, 24 hours later, the animals return to normal feeding. In many cases there is a transient diarrhea 24 hours after the overdose. Within 12 hours the diarrhea resolves without treatment. The first death loss may not be seen until 72 hours after the overdose. The death loss starting 3 days after the overdose may not be accompanied by any clinical signs. An animal may just be found dead without any previous clinical signs. In many cases the animals will all come to the feed bunk to eat feed but are found hours later in the pen, acutely dead. The peak death loss after a toxic dose of ionophores in cattle is 5 to 10 days.

Clinical signs observed after the death loss starts includes signs consistent with congestive heart failure. The clinical signs include weakness, incoordination, ataxia, hyperpnea, tachycardia, hyperventilation, dyspnea, dilated jugular vein, subcutaneous edema, nasal discharge, recumbency, and death.[4,47,53,57]

On necropsy edematous lungs may be observed. The wet heavy lungs are often mistaken for a bronchopneumonia. The initial diagnosis is a viral or bacterial pneumonia. When several animals die and there is diarrhea, an enteritis is often diagnosed. The initial clinical signs can be confusing. There is a steep death loss curve peaking at 5 to 10 days postingestion of the toxic dose of ionophore that does not follow the normal time line of bronchopneumonia in a group of cattle.

The clinical syndrome of ionophore toxicosis in cattle varies from decreased feed intake to severe heart and skeletal muscle damage. Decreased total daily dry matter intake is a fairly common sign first observed with ionophore poisoning[55,58] Intravenous monensin caused ataxia, hyperpnea, polyuria, and anorexia.[25] Lasalocid- and monensin-poisoned steers developed anorexia, tachycardia, hyperventilation, dyspnea, watery diarrhea, muscle tremors, weakness, and incoordination.,[4,52–54,57,58] Early rumen atony, diarrhea, and subsequent dehydration were also common findings in the affected steers. In studies of monensin toxicosis, calves developed anorexia, depression, and diarrhea early and had delayed onset of depression, diarrhea, tachypnea, and ataxia.[55] The severity of the clinical signs seemed to be dose related. Similar findings were reported from field cases of ionophore poisonings.[4,20,43,56,57,59] Additional signs reported from field cases include pica, prominent jugular pulses, subcutaneous edema, nasal discharge, recumbency, and deaths that were often delayed several days.

CLINICAL CHEMISTRY

Clinical chemistry changes in cases of ionophore toxicosis are consistent with muscle damage. Creatinine kinase may be elevated but this is not pathognomonic for ionophore toxicosis. Once ruminants become recumbent, the creatinine kinase will increase rapidly. Other elevations in aspartate aminotransferase, serum protein, urea nitrogen, urine protein, and glucosuria and decreases in serum potassium, serum sodium, serum calcium, urine pH, and urine specific gravity have been observed.[54,60–62] Measurement of serum troponins is helpful if taken within 7 days of the initial myocardial damage.[63–68] Measurement of cardiac troponin I (cTnI) is the gold standard for noninvasive diagnosis of myocardial injury in people and small animals.[67] This is a good marker for myocardial injury in cattle also.

Clinicopathologic changes in steers with lasalocid or monensin toxicosis are consistent with dehydration, electrolyte change, and muscle damage. Increased aspartate aminotransferase, creatine kinase, serum protein, urea nitrogen, creatinine, total bilirubin, urine protein, glucosuria, and myoglobinuria; decreased serum potassium, serum sodium, serum calcium, urine pH, and urine specific gravity; and leukocytosis were reported with monensin toxicosis.[54,60,62,69] The severity of the clinicopathologic changes was somewhat dose dependent but more dependent on the day of the sample collection. Increased creatine kinase, lactate dehydrogenase, urea nitrogen, creatinine, total bilirubin, and sorbitol dehydrogenase were reported with lasalocid poisonings.[39,52–54] The animals within a group are generally not uniform in their clinicopathologic changes. Dramatic increases in aspartate aminotransferase and creatine kinase were found only within 1 day of death in one group of calves with monensin toxicosis.[62]

GROSS PATHOLOGY

The gross pathology of ionophore toxicosis in cattle can look similar to bronchopneumonia. If the animal is in heart failure there can be edema in the lungs. Grossly the lungs will seem to be similar to a viral or bacterial bronchopneumonia. If only the lungs are submitted to the diagnostic laboratory the only pathology seen may be the interstitial fluid observed. Formalin-fixed myocardial and skeletal muscle must be submitted as well as other fixed and fresh tissues to increase the likelihood of getting a diagnosis of ionophore toxicosis. There may be pale areas in the myocardium and skeletal muscle as well as hemorrhage on the epicardium.[4,53,57,59,70] In many cases of ionophore toxicosis there may not be any gross lesions. Submission of appropriately fixed and fresh tissue is critical to a diagnosis. With congestive heart failure a swollen liver, increased pericardial and thoracic fluid, ascites, and subcutaneous edema may be observed. Pale streaking on the epicardium is sometimes confused with normal epicardial fat.

Cattle that die from ionophore overdoses reportedly have evidence of heart failure or skeletal muscle damage, but it is not uncommon for no lesions to be observed in animals that die acutely. In one study, calves dosed with monensin and killed over a

4-day period had no observed gross lesions, but calves killed over a 11-day period had yellowish-brown areas in the ventricular myocardium and occasional areas of paling of the myocardium. Petechia and ecchymosis of the myocardium also have been reported. Other observations that can be identified include froth in trachea and bronchi; pulmonary congestion; streaking or paling of the skeletal or cardiac musculature; occasional interlobular pulmonary edema; and occasional findings of swollen liver, increased pericardial and thoracic fluid and ascites, and subcutaneous edema.[4,53,56,57,59,60]

HISTOPATHOLOGY

Microscopic examination of appropriately submitted tissue is necessary for a definitive diagnosis of ionophore toxicosis. Myocardial pathology is most often observed with ionophore toxicosis and in many cases skeletal muscle pathology is also observed. Centrilobular hepatic necrosis is observed when there is congestive heart failure. Animals can die acutely and have no microscopic lesions. Myocardial lesions follow a timeline from the acute ionophore toxicosis. Initially disruption of the myofibrils is seen, an increased eosinophilic appearance, then contraction bands and an infiltrate of inflammatory cells are seen. There is hyaline and vacuolar degeneration, moderate to severe swelling of myocardial fibers with variable interstitial predominantly neutrophilic cellularity, and multifocal to diffuse myocardial necrosis.[4,57,59] This will progress to fibrin between the myofibers, necrosis of the myofibers, and mineralization where there were necrotic myofibers.

Histologic evidence of skeletal and cardiac muscle damage and changes secondary to heart failure and hepatocellular damage are the lesions reported in cattle poisoned with ionophores, but animals that die acutely may have no lesions. With monensin, maduramicin, and lasalocid, skeletal and cardiac muscle lesions of sarcoplasmic vacuolation were seen as early as 24 hours postexposure, whereas degeneration, necrosis with contraction bands, and occasional mononuclear infiltrate were seen in animals that died later.[4,53,56,57,59,61] Lesion severity tends to be somewhat dose dependent when evaluating a group with wide individual variability in occurrence and severity. Occasional histologic findings of Purkinje cell degeneration, centrilobular hepatic necrosis, alveolar and septal edema of the lungs, and fatty change in the liver may be observed. An unusual finding for both monensin and lasalocid was that all animals dying within 3 days of dosing had a noticeable lack of zymogen granules in the otherwise normal pancreas. For animals that live long enough after being poisoned, the most prominent lesion is increased fibrous connective tissue scarring of cardiac and skeletal muscles.[59] Also, skeletal, but not myocardial, lesions have been present even when there were secondary lesions that suggest heart failure.[60] Ultrastructural lesions in cattle associated with ionophore toxicosis are associated with organelle damage. Progression of lesions observed included pyknotic nuclei, disruption of contractile material, myocardial degeneration with sarcoplasmic vacuolization, lipid droplet accumulation, compact myelin figures, and mitochondrial swelling with disruption of the cristae.[61,69] Within single myocytes, affected mitochondria often have normal mitochondria adjacent to them.

DIAGNOSIS

To diagnose an ionophore toxicosis the history, clinical signs, serum chemistry, gross and microscopic changes, and analytical chemistry findings should agree. Because of the delay from ingestion of a toxic concentration of feed and development of clinical signs may be days, collection of feed at the time that animals become sick or dying it not always rewarding. It is uncommon to obtain the mis-mixed feed that was at a toxic concentration because retained feed samples are rarely kept. Identifying a toxic concentration of the ionophore in the feed is not necessary for the diagnosis of iono-phore toxicosis. Identifying the presence of an ionophore in the rumen content of a dead animal is usually not rewarding. Typically, an animal has been anorexic several days before death so if they are consuming feed it would be at a normal inclusion rate or possibly not present at all. Typically, there is a one-time mis-mix of the feed, then all subsequent feeding will contain a normal concentration of the ionophore.

Evaluating the myocardial damage by ultrasound, electrocardiographic analyses, or other diagnostic modalities is usually not rewarding. Animals have died months to years after permanent myocardial damage from an ionophore toxicosis when all the diagnostic tests to determine myocardial damage were normal.

Diagnosis of ionophore poisoning involves a coordination of the overall case. Sam-ples of the suspected diet should be analyzed for the presence of ionophores, but the collected feed may not be representative of the feed ingested. In addition to the feed analysis, rumen content should be assayed for ionophores; however, the concentra-tion identified may be lower than that of the feed originally ingested because of ab-sorption or breakdown. In addition to the analytical evidence, one must evaluate the clinical syndrome, gross pathology, and histopathology. Often, with groups of ionophore-poisoned animals, only a few of the possible clinical signs and lesions are present in an individual animal. When evaluating the overall case, consider the occurrence of signs and lesions in the group. Although abnormalities may not be iden-tified, electrocardiographic analyses may provide additional evidence of effects in the animals that survived the initial syndrome. Random evaluation demonstrated abnormal ST segments or QRS complexes in 3 bulls of a group that survived a case of monensin toxicosis.[59] In a dosing study, evidence of QT interval prolongation, QRS complex prolongation, first-degree heart block, infrequent premature atrial beats, and increased T wave amplitude developed in a few of the animals 2 to 7 days postdosing.[61]

TREATMENT

There is no specific treatment of ionophore toxicosis. Typically, there is a one-time mis-mix of the feed, then all subsequent feeding will contain a normal concentration of the ionophore. Once there is a myopathy in the cardiac or skeletal muscle the myo-fibers are not repaired. There is replacement of the damaged myofibers by fibrous tis-sue or mineralization. Death loss can occur for a month or longer after the initial myofibers are damaged, and permanent heart damage may be present. General sup-portive care can be attempted; however, deaths can occur for extended periods after exposure has stopped, and permanent heart damage may be present.

SUMMARY

An ionophore toxicosis in cattle can initially be a difficult diagnosis. A definitive diag-nosis can be made using a thorough diagnostic plan. If an ionophore toxicosis occurs in a feedlot it can be easier to assess the financial effects of the long-term damage to an animal or group of animals. A cost of the loss of gain can be determined by comparing the close-out costs of an affected pen of calves versus and unaffected group.

If an ionophore toxicosis occurs in a group of breeding animals, determining the long-term cost of the extent of a permanent damage is difficult. There can be a wide range in the pathology observed in the myocardium and skeletal muscle in an animal that is going to be used for reproduction.

DISCLOSURE

The author has nothing to disclose.

REFERENCE

1. Berger J, Rachlin A, Scott W, et al. The isolation of three new crystalline antibiotics from streptomyces1. J Am Chem Soc 1951;73:5295–8.
2. Shirling EB, Gottlieb D. Cooperative description of type strains of streptomyces: V. additional descriptions1. Int J Syst Evol Microbiol 1972;22:265–394.
3. Benz DA, Byers FM, Schelling GT, et al. Ionophores alter hepatic concentrations of intermediary carbohydrate metabolites in steers. J Anim Sci 1989;67:2393–9.
4. Blanchard PC, Galey FD, Ross F, et al. Lasalocid toxicosis in dairy calves. J Vet Diagn Invest 1993;5:300–2.
5. Pressman BC. Induced active transport of ions in mitochondria. Proc Natl Acad Sci U S A 1965;53:1076.
6. Cann I, Kobayashi Y, Onoda A, et al. Effects of some ionophore antibiotics and polyoxins on the growth of anaerobic rumen fungi. J Appl Bacteriol 1993;74: 127–33.
7. Benz D, Byers F, Schelling G, et al. Ionophore, diet, nutritional state and level of intake effects on vital organ mass and hepatic fructose 2, 6-bisphosphate levels in growing animals. Nutr Rep Int 1988;38:57–67.
8. Bergen WG, Bates DB. Ionophores: their effect on production efficiency and mode of action. J Anim Sci 1984;58:1465–83.
9. Nagaraja T, Taylor M. Susceptibility and resistance of ruminal bacteria to antimicrobial feed additives. Appl Environ Microbiol 1987;53:1620–5.
10. Andersen MA, Horn GW. Effect of lasalocid on weight gains, ruminal fermentation and forage intake of stocker cattle grazing winter wheat pasture. J Anim Sci 1987; 65:865–71.
11. Hillaire MC, Jouany JP, Gaboyard C, et al. In vitro study of the effect of different ionophore antibiotics and of certain derivatives on rumen fermentation and on protein nitrogen degradation. Reprod Nutr Dev 1989;29:247–57.
12. Nagaraja T, Avery T, Bartley E, et al. Effect of lasalocid, monensin or thiopeptin on lactic acidosis in cattle. J Anim Sci 1982;54:649–58.
13. Nagaraja T, Avery T, Galitzer S, et al. Effect of ionophore antibiotics on experimentally induced lactic acidosis in cattle. Am J Vet Res 1985;46:2444–52.
14. Olumeyan DB, Nagaraja TG, Miller GW, et al. Rumen microbial changes in cattle fed diets with or without salinomycin. Appl Environ Microbiol 1986;51:340–5.
15. Pressman BC. Biological applications of ionophores. Annu Rev Biochem 1976; 45:501–30.
16. Spears JW, Harvey RW. Lasalocid and dietary sodium and potassium effects on mineral metabolism, ruminal volatile fatty acids and performance of finishing steers. J Anim Sci 1987;65:830–40.
17. Kitame F, Utsushikawa K, Koama T, et al. Laidlomycin, a new antimycoplasmal polyether antibiotic. J Antibiot 1974;27:884–8.
18. Stipkovits L, Kobulej T, Varga Z. Efficacy of lasalocid sodium against mycoplasmas (preliminary communication). Acta Vet Hung 1984;32:127–9.
19. Stipkovits L, Kobulej T, Varga Z, et al. In vitro testing of the anti-mycoplasma effect of some anti-coccidial drugs. Vet Microbiol 1987;15:65–70.

20. Hammond AC, Bray TM, Cummins KA, et al. Reduction of ruminal 3-methylindole production and the prevention of tryptophan-induced acute bovine pulmonary edema and emphysema. Am J Vet Res 1978;39:1404–6.
21. Hammond AC, Carlson JR. Inhibition of ruminal degradation of L-tryptophan to 3-methylindole, in vitro. J Anim Sci 1980;51:207–14.
22. Nocerini MR, Honeyfield DC, Carlson JR, et al. Reduction of 3-methylindole production and prevention of acute bovine pulmonary edema and emphysema with lasalocid. J Anim Sci 1985;60:232–8.
23. Pressman B-C, Guzman N. New ionophores for old organelles. Ann N Y Acad Sci 1974;227:380–91.
24. Spears JW. Ionophores and Nutrient Digestion and Absorption in Ruminants. J Nutr 1990;120:632–8.
25. Armstrong JD, Spears JW. Intravenous administration of ionophores in ruminants: effects on metabolism independent of the rumen. J Anim Sci 1988;66:1807–17.
26. Reffett-Stabel J, Spears JW, Harvey RW, et al. Salinomycin and lasalocid effects on growth rate, mineral metabolism and ruminal fermentation in steers. J Anim Sci 1989;67:2735–42.
27. Spears JW, Harvey RW. Performance, ruminal and serum characteristics of steers fed lasalocid on pasture. J Anim Sci 1984;58:460–4.
28. Mollenhauer HH, Rowe L, Cysewski S, et al. Ultrastructural observations in ponies after treatment with monensin. Am J Vet Res 1981;42:35–40.
29. Sakuragawa N, Mito T, Kawada A. Niemann-Pick disease: Coupling and uncoupling of inhibited sphingomyelinase activity and exogenous cholesterol esterification in fibroblasts by ionophore treatment. Biochim Biophys Acta 1994;1213: 193–8.
30. Wagner D. Ionophore cmparisons for feedlot cattle. Bov Pract 1984;19:151–4.
31. Anderson KL, Nagaraja TG, Morrill JL, et al. Performance and ruminal changes of early-weaned calves fed lasalocid. J Anim Sci 1988;66:806–13.
32. Dye BE, Amos HE, Froetschel MA. Influence of lasalocid on rumen metabolites, milk production, milk composition and digestibility in lactating cows; Influence du lasalocide sur les métabolites du rumen, la production laitière, la composition du lait et la digestibilité chez les vaches en lactation. Nutr Rep Int 1988;38: 101–15.
33. Zinn RA. Influence of forage level on response of feedlot steers to salinomycin supplementation. J Anim Sci 1986;63:2005–12.
34. Zinn RA. Effect of salinomycin supplementation on characteristics of digestion and feedlot performance of cattle. J Anim Sci 1986;63:1996–2004.
35. Quigley JD III, Boehms SI, Steen TM, et al. Effects of lasalocid on selected ruminal and blood metabolites in young calves. J Dairy Sci 1992;75:2235–41.
36. Bagley CP, Feazel JI, Morrison DG, et al. Effects of salinomycin on ruminal characteristics and performance of grazing beef steers. J Anim Sci 1988;66:792–7.
37. Morris FE, Branine ME, Galyean ML, et al. Effect of rotating monensin plus tylosin and lasalocid on performance, ruminal fermentation, and site and extent of digestion in feedlot cattle. J Anim Sci 1990;68:3069–78.
38. Galyean ML, Malcolm KJ, Duff GC. Performance of feedlot steers fed diets containing laidlomycin propionate or monensin plus tylosin, and effects of laidlomycin propionate concentration on intake patterns and ruminal fermentation in beef steers during adaptation to a high-concentrate diet. J Anim Sci 1992;70:2950–8.
39. Hubbell DS, Goetsch AL, Galloway DL, et al. Digestion and performance responses to lasalocid and concentrate supplements by beef cattle fed bermudagrass hay. Arch Tierernahr 1992;42:79–92.

40. Steen TM, Quigley JD, Heitmann RN, et al. Effects of lasalocid and undegradable protein on growth and body composition of holstein heifers. J Dairy Sci 1992;75: 2517–23.
41. Dennis S, Nagaraja T, Bartley E. Effect of lasalocid or monensin on lactate-producing or using rumen bacteria. J Anim Sci 1981;52:418–26.
42. Katz MP, Nagaraja TG, Fina LR. Ruminal changes in monensin- and lasalocid-fed cattle grazing bloat-provocative alfalfa pasture. J Anim Sci 1986;63:1246–57.
43. Thivend P, Jouany J-P. Effect of lasalocid sodium on rumen fermentation and digestion in sheep. Reprod Nutr Dev 1983;23:817–28.
44. Rumpler WV, Johnson DE, Bates DB. The effect of high dietary cation concentration on methanogenesis by steers fed diets with and without ionophores. J Anim Sci 1986;62:1737–41.
45. Herod E, Bartley E, Davidovich A, et al. Effect of adaptation to monensin or lasalocid on rumen fermentation in vitro and the effect of these drugs on heifer growth and feed efficiency. J Anim Sci 1979;49:374–81.
46. Benz G, Ernst J. Efficacy of salinomycin in treatment of experimental Eimeria bovis infections in calves. Am J Vet Res 1979;40:1180–6.
47. Merchen NR, Berger LL. Effect of salinomycin level on nutrient digestibility and ruminal characteristics of sheep and feedlot performance of cattle. J Anim Sci 1985;60:1338–46.
48. Eicher-Pruiett S, Morrill J, Nagaraja T, et al. Response of young dairy calves with lasalocid delivery varied in feed sources1. J Dairy Sci 1992;75:857–62.
49. Stromberg B, Schlotthauer J, Armstrong B, et al. Efficacy of lasalocid sodium against coccidiosis (Eimeria zuernii and Eimeria bovis) in calves. Am J Vet Res 1982;43:583–5.
50. Fitzgerald P, Mansfield M. Effects of inoculations with Eimeria zuernii on young calves treated with decoquinate or narasin with or without dexamethasone. Am J Vet Res 1989;50:1056–9.
51. Hammond AC, Carlson JR, Breeze RG. Effect of monensin pretreatment on tryptophan-induced acute bovine pulmonary edema and emphysema. Am J Vet Res 1982;43:753–6.
52. Galitzer S, Bartley E, Oehme F. Preliminary studies on lasalocid toxicosis in cattle. Vet Hum Toxicol 1982;24:406–9.
53. Galitzer S, Kruckenberg S, Kidd J. Pathologic changes associated with experimental lasalocid and monensin toxicosis in cattle. Am J Vet Res 1986;47:2624–6.
54. Galitzer S, Oehme F, Bartley E, et al. Lasalocid toxicity in cattle: acute clinicopathological changes. J Anim Sci 1986;62:1308–16.
55. Potter EL, VanDuyn RL, Cooley CO. Monensin Toxicity in Cattle. J Anim Sci 1984; 58:1499–511.
56. Fourie N, Bastianello SS, Nel P, et al. Cardiomyopathy of ruminants induced by the litter of poultry fed on rations containing the ionophore antibiotic, maduramicin. 1. Epidemiology, clinical signs and clinical pathology. Onderstepoort J Vet Res 1991;58(4):291–6.
57. Janzen ED, Rodostits OM, Orr JP. Possible monensin poisoning in a group of bulls. Can Vet J 1981;22:92.
58. Thonney M, Heide E, Duhaime D, et al. Growth, feed efficiency and metabolite concentrations of cattle fed high forage diets with lasalocid or monensin supplements. J Anim Sci 1981;52:427–33.
59. Schweitzer D, Kimberling C, Spraker T, et al. Accidental monensin sodium intoxication of feedlot cattle. J Am Vet Med Assoc 1984;184:1273–6.

60. Geor RJ, Robinson WF. Suspected monensin toxicosis in feedlot cattle. Aust Vet J 1985;62:130–1.
61. Van JV, Amstutz H, Weirich W, et al. Clinical, clinicopathologic, and pathologic alterations in acute monensin toxicosis in cattle. Am J Vet Res 1983;44:2133–44.
62. Van Vleet JF, Amstutz HE, Rebar AH. Effect of pretreatment with selenium-vitamin E on monensin toxicosis in cattle. Am J Vet Res 1985;46:2221–8.
63. Fraser BC, Anderson DE, White BJ, et al. Assessment of a commercially available point-of-care assay for the measurement of bovine cardiac troponin I concentration. Am J Vet Res 2013;74:870–3.
64. Labonté J, Roy J-P, Dubuc J, et al. Measurement of cardiac troponin I in healthy lactating dairy cows using a point of care analyzer (i-STAT-1). J Vet Cardiol 2015; 17:129–33.
65. Serra M, Papakonstantinou S, Adamcova M, et al. Veterinary and toxicological applications for the detection of cardiac injury using cardiac troponin. Vet J 2010;185:50–7.
66. Varga A, Schober KE, Holloman CH, et al. Correlation of serum cardiac troponin i and myocardial damage in cattle with monensin toxicosis. J Vet Intern Med 2009; 23:1108–16.
67. Varga A, Schober KE, Walker WL, et al. Validation of a commercially available immunoassay for the measurement of bovine cardiac troponin I. J Vet Intern Med 2009;23:359–65.
68. Willis MS, Snyder JA, Poppenga RH, et al. Bovine cardiac troponin T is not accurately quantified with a common human clinical immunoassay. J Vet Diagn Invest 2007;19:106–8.
69. Van Vleet J, Ferrans V. Ultrastructural myocardial alterations in monensin toxicosis of cattle. Am J Vet Res 1983;44:1629.
70. Collins E, McCrea C. Monensin sodium toxicity in cattle. Vet Rec 1978;103:386.

Biofuels Co-Products Tolerance and Toxicology for Ruminants: An Update

Steve Ensley, DVM, PhD

KEYWORDS

• Biofuels • Co-products • Toxicology • Ruminants

KEY POINTS

- Total dietary sulfur concentration is used to assess risk to develop sulfur toxicosis in ruminants.
- Because of the elevated sulfur concentrations in feed and the subsequent rapid death, polioencephalomalacia (PEM) may only be observed in 30% of the cases of sulfur toxicosis.
- PEM caused by sulfur toxicosis has been diagnosed by the clinical signs observed in addition to microscopic lesions of laminar cortical necrosis, neuronal damage, gliosis, and spongiosis.

The rapid growth of the biofuels industry in the Midwest in the last 40 years has created an increased supply of corn co-product feed for animals.[1,2] When starch-based ethanol production started to rapidly increase, it was thought that cellulosic ethanol production would soon follow. This did not occur because the technology to find enzymes able to break down cellulose into a product that can be fermented into ethanol never occurred. The adoption of the renewable fuel standard in 2005 mandated that ethanol be used as a fuel. This mandate is what created the ethanol industry that we have today. Production of ethanol has decreased our reliance on imported oil. Since 2012 approximately 80% of dried distillers grain with solubles (DDGS) have some of the oil removed. The co-product of the ethanol industry we use for animal feeds will continue to change.

Corn co-products are a co-product of the dry and wet corn-milling ethanol manufacturing. The dry mill corn co-product includes distillers grain and soluble feedstuffs. Distillers grain can be further categorized into dry distillers grains (DDG), DDGS, wet distillers grains with solubles (WDGS), modified WDGS, and corn syrup (solubles). Wet mill ethanol production produces 2 main feed stuffs: corn gluten (wet and dry) and heavy steep water. A second type of biofuel, biodiesel, has a feed by-product called glycerol, which can also be used for cattle feed.[3]

Anatomy & Physiology, Kansas State University, 1800 Dension Avenue, P217 Mosier Hall, Manhattan, KS 66506, USA
E-mail address: sensley01@ksu.edu

Vet Clin Food Anim 36 (2020) 653–659
https://doi.org/10.1016/j.cvfa.2020.08.010
0749-0720/20/© 2020 Elsevier Inc. All rights reserved.

CORN CO-PRODUCTS

During production of ethanol from corn, sulfuric acid is added during fermentation to balance the pH of the fermentation process. Sulfuric acid also is used periodically to flush the distillation columns to keep them clear of precipitate. This added sulfur can increase sulfur concentration in corn co-products to a level that can increase the incidence of sulfur toxicosis in ruminants. Exposure to high levels, greater than 0.4% dietary sulfur, can induce polioencephalomalacia (PEM) in ruminants.[4-12] Total dietary sulfur concentration is used to assess risk to develop sulfur toxicosis in ruminants. This includes sulfur in feed and water sources.

The daily sulfur requirement for growing and adult beef cattle is 1500 to 2000 ppm of the ration on a dry matter basis. Recommended dietary sulfur concentrations are 0.20% of diet dry matter for most dairy cattle (NRC 2001). Higher amounts (0.29%) are recommended for calves consuming milk or milk replacers. The maximum tolerated dietary sulfur concentration is 0.4% of the diet in cattle other than feedlot cattle (NRC 2001). Feedlot cattle should have a diet with sulfur less than 0.3% of the diet.

PEM is a descriptive term of the lesions observed in the brain but is not pathognomonic for sulfur toxicosis. This lesion can be caused by lead poisoning, water deprivation as well as excess dietary sulfur. Grain overload has also been associated with PEM.[13,14] Historically PEM was thought to be caused solely by thiamine deficiency.[15-19] Now that the association has been made with sulfur toxicosis and PEM, the explanation of PEM being solely induced by thiamine deficiency is not correct. Reports of PEM or cerebrocortical necrosis have been in the veterinary literature since the 1950s. Impaired thiamine metabolism in ruminants was investigated as the cause for PEM in the 1970s. Research was done during this time to determine if thiaminase compounds in plants or pharmaceuticals such as Amprolium could contribute to thiamine deficiency resulting in the development of PEM. It was not until the 1980s that elevated dietary sulfur was linked to PEM. Investigators in Missouri discovered when sulfate salts used as feed limiters were removed from herds and feedlots experiencing PEM, cases of PEM decreased.[16] At that time it was not known if PEM was caused by the sulfur in the diet or if the sulfur in the diet was blocking thiamine production in the rumen or if there was something toxic present in the sulfate salt used in the feed.[15] Since this original observation several investigators have clearly demonstrated that PEM can be caused by the direct action of elevated rumen sulfur.[16] Many historical cases of blind staggers in Colorado and Wyoming, starting in the 1930s, have now been recognized to have most likely been caused by elevated dietary sulfur and not selenium.[20]

SULFUR TOXICOSIS

Hydrogen sulfide inhibits the electron transport chain and interferes with metabolism in the mitochondria.[17] Hydrogen sulfide blocks cytochrome aa3, which blocks adenosine triphosphate.[21,22] The brain is the target organ of sulfur toxicosis because of the high energy demand, high lipid content, and low amount of antioxidants.[23] The laminar cortical necrosis associated with PEM can sometimes be detected grossly using fluorescence from an ultraviolet light at 365 nm. The fluorescence is due to ceroid lipofuscin present in areas of the brain that are damaged. Fluorescence is not always observed with PEM but is helpful if observed. The damage in the brain is at the junction of white and gray matter in the cortex. Sulfides are also potent oxidants and can bind superoxide dismutase and glutathione peroxidase. The gas, hydrogen sulfide, can also cause a rapid respiratory paralysis associated with inhalation of hydrogen sulfide and is due to paralysis of the carotid body. Death can occur with one inhalation of hydrogen sulfide.[24] Because of the elevated sulfur concentrations in feed and the subsequent rapid death, PEM can only be observed in 30% of the cases of sulfur toxicosis.

RUMINAL SULFUR METABOLISM

Bacteria in the rumen can metabolize sulfur as elemental, inorganic, and organic sulfur. Sulfur metabolizing bacteria have been classified as assimilatory or dissimilatory.[8] Assimilatory bacteria reduce sulfate (SO_4) and produce amino acids containing sulfur. Dissimilatory bacteria use sulfur for an energy source but produce sulfide instead of amino acids. Dissimilatory bacteria include *Desulfovibrio* and *Desulfotomaculum*.[25,26] Most of the sulfide production in the rumen is from dissimilatory bacteria. The amount of hydrogen sulfide production in the rumen is limited by the amount in the rumen gas cap. This has been demonstrated *in vitro* using hydrogen sulfide generation tubes and measuring the gas in the headspace. As the gas cap is eliminated in the tubes, the bacteria are able to produce more hydrogen sulfide; this would suggest that as rumen gas is eructated more hydrogen sulfide will be produced in the rumen. The numbers of dissimilatory bacteria do not increase but their ability to produce more sulfide does. Nonsulfate reducing rumen bacteria include *Veillonella, Megasphaera, Wolinella, Selenomonas, Anaerovibrio,* and *Clostridium* sp. These bacteria contain cysteine desulfhydrase, an enzyme that metabolizes sulfur-containing proteins and produces sulfide.

To summarize hydrogen sulfide metabolism in the rumen, there is oxidation to sulfate (SO_4), methylation of sulfate, and reaction with metalloproteins. Dissimilatory bacteria use inorganic sulfur for energy and produce sulfide(S^{-2}), which can then be used by assimilatory bacteria to produce sulfur-containing amino acids and sulfide. Other rumen bacteria can use these sulfur-containing amino acids to produce sulfide. Hydrogen sulfide (H_2S) is absorbed across the rumen wall or absorbed via the lungs, enters the portal circulation, and then disassociates to hydrogen and HS. HS is oxidized by heme to H2O and S, which is converted back to sulfate (SO_4) by sulfide oxidase in the liver. The major route of excretion of sulfide is metabolism in the liver and excretion in the urine.

The hydrogen sulfide metabolites present in the rumen are HS, HSO3, S^{-2}, and S. These metabolites are affected by rumen pH.[27,28] One-third of H_2S is undissociated at pH 7.4. H_2S has a pKa of 7.04 for the first dissociation and 11.96 for the second.[24] As rumen pH drops, the amount of hydrogen sulfide in the rumen increases. This is an explanation for the increase in PEM observed in cattle on elevated grain rations.[29]

CLINICAL SIGNS OF SULFUR TOXICOSIS

There are 2 clinical syndromes associated with sulfur toxicosis. One is an acute syndrome where the first signs observed are animals that are recumbent and comatose. These animals respond poorly to treatment and may have minimal brain pathology because of the rapid death. A second syndrome is a delayed or more chronic response. Clinical signs include cortical blindness, stupor, bruxism, ataxia, and fine muscle tremors of the face and head. Cortical blindness means the menace reflex is absent but the palpebral reflex is present and the pupils respond to light. Animals may progress to lateral recumbency, convulsions, and death. The longer an animal is affected by sulfur toxicosis the more likely lesions will be observed. There are a wide range of clinical signs observed with PEM, not just blindness or seizuring.

DIAGNOSIS OF POLIOENCEPHALOMALACIA

PEM caused by sulfur toxicosis has been diagnosed by the clinical signs observed in addition to microscopic lesions of laminar cortical necrosis, neuronal damage, gliosis, and spongiosis. Blood vessels in the area of damage increase in size and can have evidence of vessel wall damage. Some of the damage observed grossly and microscopically is due to brain swelling and herniation of the midbrain and brainstem into the foramen magnum. There has been some discussion about whether sulfides damage the vessel walls and the resulting lesions are due to interference with blood supply to these local areas or the initial damage is to neurons. Evaluation of the diet for the total dietary sulfur intake can be helpful in diagnosis.

Differential diagnosis when PEM is suspected should include lead toxicosis, water deprivation-sodium ion toxicosis, TEME, *Listeria*, rabies, magnesium deficiency, and rumen acidosis.

TREATMENT

Treatment of PEM is symptomatic because there is no specific antidote for sulfur toxicosis. Removing the animal from more exposure to the toxin is always one of the first intervention steps to take. Sulfur toxicosis is still a thiamine responsive condition even though it is not a thiamine deficiency.[30] The more rapid the treatment is initiated the more likely there will be a response to treatment. Thiamine at 10 mg/kg BID for 3 days can be effective. A broad spectrum antibiotic and steroids are also used as adjunctive therapy.

BIOFUELS AND MYCOTOXINS

During ethanol production the concentration of mycotoxins increase 3 times in the final product.[31] One-third of the corn is used for ethanol production, one-third produces carbon dioxide, and the remaining one-third produces the corn co-product. Mycotoxin concentration in corn co-products can be a significant issue when mycotoxins are elevated in the corn that is used to produce ethanol. With wet corn co-products there is the possibility of production of mycotoxins when they are stored on the producer's site; this is called postproduction of mycotoxins. Corn co-products are good substrates for mycotoxin growth especially when the moisture concentration is elevated.

BIOFUELS AND ANTIBIOTIC RESIDUE

Why is antibiotic residue an issue in corn co-products? Ethanol fermentation containers can become contaminated with bacteria and interfere with the yeast production of ethanol. The lactic acid–producing bacteria that includes *Lactobacillus*, *Pediococcus*, *Leuconostoc*, and *Weissella* can affect ethanol yields significantly. Yeast converts starch to ethanol, but bacteria convert those same sugars to lactic or acetic acid. Ethanol production yields can drop up to 5%, which causes economic problem for ethanol producers. Virginiamycin is the only antibiotic that is approved to be used during ethanol fermentation.[32,33] Analysis of corn co-products by the Food and Drug Administration (FDA) has shown the presence of virginiamycin, penicillin, tylosin, and tetracyclines. In 2008, the FDA tested 60 DDGS samples for residues of virginiamycin, tylosin, and erythromycin. Of the 45 samples analyzed, 24 came back positive, according to Dr Daniel McChesney, director of the FDA/Center for Veterinary Medicine's Office of Surveillance and Compliance. Fifteen of the samples contained virginiamycin, 12 contained erythromycin, and 5 contained tylosin. Some were detected at levels exceeding 0.5 ppm, the limit established for virginiamycin, the only antibiotic the FDA regulates in corn co-products. Dr Linda Benjamin of FDA/CVM indicated that in this survey Distillers Dry Grains contained residues in17/27 samples. In the 17 samples, 10 contained virginiamycin, 7 contained erythromycin, and 4 of the 17 samples also contained tylosin. In wet distillers grains 6 of the 14 contained residues. Five of the samples contained virginiamycin, and 1 contained erythromycin. In 4 samples of corn solubles1 out of the 4 samples contained tylosin.

There are many alternatives to the use of antibiotics during fermentation to control bacterial growth. Most ethanol producers do not have antibiotic residue in their corn co-products.

BIODIESEL BY PRODUCT TOXICOSIS

Glycerol is a byproduct of the production of biodiesel via transesterification. Triglycerides are reacted with an alcohol such as ethanol or methanol with a catalytic base to give ethyl esters of fatty acids and glycerol. There are 2 forms of glycerol on the market: crude and purified. Crude glycerol, which is used in livestock feed, is 85% glycerin and 15% other impurities.[34] Purified glycerol, which is more expensive, is used for human products. Methanol is included in the impurities found in glycerol. Methanol is a substance used in the production of biodiesel. Additional impurities include salts and heavy metals. Methanol is toxic, and FDA does not recognize glycerol with more than 150 parts per million to be generally recognized as safe. Generally recognized as safe (GRAS) means the FDA recognizes a given substance as safe for its intended use. Crude glycerol is GRAS for use in livestock feed, but only if methanol levels are at or less than 150 parts per million (ppm). Crude glycerol has been shown to be a safe feed additive for cattle.[34]

DISCLOSURE

The author has nothing to disclose.

REFERENCES

1. Clemens RL. Steady supplies or stockpiles? Dried distillers grains and US beef production. Iowa Ag Review 2015;14:2.
2. Winterholler S, Holland B, McMurphy C, et al. Use of dried distillers grains in preconditioning programs for weaned beef calves and subsequent impact on wheat pasture, feedlot, and carcass performance. The Professional Animal Scientist 2009;25:722–30.
3. Bart JC, Palmeri N, Cavallaro S. Biodiesel science and technology: from soil to oil. Boca Raton (FL): CRC press; 2010.
4. Maxie G, Youssef S. Polioencephalomalacia of ruminants. In: Jubb KVF, Kennedy PC, Palmer N, editors. Jubb, Kennedy and Palmer's pathology of domestic animals. 5th edition. Philadelphia: Elsevier; 2007. p. 351–4.
5. Niles G, Morgan S, Edwards W. Sulfur-induced polioencephalomalacia in stocker calves. Vet Hum Toxicol 2000;42:290–1.
6. Niles G, Morgan S, Edwards W, et al. Effects of increasing dietary sulfur concentration on the incidence and pathology of polioencephalomalacia in weaned beef calves. Oklahoma State Univ Anim Sci Res Rep 2000;55–60.
7. Gould DH. Polioencephalomalacia. J Anim Sci 1998;76:309–14.
8. Gould DH. Update on sulfur-related polioencephalomalacia. Vet Clin North Am Food Anim Pract 2000;16:481–96, vi-vii.

9. Gould DH, Cummings BA, Hamar DW. In vivo indicators of pathologic ruminal sulfide production in steers with diet-induced polioencephalomalacia. J Vet Diagn Invest 1997;9:72–6.

10. Gould DH, Dargatz DA, Garry FB, et al. Potentially hazardous sulfur conditions on beef cattle ranches in the United States. J Am Vet Med Assoc 2002;221:673–7.

11. Gould DH, McAllister MM, Savage JC, et al. High sulfide concentrations in rumen fluid associated with nutritionally induced polioencephalomalacia. Am J Vet Res 1991;52:1164–9.

12. Hamlen H, Clark E, Janzen E. Polioencephalomalacia in cattle consuming water with elevated sodium sulfate levels: A herd investigation. Can Vet J 1993;34:153.

13. Brent B. Relationship of acidosis to other feedlot ailments. J Anim Sci 1976;43:930–5.

14. Owens F, Secrist D, Hill W, et al. Acidosis in cattle: a review. J Anim Sci 1998;76:275–86.

15. Niles G, Morgan S, Edwards W. The relationship between sulfur, thiamine and polioencephalomalacia-a review. Bovine Pract 2002;36:93–100.

16. Raisbeck M. Is polioencephalomalacia associated with high-sulfate diets? J Am Vet Med Assoc 1982;180:1303–5.

17. Nyack B, Mobini S, Padmore C, et al. Polioencephalomalacia (thiamine deficiency) in a calf. Edwardsville (KS): VM SAC veterinary medicine and small animal clinician; 1983.

18. Loew F, Dunlop R. Induction of thiamine inadequacy and polioencephalomalacia in adult sheep with amprolium. Am J Vet Res 1972;33:2195.

19. Loew F, Dunlop R. Blood thiamin concentrations in bovine polioencephalomalacia. Can J Comp Med 1972;36:345.

20. O'Toole D, Raisbeck M, Case J, et al. Selenium-induced "blind staggers" and related myths. A commentary on the extent of historical livestock losses attributed to selenosis on western US rangelands. Vet Pathol 1996;33:104–16.

21. McAllister M, Gould D, Hamar D. Sulphide-induced polioencephalomalacia in lambs. J Comp Pathol 1992;106:267–78.

22. McAllister M, Gould D, Raisbeck M, et al. Evaluation of ruminal sulfide concentrations and seasonal outbreaks of polioencephalomalacia in beef cattle in a feedlot. J Am Vet Med Assoc 1997;211:1275–9.

23. Olkowski A. Neurotoxicity and secondary metabolic problems associated with low to moderate levels of exposure to excess dietary sulphur in ruminants: a review. Vet Hum Toxicol 1997;39:355.

24. Beauchamp R, Bus JS, Popp JA, et al. A critical review of the literature on hydrogen sulfide toxicity. CRC Crit Rev Toxicol 1984;13:25–97.

25. Cummings B, Caldwell D, Gould D, et al. Identity and interactions of rumen microbes associated with dietary sulfate-induced polioencephalomalacia in cattle. Am J Vet Res 1995;56:1384–9.

26. Haven T, Caldwell D, Jensen R. Role of predominant rumen bacteria in the cause of polioencephalomalacia (cerebrocortical necrosis) in cattle. Am J Vet Res 1983;44:1451.

27. De Oliverira L, Jean-Blain C, Komisarczuk-Bony S. Microbial Thiamin Metabolism in the Rumen Simulating Fermenter (rusitec); The effect of Acidogenic Conditions, A High Sulfur Level and Added Thiamine. Br J Nutr 1997;78:599–613.

28. Kung L, Bracht J, Hession A. High Sulfate Induced PEM in Cattle Examined. Feedstuffs 1998;16:12–7.

29. De Oliveira LA, Jean-Blain C, Komisarczuk-Bony S, et al. Microbial thiamin metabolism in the rumen simulating fermenter (RUSITEC): the effect of acidogenic conditions, a high sulfur level and added thiamin. Br J Nutr 1997;78:599–613.

30. Amat S, Olkowski AA, Atila M, et al. A review of polioencephalomalacia in ruminants: is the development of malacic lesions associated with excess sulfur intake independent of thiamine deficiency. Vet Med Anim Sci 2013;1:1.

31. Zhang Y, Caupert J, Imerman PM, et al. The Occurrence and Concentration of Mycotoxins in U.S. Distillers Dried Grains with Solubles. J Agric Food Chem 2009;57:9828–37.

32. Compart DP, Carlson A, Crawford G, et al. Presence and biological activity of antibiotics used in fuel ethanol and corn co-product production. J Anim Sci 2013;91: 2395–404.

33. Perati PP, De Borba BM, Rohrer JS. Determination of virginiamycin, erythromycin, and penicillin in dried distillers grains with solubles. Thermo Fisher Scientific, Sunnyvale, CA, Application notes 1055.

34. Parsons GL, Shelor MK, Drouillard JS. Performance and carcass traits of finishing heifers fed crude glycerin. J Anim Sci 2009;87:653–7.

Identifying Plant Poisoning in Livestock in North America

Bryan L. Stegelmeier, DVM, PhD*, T. Zane Davis, PhD,
Michael J. Clayton, DVM, Dale R. Gardner, PhD

KEYWORDS

- Poisonous plants • Livestock • Poisoning • Diagnosis
- Veterinary diagnostic laboratory

KEY POINTS

- This framework will help livestock producers, veterinarians, and diagnosticians arrive at the most accurate and definitive diagnosis of toxic plant-induced disease.
- Animal emergency response teams or animal health alert networks are available to help identify animal disease outbreaks and develop methods to minimize their spread and impact.
- Plant sampling is critical to identify plants, determine their toxicity, and evaluate the risk they may pose for animal health.
- Plant toxins or metabolites are detected in ingesta, tissues, or blood, but these results should be interpreted with supporting clinical and pathologic findings.

INITIAL STEPS

Many toxic plants produce subtle changes in animal behavior, appetite, and movement that might not be apparent to observers that are unfamiliar with individual animals. Livestock producers, riders, herders, and shepherds often recognize such changes, and although they may initially seem unimportant. All these should be noticed and be appropriately recorded. For example, chronic dehydropyrrolizidine (DHPA) poisoning often results in chronic liver damage resulting in anorexia, rough appearance, and minimal yellow discoloration (icterus) of conjunctiva and mucosal membranes. These changes are often subtle and may barely be apparent because they develop days or weeks before obvious liver failure and overt clinical signs. Keen observers that are familiar with the animals can easily recognize these early signs indicative of liver disease. This understanding is key to obtain the time of exposure and the nature of the disease. To ensure precise recollection one can use a herd book, health records, or an electronic calendar with notes help to record observations;

USDA/ARS Poisonous Plant Research Laboratory, 1150 East 1400 North, Logan, UT 84341, USA
* Corresponding author.
E-mail address: Bryan.Stegelmeier@USDA.GOV

documenting when and where these clinical signs occurred; observed plant exposures, abundance, and phenotypes; and the ages, condition, and source of affected animals.

Because many infectious, degenerative, and immunologic diseases produce clinical signs, biochemical changes, and lesions identical to those caused by poisonous plants, careful exclusion of these alternative causes is needed. Sorting all this out is much easier with expert help and guidance. Extension agents, including local pasture or range scientists, toxicologists, diagnosticians, and pathologists, are great resources. Some may not be available locally, but with current electronic and Internet communication, they are often just a click away and they are made available for consultation. The ultimate goal is to narrow the initial list of potential causes, identify the best diagnosis, map out a treatment plan, and define strategies to avoid future poisoning.

Local veterinarians are an essential resource and should always be involved in these investigations. They are familiar with regional livestock management practices, local livestock diseases, and many endemic plants. In addition to having experience in identifying and describing disease clinical signs, lesions, and disease progression, they also are trained and routinely perform physical examinations, necropsies, or other diagnostic sample collections (**Box 1**). Blood hematology, serum biochemical, and serologic studies can help rule out many infectious and metabolic diseases. Some plant toxins produce characteristic damage to specific organ systems that result in characteristic biochemical changes. For example, DHPA-damaged livers typically result in increased serum activities of liver specific enzymes. The increased enzymes profiles differ from those characteristic of other diseases. Such biochemical changes are useful to identify damaged tissues, determine subsequent diagnostic tests, and ultimately support a specific diagnosis. Additionally, local veterinarians in collaboration with the state veterinarian are essential in enlisting additional state and federal diagnostic efforts.

Many states have organized animal emergency response teams or animal health alert networks. These response teams respond to animal disease outbreaks within a state or within cooperating adjacent states. The teams include plant, animal, and public health experts that can expedite the identification of the problem and implement control measures to limit the spread of livestock and wildlife diseases. The goal is to minimize the economic effects and ensure quality and healthy animal production and products. When needed many networks may also provide public funding to lessen the economic impact of expensive diagnostics on veterinarians and livestock producers. Technology has this process because these are often virtual teams of experts who collaborate electronically. The team director (usually the state veterinarian) identifies a problem, determines whether it should be addressed by the team and informs and activates appropriate work group, makes work assignments, organizes results, and outlines directives to minimize the problem. To best use these resources, detailed descriptions and early characterization of the outbreak is essential. The team can then formulate differential diagnoses, put in motion a plan to identify the cause, and develop local and regional strategies to control and minimize the disease effects.

DIAGNOSTIC STEPS
Field Investigations

Field studies are an essential component of the poisonous plant investigation. Some veterinarians are good at identifying toxic plants, others are anxious to learn more, and all are quick to suggest that others with more training be involved. State and county

---

Box 1
Components essential for diagnosing a suspected plant poisoning

History and Clinical Disease:
 Pertinent facts: breed, sex, age, number, condition, vaccination status, mineral supplements, feeding or pasture changes, and other treatments.
 Clinical disease: number affected, signs, clinical course and progression, lesions, mortality.
 Clinical tests: blood tests to evaluate inflammation, organ function, and evaluate immunologic responses to infectious agents (blood cell counts and serum element, metabolite and biochemical analyses, and serologic tests).

Field Studies:
 Animals: condition, unusual behaviors, clinical signs, lesions. Additional clinical tests may be indicated: blood tests or chemical tests for plant toxins or metabolites in the tissues, blood, urine, or feces.
 Pasture:
 1. Determine forage availability, plant species composition, and evidence of grazing patterns.
 2. Collection of potential problem plants or unidentified plants (dried samples for identification, frozen samples for chemical analysis).
 3. Note weather conditions and its effect on forage and forage availability.
 Prepared feeds: hay, silage, or concentrate feed samples (frozen for analysis).
 Water, salt, and mineral supplements including location and use (samples frozen for analysis).
 Physical location: weather at time of incident, and other obstacles or pressures.
 Check for other potential hazards, such as old batteries, pesticide-laced feed, and so forth.

Postmortem Examination:
 Animal condition and lesions.
 Rumen and gastrointestinal tissues and contents.
 Tissues for histologic studies fixed in 10% neutral buffered formalin (brain, lung, heart, liver, spleen, gastrointestinal tract, kidney, skeletal muscle, and any gross lesions).
 Tissues for chemical or microscopic studies stored in plastic bags and frozen (rumen and gastrointestinal contents, feces [from live animal] complete eye, liver, kidney, serum, whole blood, body fat, bone, urine, milk if lactating).

From Stegelmeier BL. Identifying plant poisoning in livestock: diagnostic approaches and laboratory tests. *Vet Clin North Am Food Anim Prac.* 2011;27:407-417; with permission.

---

extension agents and weed control specialists often are trained and experienced in plant identification. If not, they can help recruit plant identification and taxonomy experts. The objective is to examine pastures and ranges and determine what plants are present in the community, what plants the animals are eating, or in fields what plants are available to contaminate prepared feeds (**Fig. 1**). Sampling is also critical because all unknown and unidentified plants or any potentially toxic plants should be collected for positive identification and possibly for chemical analysis. If the incident involves prepared forages, the investigation become more difficult. Identifying toxic plants in hay and other forages as discussed later is challenging. Appropriate sampling of potentially contaminated feed is essential. Certainly experts should be consulted to ensure adequate samples are collected and preserved.

Plant Identification/Plant and Feed Analysis

To facilitate plant identification, the entire plant should be collected if possible. Flowering plants are most readily identified. Plant samples quickly degrade if placed in plastic bags and rotten plant samples are difficult to identify, and because their toxins may also degrade and become difficult to chemically identify. If collected plants cannot

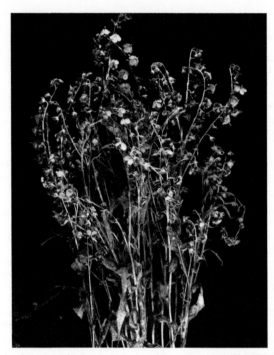

Fig. 1. Photograph of mature dry houndstongue (*Cynoglossum officinale*). Houndstongue is a biennial native to Eurasia that is often considered a noxious weed that has invaded many countries including North America. The first year it forms a rosette that generally stays close to the ground. The second year it grows from 20 to 75 cm tall. It has rough, rosette-shaped, alternate leaves with smooth edges and well-defined veins. It has reddish-purple flowers that develop into burr-covered nutlets that adhere to hair and clothing. Houndstongue is invasive and often spreads along roads and fences in disturbed areas. It often spreads into fields where it can contaminate hay and crops. Animals generally do not find houndstongue palatable and poisoning generally occurs when animals eat contaminated hay.

be put immediately in a plant press, it is best to put them in individual paper bags. Paper allows the plants to dry and the date, collection location, and likely identification can be written on the bag. When various plants are combined in a bag, it is easy to confuse collection sites and mix plant parts. Plants to be identified or submitted as herbarium vouchers have to be pressed. Using a plant press is optimal and they are easy and inexpensive to make with many different examples available on the Internet. If a plant press is not available, a convenient alternative is to press the plants flat for several days between two newspapers using cardboard spacers under a couple of heavy books. Pressed plants are easily mailed in a large envelope taped to a sheet of cardboard. Most state land grant or agricultural colleges have a plant herbarium or other plant taxonomy experts who are available to provide definitive plant identification (**Box 2**).

Plant toxin concentrations and subsequent toxicity are highly variable. For example, the concentrations of DHPA-riddelliine from sequential collections of the same population and phenotype of *Senecio riddellii* varied between two sequential years from 0.3% to nearly 15% of plant dry weight.[1] This indicates that some years only grams of plant would be required to obtain a lethal dose in susceptible species.

Box 2
Resource list

USDA/ARS Poisonous Plant Research Laboratory
1150 East 1400 North
Logan UT 84341
435-752-2941
http://www.pprl.ars.usda.gov/

State Agricultural Extension Service
http://www.csrees.usda.gov/Extension/

State Animal Disease Diagnostic Laboratory
Contact your local or state veterinarian
http://www.aavld.org/mc/page.do?sitePageId=33930&orgId=aavld (laboratories accredited by American Association of Veterinary Diagnostic Laboratories)

Local herbarium
Contact your local county agent or your land grant college or university
http://herba.msu.ru/mirrors/www.helsinki.fi/kmus/botmus.html (lists of public herbaria throughout the world)

Microscopic analysis of feces and ingesta
Texas Veterinary Medical Diagnostic Laboratories
888-646-5623
http://tvmdlweb.tamu.edu/

Toxic Plants of North America (2001) George E. Burrows and Ronald J. Tyrl, Wiley-Blackwell, 1340 pages. ISBN-10: 0813822661. $229.99 http://www.wiley.com/WileyCDA/WileyTitle/productCd-0813822661.html

A Guide to Plant Poisoning of Animals in North America (2001) Anthony P. Knight and Richard Walter. Teton New Media. 1st Edition, 367 pages. ISBN-10: 1893441118. $75.00 http://www.tetonnm.com/cgi-bin/shopper.cgi?preadd=action&key=00031893441113

Modified from Stegelmeier BL. Identifying plant poisoning in livestock: diagnostic approaches and laboratory tests. *Vet Clin North Am Food Anim Prac* 2011;27:407-417; with permission.

Consequently, it is difficult to estimate the potential risk of *Senecio* poisoning without chemical analysis of current plant populations. For quality chemical analysis plant collections should be carefully labeled (location, collection date, and species) and dried in a paper bag. If shipping and delivery are prompt, freshly collected plant samples are frozen and shipped in plastic bags. If shipping delays are likely, shipping plants partially dried is the safest option. This is best done by drying the plant in the paper bag in an oven at 150°F (65°C) for 10 to 12 hours. Do not microwave plant samples. Similarly, refrigerated samples quickly degrade, mold, and rot. Because most laboratories have specific submission requirements, contacting the laboratory before submission is recommended to ensure the sample is properly prepared and adequate sample sizes are sent (see **Box 2; Table 1**).

Some field studies may include evaluation of prepared feeds or forages. Because many feeds are not homogeneous, multiple samples are required to obtain representative results. As suggested previously, this is especially true for hay. Although bales can be taken apart and examined, patchy contamination often results in false-negative findings. Examining more bales may increase the chance of finding a contaminating plant. However, it is often more productive to examine the area where the hay or feed was harvested. Additionally, some symptoms of toxic plant ingestion are not manifested for days or even months after exposure. During the delay between ingestion and the development of symptoms, the contaminated feed may be consumed

Table 1
Partial list of tests, samples, sample size, and preservation for investigation of potential poisonous plant poisoning[1,2]

Test	Sample	Size	Shipping
Blood counts	Purple top blood tube	3–5 mL	Chilled shipped on ice
Serum biochemistries	Red top blood tube	5–10 mL	Chilled on ice or if frozen serum should be separated from the cells
Microscopic evaluation of tissues	Various tissues (see **Box 1**)	1 × 1 × 2 cm pieces	Fixed in formalin
Postmortem or necropsy	Dead or moribund animal	Whole animal	Fresh
Chemical evaluation of serum, blood, urine, or milk	Serum, whole blood, urine, or milk	20 mL	Stored in plastic tubes and shipped on ice or frozen
Chemical evaluation of tissue	Various tissues (the complete eye is the best tissue to analyze for nitrate poisoning)	2 × 2 × 4 cm pieces	Stored in plastic bags and shipped frozen
Chemical evaluation of feces or gastrointestinal contents	Feces or ingesta	5–6 g (about a sandwich bag full)	Stored in plastic bags and shipped frozen
Plant identification[a]	Whole plant	Whole plant including flowers, pods, leaves, stems, and roots	Fresh if delivered that day, dried if hand delivered later, pressed and dried if sent through the mail
Plant chemical analysis	Whole plants	5 or 6 whole plants	Fresh if delivered that day, dried if mailed or frozen if they can be maintained frozen during shipping
Hay for weed contamination and weed identification	Stored baled hay	5 or 6 bales	Dry
Hay for nitrate analysis	Hay	Several representative samples; these can be core samples, 5–6 g	Dry

(continued on next page)

Table 1 (continued)			
Test	Sample	Size	Shipping
Prepared feeds	Feeds	Representative feed samples, such as cubed feed, 5–6 g	Dry
Silage or green chopped feed	Feeds	Representative feed samples, 10–20 g	Frozen

[a] Be sure to check with the laboratory because they often require specific sampling, sample preparation, and shipping. Label all materials with indelible ink; provide date, owner, location, and contact information.

Modified from Stegelmeier BL. Identifying plant poisoning in livestock: diagnostic approaches and laboratory tests. *Vet Clin North Am Food Anim Prac* 2011;27:407-417; with permission.

making it unavailable for sampling. Close examination of the hay field before cutting the first crop provides the best indication of contamination. This also facilitates collecting plant samples for identification and chemical analysis. If field examination is not possible, multiple randomly collected samples are required. For example, hay submissions should include submission of at least five or six intact bales to maximize the chance of finding contaminating plants. Because many toxic plants are not highly palatable, examination of refused feed is also helpful. Core samples of hay are often used for nitrate or nutrient analysis, but they destroy plant morphology and therefore are of minimal use for plant identification. When more intensely prepared feed, such as pellets, are submitted for analysis, they should be randomly sampled, dried at low temperatures, and stored in paper bags so they do not mold.

Biologic Samples and Necropsy

The field studies, clinical presentation, and serum biochemical studies often lead to a list of possible causes of the observed animal disease. This is called a differential diagnosis and the goal now is to prove which diagnosis is the most likely cause. This is often a process of exclusion that may necessitate additional field investigations, plant collections, chemical analysis, and collection of blood or tissue samples. Necropsy is an extremely valuable tool to collect tissues and information.

Livestock producers often complain that the most expensive animals are the first to be poisoned and die. Producers should be reminded that if these early fatalities are used to prevent further losses, they indeed are the most valuable. A good postmortem examination, or necropsy, often provides the best information needed to formulate a definitive diagnosis. At times field necropsies are the only option; however, the best and most complete samples are obtained when animals are submitted whole to a veterinary diagnostic laboratory. For example, liver necrosis is often seen in animals poisoned with hepatotoxic plants, such as houndstongue (*Cynoglossum officinale*) (**Fig. 2**).[2] At necropsy hepatic necrosis is easily identified and a differential diagnosis will be generated and further studied. Rotten carcasses provide little information because toxins may degrade, tissues become difficult to identify, and collected samples are unsuitable for microscopic evaluation. Submission of freshly dead or moribund animals to a diagnostic laboratory can increase diagnostic speed and accuracy. Nearly all states have animal diagnostic laboratories that specialize in postmortem examinations and diagnosing animal diseases. State agriculture departments usually support these services and fees are minimal. The veterinary pathologists at

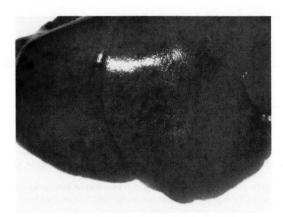

Fig. 2. Liver from a 28-day-old pig that was dosed for 10 days with purified riddelliine from Riddell groundsel or ragwort (*Senecio riddellii*). Notice the swollen liver with small red foci that make the tight lobular patterns apparent grossly. The entire liver is yellow and there was systemic icterus. *S riddellii* is a perennial small shrub 30 to 90 cm tall with small hairless bright green leaves. It has bright yellow flowers in late summer or fall. Riddell groundsel is unique because its toxic alkaloid is primarily a single dehydropyrrolizidine alkaloid known as riddelliine and its *N*-oxide. Riddelliine concentrations can vary within the same population because concentrations of nearly 14% were detected 1 year and the same plant populations and phenotype were less than 0.5% the subsequent year.[1]

these facilities have the experience and instrumentation to recognize, sample, and analyze postmortem tissue samples (see **Box 2**).

At necropsy (either a field necropsy or one performed in a diagnostic laboratory), animal tissue samples should be collected for microscopic studies (see **Box 1, Table 1**). These tissues should be small (1 × 1 × 2 cm) and preserved in fixative (10% neutral buffered formalin with volumes of about 10 times the volume of the tissues). Microscopic evaluation of animal tissues is helpful in identifying many disease and some plant-induced lesions. However, most of the plant-induced microscopic lesions are not specific for plant toxins. For example, DHPAs are potent hepatotoxins and would certainly be included in the differential diagnosis for liver necrosis. Microscopically HDPAs produce fibrosis and biliary hyperplasia (**Fig. 3**). Chronic poisoning with prolonged durations often result in altered cellular mitosis and megalocytosis (**Fig. 4**). These changes are highly suggestive of DHPA poisoning and narrow the differential diagnosis and direct the investigation to additional assays to support that as the most likely cause.[3] If there are no microscopic lesions or if information from microscopic studies does not specifically identify the cause, the results can always be used to exclude those toxins and other types of diseases that would have produced lesions. For example, the absence of characteristic liver disease and hepatic lesions makes DHPA poisoning unlikely.

Plant Fragment, Toxin, or Metabolite Analysis

Some toxic plants are good forages and they are palatable and readily consumed by livestock. With these plants poisoning occurs when animals ingest a toxic dose either by eating too much too quickly or when toxic plants are eaten by susceptible animals. Consequently ingesta, tissues, urine, and blood collected from nonpoisoned animals, clinically healthy animals, or even animals that died of some other disease may contain poisonous plant parts and toxins. These false-positives are confusing, but when

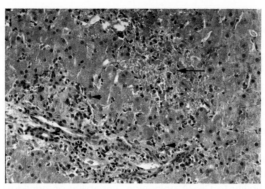

Fig. 3. Photomicrograph of the liver of a cow dosed with dried, ground tansy ragwort (*Senecio jacobea*). Notice the focal hemorrhagic necrosis (*arrow*). There is also extensive oval cell and biliary epithelial cell proliferation (*arrowheads*) with mild fibrosis and lymphocytic inflammation. Tansy ragwort is a widely distributed perennial that has invaded and poisoned animals in Western Europe, South Africa, Australia, New Zealand, and North America. It is a 50 to 150 cm plant with large variably sized leaves with two or three pinnate divisions. It has upright inflorescences with composite yellow flowers that develop into thousands of wind-dispersed seeds. It has spread and dominated many pastures and ranges resulting in livestock and wildlife poisoning (hematoxylin-eosin stain with original magnification of 100X).

interpreted with supporting clinical signs, and gross and microscopic lesions, they are usually easily sorted out and identified. Because plant toxin concentrations are likely to be highest in rumen and upper gastrointestinal ingesta and blood, at necropsy, gastrointestinal contents and blood should be collected and preserved for later physical, microscopic, and chemical evaluations if they are indicated. Many plants have characteristic leaves or cellular structures that are recognized in the ingesta. These morphology studies are technically challenging and a highly specialized skillful and experienced technician is required. Currently the best analysis is available through the Texas Veterinary Medical Diagnostic Laboratory (see **Box 2**).

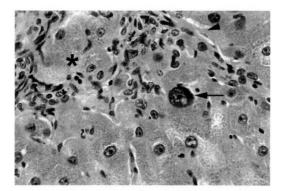

Fig. 4. Photomicrograph of a liver biopsy from horse treated with ground, dried houndstongue (*Cynoglossum officinale*) at a rate of 5 mg total dehydropyrrolizidine alkaloids/kg body weight for 10 days and allowed to recover for 45 days. Notice the large swollen hepatocytes (*asterisk*) and megalocytosis: large hepatocyte with a huge nucleus with prominent nuclear vacuolation (*arrow*) (hematoxylin-eosin stain with initial magnification of 400X).

Plant toxins or metabolites can also be identified in blood, serum, tissues or gastro-intestinal ingesta. For example, DHPAs are metabolized into potential alkylating agents called pyrroles that quickly react with liver tissues resulting in hepatic necrosis and liver failure. Recently testing has become available to identify and quantitate pyrroles in DHPA damaged liver (**Fig. 5**). Pyrrole detection provides definitive evidence of exposure and consumption, but it does not indicate DHPAs are the cause of either disease or death.[4] However, when a positive pyrrole result is combined with supporting clinical signs and histologic lesions consistent with DHPA poisoning, the diagnosis easily become the most likely cause. **Fig. 5** also clearly identifies a positive correlation ($R = 0.90$) of pyrrole concentrations with DHPA dose. This indicates that hepatic pyrrole concentrations are dose related. However, there is no pyrrole concentration that definitively indicates DHPA toxicity and disease. This is caused by marked variability of animal susceptibility to DHPA poisoning, variability of individual alkaloid toxicity, and DHPA-specific pyrrole production. Similar diagnostic challenges occur with toxin analysis for many other poisonous plants. With the exception of extremely toxic plants, such as Japanese yew (*Taxus* spp), or fluoroacetate-containing plants, chemical identification of plant toxins or metabolites is only indicative of exposure. False positives and overinterpretation can be avoided by carefully correlating these chemical results with clinical disease, postmortem findings, and microscopic findings. This is generally not too difficult if there are evidence of exposure, clinical signs, and pathologic lesions suggestive of a specific intoxication. However, these false positives become problematic when supporting evidence is not available. Some diagnostic laboratories have developed panels of plant alkaloid screens. These may also have false positives and should not be interpreted without supporting exposure, clinical signs, or pathologic lesions. Most plant toxins are unique and specific instruments and conditions are required to analyze and specifically quantitate each toxin. In any case if the cause is unknown, it is always good to collect potential samples and preserve them until a likely cause is established and specific assay can be used. Most samples are easily stored by freezing with exceptions of whole blood, which should be refrigerated, or tissues for microscopic analysis that should be fixed in formalin (see **Box 1**). Care should

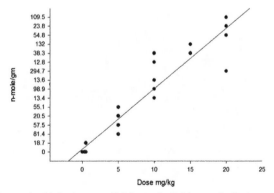

Fig. 5. Graph of pyrrole (dehydropyrrolizidine alkaloid metabolite) concentration in the liver of pigs that were dosed with purified riddelliine. As seen with the regression there is a positive correlation with dose that was significant with $r^2 = 0.90$. Pyrrole analysis was done following previously described techniques.[4] The animal work was also previously reported.[5] Similar positive correlations of pyrrole concentrations with PA dose have been seen in other species with variations relating duration and recovery time.

also be taken to ensure samples are properly shipped in a timely fashion that does not result in thawing during transport or delivery.

INTERPRETATION AND CONCLUSIONS

When all information is accumulated and probable diagnoses are evaluated and compared, the information often identifies a most likely diagnosis. This is challenging because some portions of the investigative results may seem contradictory. It is possible that no definitive diagnosis will emerge. Despite the contradictions, a most likely diagnosis or short list needs to be determined to formulate recommendations and treatment. From these consultations, a plan should be formulated to avoid additional poisoning and livestock losses. This step is often easy and inexpensive. For example, many PA-containing plants are controlled with herbicides and contaminated hay can be discarded or fed to resistant species. Other solutions may involve changes in grazing or animal management, herbicidal control, or a variety of other options.

Correctly organizing, collecting, and preserving materials, and enlisting the proper experts and techniques in the correct manner are essential in arriving at accurate diagnoses and formulating practical solutions for livestock poisoning by toxic plants. A rapid and accurate diagnosis not only aids in avoiding future losses, but provides a valuable guide to avoiding animal disease and suffering and to ensuring safe and high-quality animal products.

DISCLOSURE

The authors have nothing to disclose.

REFERENCES

1. Johnson AE, Molyneux RJ, Ralphs MH. Senecio: a dangerous plant for man and beast. Rangelands 1989;11:261–4.
2. Stegelmeier BL, Gardner DR, James LF, et al. Pyrrole detection and the pathologic progression of *Cynoglossum officinale* (houndstongue) poisoning in horses. J Vet Diagn Invest 1996;8:81–90.
3. Stegelmeier BL. Pyrrolizidine alkaloid-containing toxic plants (*Senecio*, *Crotalaria*, *Cynoglossum*, *Amsinckia*, *Heliotropium*, and *Echium* spp.). Vet Clin North Am Food Anim Pract 2011;27:419–28, ix.
4. Brown AW, Stegelmeier BL, Colegate SM, et al. The comparative toxicity of a reduced, crude comfrey (*Symphytum officinale*) alkaloid extract and the pure, comfrey-derived pyrrolizidine alkaloids, lycopsamine and intermedine in chicks (Gallus gallus domesticus). J Appl Toxicol 2016;36:716–25.
5. Stegelmeier BL, James LF, Panter KE, et al. Toxicity of a pyrrolizidine alkaloid, riddelliine, in neonatal pigs. In: Acamovic T, Stewart CS, Pennycott TW, editors. Poisonous plants and related toxins. Wallingford (United Kingdom): CABI; 2004. p. 44–9.

Neurotoxic Plants that Poison Livestock

Bryan L. Stegelmeier, DVM, PhD*, T. Zane Davis, PhD, Michael J. Clayton, DVM

KEYWORDS

- Poisonous plants • Neurotoxic plants • Livestock • Poisoning • Diagnosis

KEY POINTS

- Locoweed poisoning requires extended exposures to produce disease.
- Chronic locoweed poisoning and nitrotoxin poisoning have similar histologic lesions and are difficult to differentiate.
- Chemical analysis and chemotyping of larkspurs are helpful in developing management strategies.
- Chemical detection of many neurotoxins—larkspur, lupine, hemlocks, and death camas— in a variety of samples and tissues can be used to confirm exposure.
- When correlated with field studies and the lack of other gross and microscopic lesions, identification of neurotoxic plant toxins can be used to obtain a most likely diagnosis.

LOCOWEED

Locoweed poisoning, or locoism, is a neurologic disease that was historically considered to be the largest poisonous plant problem in the western United States.[1,2] Nearly a century ago, resources were first appropriated to provide livestock producers solutions to locoism. Despite huge advances in understanding and managing the disease, many problems persist and additional solutions to avoid poisoning are needed. Poisoning initially was described in horses, cattle, sheep, and goats. From this work, it became obvious that several plants were the cause of poisoning. These were commonly referred to as locoweeds and they included approximately 20 species of the *Astragalus* and *Oxytropis* genera.[1] The next 4 or 5 decades did little other than to map locoweed populations, characterize the extent of their toxicity, and educate livestock producers to avoid using contaminated ranges. In the 1960s and 1970s, more detailed publications were produced to better characterize both the clinical and histologic changes of poisoning. Extensive visceral and neuronal vacuolation of certain cell populations were identified. Additionally, this vacuolation was found to be similar to livestock poisoning caused by Australian *Swainsona* species.[3] Subsequent

USDA/ARS Poisonous Plant Research Laboratory, 1150 East 1400 North, Logan, UT 84341, USA
* Corresponding author.
E-mail address: Bryan.Stegelmeier@USDA.GOV

Vet Clin Food Anim 36 (2020) 673–688
https://doi.org/10.1016/j.cvfa.2020.08.002
0749-0720/20/Published by Elsevier Inc.

collaboration with Australian researchers found that the locoweeds also contained the *Swainsona* toxin, swainsonine.[4] Swainsonine is an indolizidine alkaloid that is produced by locoweed-specific endophytes.[5] It later was discovered that swainsonine inhibits lysosomal α-mannosidase and mannosidase II, which results in lysosomal accumulation of mannose-rich oligosaccharides. Microscopically, this is seen as characteristic visceral and neuronal vacuolation due to lysosomal accumulation of mannose-rich oligosaccharides. The resulting induced storage disease is biochemically, morphologically, and clinically indistinguishable from genetic mannosidosis.[6] Swainsonine and similar induced storage and neurologic disease subsequently have been identified in other toxic plants, including certain *Swainsona, Ipomoea, Turbina*, and *Sida* spp.[7]

Natural and experimental locoweed or swainsonine intoxication has been documented in sheep, cattle, goats, horses, rats, hamsters, mice, guinea pigs, rabbits, chickens, pigeons, elk, and deer.[8,9] Poisoning requires continuous inhibition of cellular mannosidases as a result of extended swainsonine ingestion. Intermittent poisoning of relatively short duration (less than 3 days) does not produce lesions or disease.[10] There is marked variability in species susceptibility to poisoning. Horses and cattle are most susceptible followed by sheep and goats. Rodents and some wildlife are relatively resistant to poisoning. Birds probably are totally resistant, although only a single species from 2 orders, Galliformes (chicken) and Columbinae (pigeons), were tested.[11] Susceptible species develop minimal signs after 10 days to 14 days of exposure. Although the early signs vary between species, all poisoned animals are reluctant to move and demonstrate loss of condition and emaciation that may occur in conditions of plentiful feed. The coat and hair appear dull and rough and do not shed during the appropriate season (**Fig. 1**). After 10 days to 14 days of poisoning, most animals develop weakness, mild proprioceptive deficits, and minimal intention tremors that are noticeable only when animals are forced to move. With continuous exposure for weeks and months, poisoned animals develop more severe neurologic signs, including depression, disorientation and obvious loss of proprioception, excitability, and irregular gait often including hypermetria and incoordination. The eyes appear dull and dry, but poisoned animals are visual, although severely affected animals may lack interest in what is seen. Some animals develop mild opisthotonos. With continued exposure, poisoned animals become anorexic and recumbent because

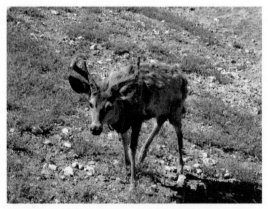

Fig. 1. Mule deer (*Odocoileus hemionus*) poisoned with locoweed (*Astragalus lentiginosus*) at a dose of 5 mg swainsonine/kg BW for 180 days. Notice the rough hair coat that has shed incompletely, with loss of body condition and dull-appearing eyes.

they often are reluctant to rise or have difficulty in rising. Poisoning generally is not fatal until the neurologically compromised animals encounter some mishap. Resistant species, such as rodents and some wildlife species, develop minimal neurologic signs although they become emaciated with extensive vacuolation of many visceral tissues.[12]

Most locoweed-poisoned animals do not have gross lesions. Some animals may have lesions attributed to secondary changes, such as heart failure, hydrops amnii, or abortion. Chronic poisoning also may have nonspecific changes related to loss of condition, such as cachexia and marked atrophy of adipose tissue.

The microscopic changes of locoweed poisoning are remarkable and characteristic of poisoning. Generally speaking, locoweed lesions can be described as widespread visceral and neurologic cytoplasmic vacuolation. The vacuolation is due to the lysosomal accumulation of incompletely processed glycoproteins and oligosaccharides. The extent and distribution of lesions are species-specific. Livestock all develop extensive neurologic vacuolation that is most severe in cerebellar Purkinje cells (the most consistent lesions are seen in the central cerebellar lobe) and large neurons of the basal ganglia (mostly gabanergic neurons) (**Fig. 2**A). Horses also develop extensive vacuolation of visceral and endocrine tissues, but the distribution is different than in other livestock. For example, equine liver has extensive vacuolation, but the thyroid epithelium has minimal change. Hepatocellular vacuolation in sheep and cattle is minimal and the thyroid is severely vacuolated. Rodents and deer have minimal neuronal vacuolation, but they have extensive vacuolation of the thyroid and pancreas. These animals develop neurologic lesions but only with high doses of very long duration (3 or more months).[9] Characteristic Purkinje cell lesions that correlate with the neurologic signs include massive cytoplasmic swelling and vacuolation with axonal dystrophy and abnormal neuritic processes, meganeurite formation at the axonal hillock, aberrant synapses, and dendritic outgrowths.[8,13,14] If poisoning is maintained for several weeks, mannose-rich glycoproteins within affected visceral epithelium and neurons can be identified by staining with biotinylated lectins.[15,16] Many of the visceral lesions are reversible, and recovery studies indicate that most resolve within weeks of discontinuing exposure.[8] Resolution of the neuronal vacuolation, however, is slower and if severe often results in neuronal necrosis. This is seen microscopically as neuronal empty baskets (**Fig. 2**B) and decreased numbers of Purkinje cells (**Fig. 2**C). Clinical poisoning generally is recurrent because animals use contaminated ranges over several years. Many locoweed populations are cyclic with increased growth and subsequent poisoning occurring in years of increased precipitation. The result of these repeated and sporadic poisonings is that affected animals slowly develop permanent neurologic deficits and disease that progress until the animal loses condition and is culled. Microscopic lesions of such chronically poisoned animals include decreased numbers of cerebellar Purkinje cells with subsequent axonal degeneration and spheroid formation (see **Fig. 2**C). Because many culled animals are necropsied when they are not actively poisoned, they may not have visceral epithelial cell vacuolation, complicating the diagnosis. Despite their poor body condition, some of these chronically poisoned animals may even be reproductively active. It is especially difficult to differentiate between the chronic neurologic lesions of locoweed and of other neurotoxins, such as the nitrotoxins.

Swainsonine poisoning damages both male and female reproductive functions. Although not all species have been evaluated, it has been shown that poisoning inhibits both spermatogenesis and spermatozoal function in sheep. Many testicular and spermatic lesions are reversible, but the time required for normal spermatozoa maturation should be considered. Severe poisoning in animals with extensive

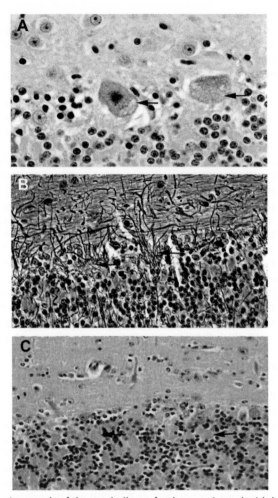

Fig. 2. (A) Photomicrograph of the cerebellum of a sheep poisoned with locoweed (*Oxytropis sericea*) to obtain swainsonine doses of 0.8 mg/kg for 30 days. Notice the extensive fine vacuolation of the Purkinje cell cytoplasm (*arrows*). This section was stained with lectin concavolin A and counter-stained with hematoxylin (the original magnification was 200X). (*B*) Silver stain of the cerebellum of a horse dosed with locoweed (*Astragalus lentiginosus*) to obtain swainsonine doses of 1.5 mg/kg for 45 days. Notice the empty baskets (*arrows*) where Purkinje cells have dropped out (original magnification 200X). (*C*) Central lobe of the cerebellum of a range cow that was poisoned repeatedly with Green River milkvetch (*Astragalus pubentissimus*). The cow was thin and emaciated with an obstinate mean attitude that made it difficult to herd and dangerous. She was lactating and she had a small, poor doing calf. Notice the lack of healthy Purkinje cells. Some eosinophilic bodies (*arrows*) that may be swollen axons or spheroids are visible in the superficial granular cell layer (hematoxylin-eosin stain, original magnification was 200X).

neurologic disease can result in the permanent loss of libido and the physical ability to breed.[17] The effects of poisoning on female reproduction include abortion and reduced fertility.[18] Studies in horses and cattle found that estrus cycles are altered as the ovaries become enlarged and cystic.[11,19] Although swainsonine does not appear to alter embryogenesis, implantation, or placentation, it probably is fetotoxic because early gestation fetuses often die, resulting in fetal and placental resorption.[20,21] Poisoned lambs that are not aborted often are born small and weak with various different arthropathies.[22,23] Transplacental and transmammary poisoning both produce fetal, neonatal, and juvenile microscopic lesions of characteristic neuro-visceral vacuolation and degeneration similar to adults. Poisoned cows also may develop placental abnormalities, such as hydrops amnii, and poisoned cattle are pre-disposed to develop altitude-related, congestive heart failure and high mountain dis-ease.[24] If neurologic damage is not extensive, many animals recover if they are removed from infested ranges. This is true especially of reproductive function and many previously poisoned animals become reproductively functional within several months.[11] Most of the neurologic lesions, however, are permanent, and severely poisoned animals may have irreversible neurologic deficits that especially precludes using permanently damaged animals for work.[8]

A diagnosis of locoweed poisoning is dependent on identifying exposure and inges-tion with supporting clinical signs and microscopic lesions. Because some locoweed populations have varying endophyte infections and subsequent swainsonine concen-tration, plant sampling and analysis may be indicated. Because endophyte infections are transmitted vertically in the seed, once populations are identified as toxic, the endophyte infection rates change little. Chemical detection of serum and tissue swain-sonine concentrations also can be used to identify animals currently ingesting loco-weeds. These assays have limited diagnostic usefulness, however, because swainsonine clearance is rapid with a half-life of approximately 20 hours. Conse-quently, samples collected from animals removed from locoweed infested ranges a couple of days prior to testing do not contain detectable serum swainsonine concen-trations. Certainly, previously poisoned animals present a diagnostic challenge that require both experience in identifying subtle microscopic changes and close compar-ison to appropriate negative controls.

NITROTOXINS

There are more than 250 nitrotoxin-containing *Astragalus* species that have been identi-fied in North America.[25,26] Nitrotoxin poisoning also is a global problem because many more toxic *Astragalus* species have been identified in Europe, Asia, and South America.[27] Additionally, there are additional species of the *Cornoilla*, *Indigofera*, *Lotus*, and *Hippo-crepis* genera and several fungi from *Arthrinium*, *Aspergillus*, and *Penicillium* genera have been shown to produce nitrotoxins.[25] Nitrotoxins generally are found in plants as glycosides. A common glycoside is miserotoxin, the β-D-glucoside of 3-nitro-1-propa-nol.[28] Glycosides are not directly toxic, but they become toxic as they are hydrolyzed in the rumen or upper gastrointestinal tract into nitropropanol and nitropropionic acid (NPA).[29] Because most clinical poisonings involve cattle, it has been suggested that non-ruminants may be less susceptible to poisoning. Poisoning has been reported, however, in monogastric livestock and laboratory animals.[25,30] NPA has been shown to irreversibly inhibit succinate dehydrogenase and subsequently block oxidative phosphorylation.[31,32] The nitrotoxins also oxidize hemoglobin, and methemoglobinemia has been used as an indicator of poisoning. Methemoglobin does not appear to be an important part of the neurologic disease because both the concentration of methemoglobin and prevention of its formation do not alter the progression of neurologic disease.[33]

Gabanergic neurons that are common in the basal ganglia appear to be especially sensitive to NPA damage. It has been suggested that NPA toxicity accentuates gluta-mate toxicity, possibly through the *N*-methyl-D-aspartate receptor.[34] Clinical and his-tologic studies, however, have documented damage to many tissues where glutamate is not a contributing factor. Poisoned cattle develop severe respiratory dyspnea, muscular incoordination and weakness, frequent urination, cyanotic mucous membranes, and collapse and eventually become recumbent. Although a nonspecific change, wasted animals with chronic NPA poisoning often are described as having rear limb incoordination, proprioceptive deficits, weakness, and altered gait, resulting in interference or clacker heels (**Fig. 3**). Lethal doses typically are fatal within 24 hours. Cattle appear to be much more susceptible than sheep. Gross lesions often are nonspecific agonal changes, including pulmonary edema and congestion with extensive interlobular edema, emphysema, and pericardial petechial hemorrhages. Histologic lesions in cattle include necrosis of the thalamus, patchy cerebellar Purkinje cell necrosis, spongiosis of the white tracts in the globus pallidus, distension of the lateral ventricles, and wallerian degeneration of the ventral and lateral columns of the spinal cord and of the sciatic nerves.[25,30,33] Rodent toxicity studies also described neuronal degeneration, axonal and dendritic swelling, and myelin degeneration of the caudate nucleus, putamen, globus pallidus, and substantia nigra. Degeneration also occurs in the hippocampus and thalamus.[32]

NPA toxicity in horses remains largely unknown. One potential NPA intoxication in horses may be Australian Birdsville disease caused by ingestion of *Indigofera linnaei*. Like poisoned cattle, affected horses are weak, depressed, and uncoordinated and may shiver, twitch, and sway when standing. The histologic changes have not been characterized completely but there also appears to be neuronal degeneration and necrosis in the basal ganglia.[35] More work is needed to determine nitrotoxin involvement because *Indigofera linnaei* also contains indospicine. Indospicine is a toxic amino acid that causes severe hepatocellular degeneration and necrosis in dogs eating indospicine contaminated meat. Indospicine does not seem to affect horses.[36,37]

Diagnosis is made largely by correlating exposure to plants with clinical and histologic changes. Chronic poisoning is especially difficult to identify microscopically because the lesion primarily affects neurons in the basal ganglia that secondarily alter cerebellar Purkinje cell populations.

LARKSPURS

The larkspurs (*Delphinium* spp) are a diverse group of plants and, although their toxicity and toxins are similar, the different larkspurs grow in different plant communities, producing different poisoning scenarios. The tall larkspurs (primarily *D barbeyi*, *D occidentale*, *D glaucescens*, and *D glaucum* [**Fig. 4**]) grow in high mountain ranges

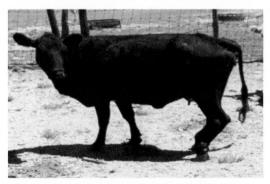

Fig. 3. Cow chronically poised with miserotoxin containing Emory milkvetch (*Astragalus emoryanus*). Notice the severe rear leg weakness with knuckling that caused interference or clacking when she moves.

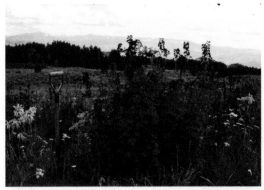

Fig. 4. Tall larkspur, *D barbeyi*, found in a mixed plant community in eastern Utah. *D barbeyi* is a perennial herb found in Arizona, Colorado, New Mexico, Utah, and Wyoming. It grows early in the spring, producing a highly toxic vegetative forb approximately 0.5 m to 1 m tall. Most cattle find this phenotype unpalatable. Later in early summer, the plant produces a tall flowering racemes that may have up to 50 flowers that have the characteristic spurlike sepal. This phenotype is moderately toxic; however, cattle find it more palatable and often cyclically consume the plant. Cattle poisoning and deaths generally occur when, under some undefined conditions, the plant becomes more palatable and animals consume lethal doses. Later in the season, tall larkspur produces seed in a 2.0-cm to 2.5-cm pod. These phenotypes are less toxic. Some management strategies include late season grazing on dense *D barbeyi* ranges after the pods have shattered and the plant toxicity is comparatively low.

and pastures where moisture is relatively abundant. They often are found on north-facing slopes, where winter snows accumulate, and the subsequent moisture consistently produces tall robust plants. These constant tall larkspur populations result in endemic cattle poisoning that in some ranges can produce yearly herd mortalities as high as 10%. Not all tall larkspur populations are toxic, however, even within the same species and general location.[38] Although most producers using larkspur-infested ranges have experience that allows them to map toxic populations, this may not be the most effective method to avoid poisoning. An alternative to using actual poisoning may be appropriate population sampling and chemical analysis. Plant chemotypes are useful tools to map toxic populations. These maps can be used to predict the risk of poisoning and to develop management strategies to minimize poisoning.

The low larkspurs (*D nuttallianum*, *D andersonii*, and *D bicolor* [**Fig. 5**]) grow in most pastures and meadows, and their populations can expand to the extent that the fields appear blue with larkspur flowers. Growing before most grasses and other forbs, low larkpsurs sprout in early spring; flower and throw seed in late spring; and shatter and senesce in early summer. So, the time when there is adequate, palatable larkspur mass to poison cattle is relatively short. Low larkspurs generally have cyclic growth patterns, with populations markedly expanding in years with above normal spring precipitation. Consequently, poisoning tends to be sporadic, with epidemic losses involving many animals, with mortalities up to 40% to 50%.[39] Such catastrophic poisoning occurs most often when hungry cattle are inadvertently put in contaminated meadow pastures or ranges. Young, naïve cattle are those poisoned most often. The signs of low larkpsur poisoning appear to progress rapidly because most animals are simply found dead. Plant toxicity and subsequently risk of poisoning drop when plants senesce and dry up. The other larkspurs (*D geyeri* [foothills larkspur] and *D virescens* [plains larkspur]) generally have more stable populations, and cattle poisoning is dependent on both population expansion and endemic plant populations.

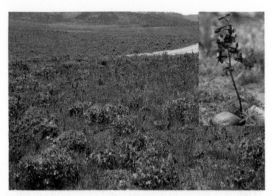

Fig. 5. Low larkspur (*D andersonii*) from southeastern Idaho. Low and foothill larkspurs grow in the early spring, commonly poisoning cattle when susceptible animals are put on infested pastures and ranges. They are erect perennials that grow up to 50 cm tall. (Inset) demonstrates an individual D andersonii that demonstrates the hairy leaves and stems and produce deep blue to purple flowers that that have the typical larkspur spur.

Cattle are uniquely sensitive to larkspur poisoning, whereas clinical poisoning in other species does not occur. The first signs of poisoning in cattle is restlessness and agitation. More severely poisoned cattle develop muscular tremors that initially are noticeable in the front limbs. Other signs include frequent urination, incomplete defecation, tachypnea, tachycardia, and severe general muscular weakness that leads to periodic collapse. Severely poisoned animals have a stiff, staggering gait and are only temporarily mobile. Often, they lapse into sternal and lateral recumbency, and if they cannot recover from lateral recumbency they bloat. Fatally poisoned animals have severe dyspnea, and death results from hypoxia caused by respiratory paralysis and bloat. Exertion or excitement hastens and exacerbates the clinical signs. Although poisoned animals often have gross lesions of rumen tympany (an esophageal bloat line may be apparent) and pulmonary lesions of severe dyspnea (emphysema and petechial serosal hemorrhages), there are essentially no specific gross or histopathologic lesions that characterize poisoning.

The larkspur alkaloids have their primary effect in cattle at the neuromuscular junction. Larkspur alkaloids are nicotinic acetylcholine (nACh) receptor antagonists that reduce synaptic efficacy and block neuromuscular transmission.[40] Specific nACh receptor studies indicated the majority of *Delphinium* alkaloids act at $\alpha7$-nACh receptors, at least in the intercardiac ganglia.[41] The alkaloid structure and subsequent binding affinity result in markedly different toxicity for the individual alkaloids. Chemical analysis and characterization of a population's alkaloid profile can be used to generate a population specific chemotype that can be used to determine poisoning potential and risk.[42] Receptor binding appears to be competitive and acetylcholinesterase inhibitors, such as neostigmine (0.02–0.04 mg/kg intramuscularly or intravenously [IV]) or physostigmine (0.04 mg/kg IV) can be used to temporarily reverse many of the clinical signs.[43] The effect is short lived and multiple treatments may be needed. The goal is to keep cattle calm and maintain sternal recumbency to reduce bloating until the toxins are excreted. In severe cases, bloat also may be alleviated by passing a stomach tube or by trocarizing the rumen to relieve the pressure. Stress and physical exertion exacerbate the progression of clinical signs and increase the risk of death; hence, treatment should be reserved until poisoning is severe and minimal restraint is required for treatment.

A definitive diagnosis is made by confirming larkspur exposure and consumption, excluding other causes of sudden death (seen as the lack of gross and histologic lesions as produced by many other causes of sudden death), and associating these findings with compatible clinical signs and clinical course. Most poisoned animals are found dead. Because the clinical course often is short, identifying poisoned animals is difficult and often requires close and frequent examination. Documenting exposure may be done by identifying consumed plants, gross or microscopic identification of larkspur plant fragments in rumen contents, or by identifying larkspur toxins in blood, tissues, or other samples. Because cattle often ingest nonlethal larkspur doses, the risk of false positives (identifying larkspur toxins in animals that have not been lethally poisoned) is likely. New analytical technology can detect larkspur toxins in a variety of animal samples, including serum, rumen contents, nasal mucous, oral fluid, aqueous humor, and ear wax.[44] Serum and rumen contents, however, are the preferred samples, because they reflect more accurately the immediate concentrations that result in poisoning. Serum and rumen contents also contain higher toxin concentrations that generally are more reliable and easily detected. There is wide variation in susceptibility between individual animals, breeds, sex, and ages of cattle. As a result, serum or rumen larkspur concentrations indicative of fatal poisoning are not available. Positive analysis and detection of larkspur toxins in any of these tissues only definitively confirms larkspur exposure and ingestion, not poisoning. Correlating clinical signs, exposure, and lack of gross and histologic changes as well as documents exposure is essential to obtain a most likely diagnosis.

CENTAUREA SPP

There are 450 to 500 species of *Centaurea* and 29 have been described in North America.[45] Most are invasive and have aggressively invaded rangelands and pastures, especially those that have been overgrazed, burned or, disturbed. Of these, only 2 are of any toxicologic significance, *C repens* (Russian knapweed) and *C solstitialis* (yellow star thistle). Both these species are only known to poison horses.

Yellow star thistle is considered a noxious invasive weed in the western United States, where in many ranges it has spread and dominated some plant communities.[45–47] Russian knapweed also invades rangelands; however, more often it is a problem in pastures and fields.[45] Although the aggressive nature of these species threatens horses, the real economic loss is due to loss of sensitive or threatened native plant species and the balance of plant biodiversity.

Poisoning has been referred to as a disease of abuse because horses must be forced by the lack of alternative feed to eat the plant for weeks or months. Several sesquiterpene lactones have been suggested as likely causes. Of these compounds, repin, subluteolide, janerin, cynaropicrin, acroptilin, and solstitialin have been screened for in vitro neuronal and fetal tissue cytotoxicity, although none has been identified as the definitive toxin. It also has been suggested that sesquiterpene lactones are unstable and they are metabolized quickly into some yet undiscovered neurotoxin.[48,49] Other investigators have suggested pathogenesis is similar to Parkinson disease, because there are aspartic and glutamic acids present in these plants that also have neuroexcitatory properties.[50]

As indicated, yellow star thistle and Russian knapweed only poison horses and these *Centaurea* species may be useful forage for sheep and goats. There are rare reports of sesquiterpene lactone toxicity, however, in other species. In South Africa, Russian knapweed fed to sheep at 600 g for 2 days caused acute digestive upset, pulmonary edema, and ascites.[51] Later in Azerbaijan, Russian knapweed was reported to cause chewing disease in buffalo similar to that described in horses. No neuropathologic microscopic findings were identified, however, and it was suggested that the reported chewing disease actually was mustard-associated wooden tongue.[52]

Poisoning occurs most often in the late summer and fall, when alternative forages are depleted and horses are forced to graze knapweed or yellow star thistle. Certain horses develop a taste for these weeds and some investigators have suggested that palatability increases when plants are treated with herbicide. Poisoning requires ingestion for several weeks or months before an abrupt onset of neurologic dysfunction. The clinical presentation is characterized first by impaired eating and drinking followed by mental depression with hypertonicity and abnormal posture of the lips and tongue. Some horses may stand with their mouth open and tongue protruding. Other may manifest nonproductive chewing motions resulting in reference to the disease as "chewing disease." The end stages of poisoning are complicated by dehydration and nutritional disease as affected horses develop locomotor and awareness deficits. Some may walk aimlessly and others appear drowsy as they continually stand with their suspensory ligaments locked and their head low as if they were sleeping. The neurologic disease is considered permanent and, once severe neurologic signs are observed, prognosis for recovery is poor and euthanasia should be considered.[53,54]

The lesions are specific and described as necrosis of the globus pallidus and the substantia nigra (nigropallidal encephalomalacia) (**Fig. 6**). The lesions are grossly evident and typically bilateral and symmetric.[53,54] The microscopic lesions are degeneration and necrosis of neurons in the nuclei, with smaller foci of degeneration and satellitosis in the adjacent pars reticularis. The necrosis generally involves the entire nuclei with proliferation of glia and capillaries within sharply defined margins of the involved nuclei. Occasionally, secondary lesions may be observed in the adjacent gray and white matter of the brain.

Yellow star thistle and Russian knapweed poisoning are unique because the clinical disease, and histologic lesions are specific for poisoning. The prognosis for recovery is poor because, even with good supportive therapy, including easy access to high-quality feed and water, supplemental vitamins, and good nursing care, most horses do not recover. Certainly, avoiding poisoning is best and when animals are first observed grazing *Centaurea* species, they should be moved immediately to pastures with adequate forage.

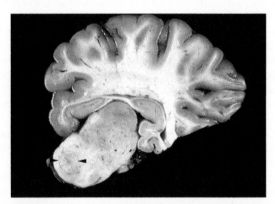

Fig. 6. Cross-section of the basal ganglia of a horse poisoned with yellow star thistle (*C solstitialis*). Notice the yellow soft zone of necrosis (*arrowheads*) that involves the globus pallidus.

HEMLOCKS

The toxic hemlocks are members of the Umbelliferae family and comprise 2 separate genera: *Conium maculatum* (poison hemlock) and *Cicuta* spp (water hemlock).

Poison hemlock is a biennial that can grow 2 m tall with white flowers and distinguishing purple spots on the stem. Both piperidine alkaloids γ-coniceine and coniine (nACh receptor agonists) have been identified in all parts of the plant. The plant mostly is unpalatable and poisoning generally occurs in the early spring, when the small early sprouts are the only green forage present and growing. Fatal poisoning results most often from feeding contaminated fresh green chopped forages. The clinical signs of poisoning include initial stimulation (nervousness), resulting in frequent urination and defecation, tachycardia, temporarily impaired vision as the nictitating membrane fails to retract, muscular weakness, muscle fasciculations, ataxia, and incoordination followed by depression, recumbency, collapse, and ultimately death from respiratory failure.[55] The mechanism of action of the *Conium* alkaloids is 2-fold. The most serious effect occurs at the neuromuscular junction, where the alkaloids act as nondepolarizing blockers like curare.[56] The systemic effects generally are less severe and include nicotinic effects, such as salivation, mydriasis, and tachycardia, followed by bradycardia. This probably is a result of their action in autonomic ganglia. Horses generally are poisoned when eating small plants that sprout early in the spring. This often presents in individuals that are weak, trembling, and recumbent. Poisoned animals often have been described as having a distinct mousy-urine smell, although, in my opinion, it is better described as an almond-like smell. If poisoned animals are allowed to calmly clear the toxin, they slowly recover in 2 hours to 4 hours. In cattle, poisoning often is fatal because they most commonly are poisoned by eating contaminated green-chopped hay. Hay is harvested later in the season when poison hemlock plants are quite large. The resulting contamination is extensive, resulting in ingestion of relatively high doses. Contaminated cured hay is less toxic, suggesting that the coniine is degraded with storage.

Water hemlock is a similar biennial plant that also grows to approximately 2 m tall. It has a carrot-like leaf, but it has tuberous, multichambered root. It requires a wet habitat and is found in streambeds and along ditch banks. The water hemlock toxin has been identified as an unsaturated alcohol, cicutoxin. It is a potent convulsant that has been shown to be an antagonist of γ-aminobutyric acid receptors.[57,58] Clinical presentation of poisoning is severe convulsive seizures that are characterized by ataxia, dyspnea, muscular tremors, and weakness that progress to spastic head and neck movements and intermittent grand mal seizures followed by periods of exhaustion with minimal relaxation. If the seizures are not controlled, death occurs due to asphyxia.[59]

The postmortem and histologic findings with both types of hemlock poisoning are nonspecific and generally related to an animal's agonal condition—dermal abrasions, bruising, and petechiae on serosal surfaces with intense convulsions. Human poisonings usually are accidental because hemlocks are misidentified as herbs or medicinal plants.[60] Hemlock toxins can be identified in serum, urine, and gastric contents, and the best diagnosis can be made by correlating exposure with the clinical signs and lack of significant lesions.

LUPINES

Lupines (*Lupinus* spp) include plants with a worldwide distribution and varying toxicity and poisoning syndromes.[61] Reproductive toxicity currently is the more common problem, but historically, lupine, quinolizidine, and piperidine lupine alkaloids were most noted for producing fatal acute neurologic disease in sheep. This has changed largely due to changing in stocking because sheep are less common and cattle use has expanded on most lupine-infested western ranges. Sheep prefer to eat the highly toxic seed pods and historically this preference was potentiated further when herders moved hungry animals onto lupine patches or when snow covered alternative feeds. The consequence was that sheep nonselectively grazed lupine pods, resulting in hundreds of deaths. Some lupines in the pod stage also were unknowingly harvested as hay to be fed in the winter. Lupine seeds are highly toxic because doses as low as 0.25% to 1.5% of their body weight are fatally toxic to sheep. The clinical signs of poisoning include nervousness, urination and defecation, depression, frothing at the mouth, ataxia, muscular fasciculations weakness, lethargy, collapse, recumbency, respiratory failure, and death.[62] As with most neurotoxins, postmortem and histologic examinations of poisoned animals are unremarkable. Neurotoxic lupine alkaloids include anagyrine and lupanine (quinolizidine alkaloids), and ammodendrine and N-methyl ammodendrine (piperidine alkaloids). All appear to be nicotinic agonists at acetylcholine receptors. Additionally, quinolizidine alkaloids have some activity at muscarinic acetylcholine receptors.[63] The lupine alkaloids can be detected chemically in serum, rumen contents, and many other tissues to confirm exposure. Because lupines are relatively good forages, they commonly are eaten at sublethal doses, and correlation of exposure with clinical signs is essential to formulate a most likely diagnosis.

DEATH CAMAS

Death camas (*Zigadenus* spp) are endogenous plants of North and Central America. They typically grow in the early spring and after flowering they quickly senesce in the early summer. Poisoning occurs when livestock eat the whole plants or bulbs. Plant populations vary with available moisture, and environmental population expansions can result in epidemic type fatalities.[64] Human poisonings occur when bulbs and tubers are confused with those of other edible plants.[65]

Zigadenus spp contain steroidal alkaloids that have been identified as germine, pertoverine, and zygadenine with their glycoside derivatives—germidine, neogermidine, neogermitrine, protoveratridine, protoveratrine, vanilloylzygadenine, vertroylzygadenine, and zygacine. Of these, zygacine is the most prevalent and often is used to monitor exposure and toxicity. Although the exact mechanism of toxicity has not been identified, these alkaloids are suspected of altering membrane action potential and homeostasis by impairing sodium transport. Although these steroidal alkaloids are found in varying combinations and concentrations in the different species, all species are considered to be toxic.

Poisoning produces frothy salivation, hypothermia, depression, nausea, vomiting, retching, colic, and grinding of teeth. As the disease progresses signs include severe trembling, incoordination, depression, and weakness. Affected animals often stand with their heads held low, ears drooped, and backs arched. Poisoning also increases intestinal peristalsis with frequent defecation and urination. Fatally poisoned animals develop tachycardia, severe dyspnea, recumbent coma, and death. All animals are susceptible to poisoning, although sheep seem to be poisoned most often. It is suggested that this is due to their grazing preferences and manner because they often pull and eat plant tuber and roots.[45,64] Cattle also may be poisoned more frequently when conditions are moist and it has been suggested this enables them to pull up and ingest the roots.[45,64] Recent findings suggest that combined poisoning with larkspur and death camas is common. Additionally it has been shown that the toxic effects of these plants are additive, despite the marked difference in mechanisms of action.[66,67] Zygacine appears to be quickly metabolized because it is not commonly detected in serum or gastrointestinal contents. Correlating field study evidence of exposure, clinical signs, and lack of gross and histologic lesions provides the most positive diagnosis. Avoiding exposure is the best way to prevent poisoning. Treatments suggested for poisoned animals include atropine, picrotoxin, and activated charcoal. Atropine and dopamine treatments are used for human poisoning, but little has been done to confirm their effectiveness in livestock.[65]

SUMMARY

Some neurotoxic plants do not produce significant clinical or microscopic lesions. Additionally, some may be consumed at sublethal doses, and subsequently plant toxins commonly are present in the serum, ingesta, and other animal tissues. Care is needed to avoid overintrepreting these results. An accurate diagnosis depends on correlating exposures as determined by field studies or identification of plant fragments or toxins in ingesta, serum, or tissues, with supporting clinical disease and lack of lesions indicative of other disease. This is contrasted by the locoweeds, nitrotoxin-containing plants, Russian knapweed, and yellow star thistle that produce significant and distinct lesions that can be definitively used to identify poisoning. This list of neurotoxic plants is incomplete and readers are directed to more extensive references for those plants considered less common for this review.[45,46]

DISCLOSURE

The authors have nothing to disclose.

REFERENCES

1. Marsh CD. Stock-poisoning plants of the range. United States Department of Agriculture. Bureau of Animal Industry. Bulletin 1245. Washington DC. 1929. p. 22–44.
2. Marsh CD. The locoweed disease of the plains. United States Department of Agriculture Bureau animal industry Bulletin, No. 112, 1909 Washington, DC. 1909.
3. Colegate SM, Dorling PR, Huxtable CR. A spectroscopic investigation of swainsonine: an alpha-mannosidase inhibitor isolated from Swainsona canescens [a plant poisonous to livestock]. Aust J Chem 1979;32:2257–64.
4. Molyneux RJ, James LF. Loco intoxication: Indolizidine alkaloids of spotted locoweed (Astragalus lentiginosus). Science 1982;216:190–1.
5. Cook D, Gardner DR, Grum D, et al. Swainsonine and endophyte relationships in Astragalus mollissimus and Astragalus lentiginosus. J Agric Food Chem 2011;59:1281–7.
6. Dorling PR, Huxtable CR, Vogel P. Lysosomal storage in Swainsona spp. toxicosis: an induced mannosidosis. Neuropathol Appl Neurobiol 1978;4:285–95.
7. Cook D, Gardner DR, Pfister JA. Swainsonine-containing plants and their relationship to endophytic fungi. J Agric Food Chem 2014;62:7326–34.
8. Stegelmeier BL, James LF, Panter KE, et al. The pathogenesis and toxicokinetics of locoweed (Astragalus and Oxytropis spp.) poisoning in livestock. J Nat Toxins 1999;8:35–45.
9. Stegelmeier BL, Lee ST, James LF, et al. The comparative pathology of locoweed poisoning in livestock, wildlife and rodents. In: Panter KE, Wierenga TL,

Pfister JA, editors. Poisonous plants global research and solutions. Cambridge (MA): CABI Publishing; 2007. p. 359–65.

10. Stegelmeier BL, James LF, Panter KE, et al. The clinical and morphological changes of intermittent locoweed (Oxytropis sericea) poisoning in sheep. In: Acamovic T, Stewart CS, Pennycott TW, editors. Poisonous plants and related toxins. Wallingford (United Kingdom): CABI Publishing; 2004. p. 431–5.

11. Stegelmeier BL, Davis TZ, Welch KD, et al. The comparative pathology of locoweed poisoning in horses and other livestock. In: Riet-Correa F, Pfister JA, Schild AL, et al, editors. Poisoning by plants, myocotoxins,and related toxins. Oxfordshire (United Kingdom): CABI; 2011. p. 309–10.

12. Stegelmeier BL, James LF, Gardner DR, et al. Locoweed (Oxytropis sericea)-induced lesions in mule deer (Odocoileius hemionus). Vet Pathol 2005;42:566–78.

13. Huxtable CR, Dorling PR, Walkley SU. Onset and regression of neuroaxonal lesions in sheep with mannosidosis induced experimentally with swainsonine. Acta Neuropathol 1982;58:27–33.

14. Walkley SU, James LF. Locoweed-induced neuronal storage disease characterized by meganeurite formation. Brain Res 1984;324:145–50.

15. Alroy J, Orgad U, Ucci AA, et al. Swainsonine toxicosis mimics lectin histochemistry of mannosidosis. Vet Pathol 1985;22:311–6.

16. Stegelmeier BL, Molyneux RJ, Elbein AD, et al. The lesions of locoweed (Astragalus mollissimus), swainsonine, and castanospermine in rats. Vet Pathol 1995; 32:289–98.

17. Panter KE, James LF, Stegelmeier BL, et al. Locoweeds: Effects on reproduction in livestock. J Nat Toxins 1999;8:53–62.

18. Balls LD, James LF. Effect of locoweed (Astragalus spp.) on reproductive performance of ewes. J Am Vet Med Assoc 1973;162:291–2.

19. Stegelmeier BL, Snyder PD, James LF, et al. The immunologic and toxic effects of locoweed (Astragalus lentiginosus) intoxication in cattle. In: Garland TR, editor. Toxic plants and other natural toxicants. Wallingford (United Kingdom): CAB International; 1998. p. 285–90.

20. Wang S, Panter KE, Holyoak GR, et al. Development and viability of bovine preplacentation embryos treated with swainsonine in vitro. Anim Reprod Sci 1999;56:19–29.

21. Furlan S, Panter KE, Pfister JA, et al. Fetotoxic effects of locoweed (Astragalus lentiginosus) in pregnant goats. In: Panter KE, Wierenga TL, Pfister JA, editors. Poisonous plants: global research and solutions. Wallingford (United Kingdom): CABI; 2007. p. 130–5.

22. James LF, Shupe JL, Binns W, et al. Abortive and teratogenic effects of locoweed on sheep and cattle. Am J Vet Res 1967;28:1379–88.

23. Astorga JB, Pfister JA, Stegelmeier BL. Maternal ingestion of locoweed: II. The ability of intoxicated ewes to discriminate their own lamb. Sm Rum Res 2006;65:64–9.

24. James LF, Hartley WF, Van Kampen KR, et al. Relationship between ingestion of the locoweed, Oxytropis sericea and congestive right-sided heart failure in cattle. Am J Vet Res 1983;44:254–9.

25. Anderson RC, Majak W, Rassmussen MA, et al. Toxicity and metabolism of the conjugates of 3-nitropropanol and 3-nitropropionic acid in forages poisonous to livestock. J Agric Food Chem 2005;53:2344–50.

26. Williams MC, Barneby RC. The occurrence of nitrotoxins in North America Astragalus (Fabaceae). Brittonia 1977;29:310–26.

27. Williams MC, Barneby RC. The occurrence of nitro-toxins in Old World and South American Astragalus (Fabacaeae). Brittonia 1977;29:327–31.

28. Stermitz FR, Norris FA, Willams MC. Miserotoxin, a new naturally occurring nitro compound. J Am Chem Soc 1969;91:4599–600.

29. Williams MC, Norris FA, Van Kampen KR. Metabolism of miserotoxin to 3-nitro-1-propanol in bovine and ovine ruminal fluids. Am J Vet Res 1970;31:259–62.

30. Williams MC, Van Kampen KR, Norris FA. Timber milkvetch poisoning in chickens, rabbits, and cattle. Am J Vet Res 1969;30:2185–90.

31. Alston TA, Mela L, Bright HJ. 3-Nitropropionate, the toxic substance of Indigofera , is a suicide inactivator of succinate dehydrogenase. Proc Natl Acad Sci U S A 1977;74:3767–71.

32. Gould DH, Gustine DL. Basal ganglia degeneration, myelin alterations, and enzyme inhibition induced in mice by the plant toxin, 3-nitropropanoic acid. Neuropathol Appl Neurobiol 1982;8:377–93.

33. James LF, Hartley WJ, Van-Kampen KR. Syndromes of Astragalus poisoning in livestock. J Am Vet Med Assoc 1981;178:146–50.

34. Albin RL. Basal ganglia neurotoxins. Neurol Clin 2000;18:665–80.

35. Carroll AG, Swain BJ. Birdsville disease in the central highlands area of Queensland. Aust Vet J 1983;60:316–7.

36. Hegarty MP, Kelly WR, McEwan D, et al. Hepatotoxicity to dogs of horse meat contaminated with indospicine. Aust Vet J 1988;65:337–40.

37. FitzGerald LM, Fletcher MT, Paul AE, et al. Hepatotoxicosis in dogs consuming a diet of camel meat contaminated with indospicine. Aust Vet J 2011;89:95–100.

38. Gardner DR, Ralphs MH, Turner DL, et al. Taxonomic implications of diterpene alkaloids in three toxic tall larkspur species (*Delphenium* spp.). Biochem Syst Ecol 2002;30:77–90.

39. Pfister JA, Gardner DR, Stegelmeier BL, et al. Catastrophic cattle loss to low larkspur (Delphinium nuttallianum) in Idaho. Vet Hum Toxicol 2003;45:137–9.

40. Dobelis P, Madl JE, Manners GD, et al. Antagonism of nicotinic receptors by Delphinium alkaloids. Soc Neruosci Abstracts 1993;631:12.

41. Green BT, Welch KD, Cook D, et al. Potentiation of the actions of acetylcholine, epibatidine, and nicotine by methyllycaconitine at fetal muscle-type nicotinic acetylcholine receptors. Eur J Pharmacol 2011;662:15–21.

42. Manners GD, Panter KE, Pelletier SW. Structure-activity relationships of norditerpenoid alkaloids occurring in toxic larkspur (Delphinium) species. J Nat Prod 1995;58:863–9.

43. Green BT, Lee ST, Welch KD, et al. The serum concentrations of lupine alkaloids in orally-dosed Holstein cattle. Res Vet Sci 2015;100:239–44.

44. Lee ST, Stonecipher CA, Dos Santos FC, et al. An Evaluation of Hair, Oral Fluid, Earwax, and Nasal Mucus as Noninvasive Specimens to Determine Livestock Exposure to Teratogenic Lupine Species. J Agric Food Chem 2019;67:43–9.

45. Burrows GE, Tyrl RJ. Toxic plants of North America. Iowa State Press; 2001.

46. Knight AP, Walter RG. A guide to plant poisoning. Jackson (WY): Teton Newmedia; 2001.

47. Panter KE. Neurotoxicity of the knapweeds (Centaurea spp.) in horses. In: James LF, Evans JO, Ralphs MH, et al, editors. Noxious range weeds. Boulder (CO): Westview Press; 1991. p. 316–24.

48. Riopelle RJ, Boegman RJ, Little PB. Neurotoxicity of sesquiterpene lactones. In: Keeler RF, Bailey EM, Cheeke PR, editors. Poisonous plants. Ames (IA): Iowa State University Press; 1992. p. 298–303.

49. Cheng CH, Costall B, Hamburger M, et al. Toxic effects of solstitialin A 13-acetate and cynaropicrin from Centaurea solstitialis L. (Asteraceae) in cell cultures of foetal rat brain. Neuropharmacology 1992;31:271–7.

50. Roy DN, Peyton DH, Spencer PS. Isolation and identification of two potent neurotoxins, aspartic acid and glutamic acid, from yellow star thistle (Centaurea solstitialis). Nat Toxins 1995;3:174–80.
51. Steyn DG. Plant poisoning in stock and the development of tolerance. Onderstepoort J Vet Sci Anim Indust 1933;1:141–3.
52. Dil'bazi GI. Poisoning of buffalos eating hay containing choking mustard. Veterinariya 1974;2:106–7.
53. Cordy DR. Nigropallidal encephalomalacia in horses associated with ingestion of yellow star thistle. J Neuropathol Exp Neurol 1954;13:330–42.
54. Cordy DR. Centaurea species and equine negropallidal encephalomalacia. In: Keeler RF, Van Kampen KR, James LF, editors. Effects of poisonous plants on livestock. New York: Academic Press; 1978. p. 327–36.
55. Panter KE, Bunch TD, Keeler RF. Maternal and fetal toxicity of poison hemlock (Conium maculatum) in sheep. Am J Vet Res 1988;49:281–3.
56. Bowman WC, Sanghvi IS. Pharmacological actions of hemlock (Conium maculatum) alkaloids. J Pharm Pharmacol 1963;15:1–25.
57. Uwai K, Ohashi K, Takaya Y, et al. Exploring the structural basis of neurotoxicity in C(17)-polyacetylenes isolated from water hemlock. J Med Chem 2000;43:4508–15.
58. Panter KE, Gardner DR, Stegelmeier BL, et al. Water hemlock poisoning in cattle: Ingestion of immature Cicuta maculata seed as the probable cause. Toxicon 2011;57:157–61.
59. Panter KE, Gardner DR, Holstege D, et al. A case of acute water hemlock (Cicuta maculata) poisoning and death in cattle after ingestion of green seed heads. In: Panter KE, Wierenga TL, Pfister JA, editors. Poisonous plants: global Research and solutions. Wallingford (United Kingdom): CABI; 2007. p. 259–64.
60. Vetter J. Poison hemlock (Conium maculatum L.). Food Chem Toxicol 2004;42:1373–82.
61. Wink M, Meibner C, Witte L. Patterns of quinolizidine alkaloids in 56 species of the genus Lupinus. Phytochem 1995;38:139–53.
62. Panter KE, James LF, Wierenga TL, et al. Research on lupine-induced 'crooked calf disease' at the poisonous plant research laboratory: past, present and future. In: Panter KE, Wierenga TL, Pfister JA, editors. Poisonous plants global research and solutions. Wallingford (United Kingdom): CABI; 2007. p. 59–65.
63. Panter KE, James LF, Gardner DR. Lupines, poison-hemlock and Nicotiana spp: toxicity and teratogenicity in livestock. J Nat Toxins 1999;8:117–34.
64. Panter KE, Ralphs MH, Smart RA, et al. Death camas poisoning in sheep: a case report. Vet Hum Toxicol 1987;29:45–8.
65. West P, Horowitz BZ. Zigadenus poisoning treated with atropine and dopamine. J Med Toxicol 2009;5:214–7.
66. Welch KD, Green BT, Gardner DR, et al. The effect of low larkspur (Delphinium spp.) co-administration on the acute toxicity of death camas (Zigadenus spp.) in sheep. Toxicon 2013;76:50–8.
67. Welch KD, Panter KE, Gardner DR, et al. The acute toxicity of the death camas (Zigadenus species) alkaloid zygacine in mice, including the effect of methyllycaconitine coadministration on zygacine toxicity. J Anim Sci 2011;89:1650–7.

Plant-Induced Myotoxicity in Livestock

T. Zane Davis, PhD, Bryan L. Stegelmeier, DVM, PhD*, Michael J. Clayton, DVM

KEYWORDS

- Poisonous plants • Myotoxic • Cardiotoxic • Selenium

KEY POINTS

- White snakeroot and *Isocoma* spp can cause myoskeletal and/or myocardial lesions in livestock when ingested over a period of 1 week to 3 weeks.
- Many plants contain cardioglycosides, which often are lethal when ingested, even in small dosages.
- Some *Senna* and *Thermopsis* species can cause extensive skeletal and myocardial lesions.
- Selenium can cause myoskeletal or myocardial lesions either by deficiency in the diet or by acute or chronic ingestion of selenium-containing plants.

CARDIOACTIVE GLYCOSIDE-CONTAINING PLANTS

Many plants contain toxic cardioglycosides (**Table 1**) that can poison livestock. Historically many of these plants, such as digoxin, have been carefully used medicinally for treatments of various heart conditions. At therapeutic doses, they inhibit sodium potassium pumps in cell membranes, ultimately resulting in increased sequestration and subsequently increased calcium release upon stimulation. This increased calcium release allows the myocyte to contract faster and more forcefully. The margin of safety is small and toxic doses are relatively low. In poisoning the imbalance of intracellular and extracellular sodium and potassium alters membrane potentials with decreased cardiac conduction, resulting in atrioventricular block and ventricular fibrillation. Most cardioglycosides are very toxic and, ingestion of relatively small amounts of toxic plant material can be lethal.

Cardioactive glycoside toxicity is affected by solubility and binding affinity that largely depends, and the chemistry of the side groups attached to the steroidal backbone and the lactone ring. Additionally, there are animal differences that contribute to susceptibility. Both species and sex differences in metabolism and Na^+/K^+-ATPase binding affinity influence toxicity.[1] All parts of these plants are poisonous to animals fresh or dried, processed, and included in stored food and feeds. Because many of these are ornamental plants, most livestock poisonings occur when animals are fed

USDA/ARS Poisonous Plant Research Laboratory, 1150 East 1400 North, Logan, UT 84341, USA
* Corresponding author.
E-mail address: Bryan.Stegelmeier@USDA.GOV

Vet Clin Food Anim 36 (2020) 689–699
https://doi.org/10.1016/j.cvfa.2020.08.005
0749-0720/20/Published by Elsevier Inc.
vetfood.theclinics.com

Table 1
List of some common cardioactive glycoside containing plants that can poison livestock

Acokanthera spp	Bushman's poison bush
Adenium multiflorum	Impala lily
Adonis microcarpa	Pheasant eye
Asclepias spp	Milkweeds
Asclepias curassavica	Red-head cotton bush
Apocynum cannabinum	Dogbane
Bryophyllum spp	Kalanchoe
Convallaria majalis	Lily of the valley
Corchorus olitorius	Jute
Cryptostegia grandiflora	Rubber vine
Digitalis purpurea	Foxglove
Euonymus spp	Eunoymus
Gomphocarpus spp	Milkweed, balloon cotton
Helleborus spp	Hellebores
Homeria flaccida and *H miniata*	One-leaf and 2-leaf cape tulip
Hyacinthus spp	Hyacinth
Kalanchoe delagoensis	Mother of millions
Nerium oleander	Oleander
Ornithogalum spp	Star of Bethlehem
Sisyrinchium spp	Blue eyed grass
Strophanthus spp	Poison rope
Thevetia peruviana	Yellow oleander
Urginea spp	Squill
Vinca major	Periwinkle

clippings. Some plants have escaped cultivation and grow along fences and road-sides where they can invade adjacent fields and contaminate forages.

Cattle are highly susceptible to poisoning and when poisoned, they most often are found dead. Poisoned animals develop various cardiac arrhythmias and heart blocks, such as ventricular tachycardia and first-degree and second-degree conduction blocks. This is seen clinically as rapid breathing, cold extremities, and a rapid, weak, and often irregular pulse. Death usually occurs within 24 hours of ingestion.

The gross and microscopic lesions are variable and seem to be related to the dose and duration of clinical signs before death. Oleander poisoning, one of the most common of the cardioglyoside-containing plants, often produces serosal hemorrhages, edema, and congestion of visceral organs and occasionally myocardial degeneration that is seen grossly as pale soft streaking in the heart. As suggested, the distinctive microscopic changes seem to relate to the duration of the disease. Some animals develop mild nonsuppurative myocardial degeneration with mononuclear inflammation. Ultrastructural changes also may vary because some myocardial cells up-regulate energy production with increased numbers of mitochondria. As with many myocardial degeneration lesions, however, most myocardial cells have swollen mitochondria, hypercontracted sarcomeres, and, occasionally, myofibrillar disruption.[2]

The treatment consists of prevention of further absorption of the poison (gastric lavage and introduction of activated charcoal) and correction of any electrolyte deficiencies. Some clinicians have attempted therapy with cardiac pacing and antidigoxin antibodies (Fab) fragments-(DigiFab) but this is expensive and has not had much success in veterinary medicine.

ISOCOMA SPP AND WHITE SNAKEROOT

White snakeroot (*Ageratina altissima*) (**Fig. 1**A) and *Isocoma* spp, including *I pluriflora* (rayless goldenrod) (**Fig. 1**B), *I acradenia*, and *I tenuisecta*, are found in the midwestern and southwestern United States, respectively. White snakeroot is an herbaceous perennial that grows 30 cm to 150 cm tall and bears loose hemispheric or flat-topped clusters of white heads at the ends of short branches during the late summer and early fall months, hence the common names white top, white sanicle, and white snakeroot. *Isocoma* spp are erect, bushy, unbranched perennial shrubs with yellow flowers at the top of their woody stems that commonly grow in alkaline and gypsic soils in riparian zones along river valleys, drainage areas, or dry plains. The main differences in *Isocoma* spp are the shapes of their leaves. Even though *Isocoma* spp and white snakeroot are distinctly different and grow in very different environments, the suspected toxins are believed to be the same. In the late 1920s, the toxin was identified as tremetol, which later was demonstrated to be a complex mixture of alcohols and ketones, including benzofuran ketones, such as tremetone, dehydrotremetone, 3-oxyangeloyl-tremetone, and 6-hydroxytremetone.[3] Tremetone has been identified as the most likely toxic compound based on in vitro studies and its common appearance in toxic plant populations.[4] Attempts to demonstrate in vivo, however, that tremetone is the toxin and to quantify its concentration in a toxic dose recently have led researchers to hypothesize that another compound may be the toxic principle or that there is another compound that interacts synergistically with tremetone.[5]

After eating the plant for several days to weeks, most livestock, including sheep, goats, cattle, and horses, develop a disease characterized by reluctance to move and fine muscle tremors of the nose, flanks, and legs, especially after exercise or activity. The affected animal often has tachypnea, tachycardia, a stiff gait, and altered posture because poisoned animals stand in an arched back position. Nursing young

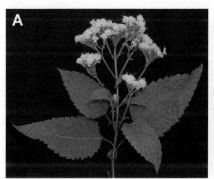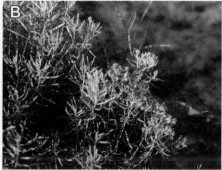

Fig. 1. (*A*) Photomicrograph of white snakeroot, a historically important plant that in the mid-1800s caused entire settlements to be abandoned due to poisoning of livestock and its toxin or metabolites being passed through the milk, causing milk sickness in humans who drank the contaminated milk. (*B*) Photomicrograph of *I pluriflora* (rayless goldenrod) that commonly is found in the southwestern United States. In the early 1900s, it was observed that it produced nearly identical clinical signs as white snakeroot when consumed by livestock.

often develop the disease before their dam as the toxins are eliminated through the milk.

White snakeroot poisoning usually occurs during the late fall when other forages have been consumed or during inclement weather when animals take shelter in wooded areas that often contain white snakeroot. Poisoning by *Isocoma* spp normally occurs during winter when snowfall covers other forages or during the transition from winter to spring when *Isocoma* plants have green vegetation before other forages begin to grow. Cases of poisoning by both plants have been reported in nearly all livestock species as well as humans who drink contaminated milk. Toxicity of plant populations is variable, and potentially toxic populations have been difficult to identify.[6]

Most animal species that are poisoned by *Isocoma* spp or white snakeroot have swelling and pallor or pale streaking of many skeletal muscles that is seen easily at necropsy. In experimental studies of *I pluriflora* toxicosis in goats, the distribution of lesions was patchy with no distinct pattern or muscle groups that were consistently damaged.[7] The large appendicular muscles (semimembranosus, semitendinosus, biceps femoris, gluteus medius, supraspinatus, and triceps brachii), however, were those damaged most frequently with extensive monophasic degeneration and necrosis. These muscles should be collected and examined closely in potential poisoning cases. The hearts of goats dosed with white snakeroot at 2% and 3% of body weight (BW) often had streaks of soft and pale myocardium. When calves were administered *I pluriflora* and *I acradenia*, they also developed lesions in the large appendicular muscles.[8] Increased serum enzyme activities of lactate dehydrogenase (LDH), asparate aminotransferase (AST), alanine aminotransferase (ALT), and especially creatine kinase (CK) have been correlated with significant histologic changes. Marked increases in cardiac troponin I concentrations also have been observed in animals with myocardial necrosis.[9] Additionally, a gas chromatography–mass spectrometry technique recently has been used to identify tremetone in the liver of a poisoned animal.[10]

The myocardium of goats that exhibited significant clinical signs had multifocal mild myocyte swelling, degeneration, and rarely necrosis. Horses appear more susceptible to the cardiotoxic effects of white snakeroot and rayless goldenrod. At necropsy, the myocardium of a horse dosed with rayless goldenrod for 10 days was pale and soft. Many of the appendicular and large apical muscles also were pale and moist. Histologically, the myocardium had extensive myocardial degeneration and necrosis with extensive fibrosis and multifocal mineralization.[9] In a clinical case[11] and an experimental produced incident[12] of white snakeroot poisoning of horses, the myocardial degeneration and necrosis appeared to be more severe than the myoskeletal lesions.

In order to prevent poisoning of livestock by *Isocoma* spp or white snakeroot, producers should be aware of the feed that animals are eating. Pastures and ranges should be maintained in good condition so that animals should always have other choices of palatable feed. When storms cover other forages or animals are pushed into wooded areas because of inclement weather, processed feed should be supplemented to the livestock or they should be moved to other areas to prevent prolonged ingestion of *Isocoma* spp or white snakeroot.

THERMOPSIS SPP

Thermopsis spp are more common in Asia but 3 species are found in North America and, of those, *T rhombifolia* has been associated with livestock poisoning.[13] *T rhombifolia*, commonly known as prairie goldenbanner, golden bean, or buffalo bean, is a hardy perennial that grows about 30 cm tall with yellow flowers and is found in the high plains of western North America. Ingestion of dried plant at a dosage of 0.6 g/kg to 2.8 g/kg body weight for several days produces disease in cattle.[14] Young plants potentially are more toxic, with toxicity decreasing as the plant matures until the seeds mature at which time toxicity peaks. Quinolizidine alkaloids, anagyrine, thermopsine, cystisine, and N-methylcytisine, are toxins that have been isolated from *T rhombifolia* var. *montana*. Semipurified alkaloids have reproduced muscle lesions when dosed and it has been suggested that the effects of the alkaloids are additive and may also produce contracture congenital defects similar to lupine-induced crooked calf disease.[15] Clinical signs of poisoned animals are muscle weakness often accompanied by recumbency, which often leads to dehydration, malnourishment, and possibly death. These signs are accompanied by marked serum biochemical changes in CK, AST, and LDH activities. Gross lesions generally are minimal, with some pallor and softening of skeletal muscle and loss of adipose tissue and body condition. Microscopically, there is prominent skeletal muscle degeneration and necrosis with patchy areas of regenerations (**Fig. 2**). Adjacent, less severely affected myofibers often are swollen with hypereosinophilia and bands of hypercontracted myofibers (hyaline degeneration). Poisoned animals may recover if fed and watered but the permanent sequelae of poisoning are unknown.

CASSIA, SENNA, OR CHAMAECRISTA SPECIES

The these species have been repeatedly reclassified changing their nomenclature and perceived toxicities several times through the years. Historically they have been used as herbal medicines even though it has been suggested that all species and plant parts are toxic. The beans have been roasted and used as coffee whereas the leaves are cooked and eaten. Generally, they are not considered palatable to livestock; however, several species have poisoned animals when conditions are right. The species involved most often in clinical poisoning include *S occidentalis* and *S obtusifolia* with occasional reports of poisoning attributed to *S roemericana*, *Chamaecrista fasciculata*, *S lindheimeriana*, and *Chamaecrista nictitans.* These plants generally are

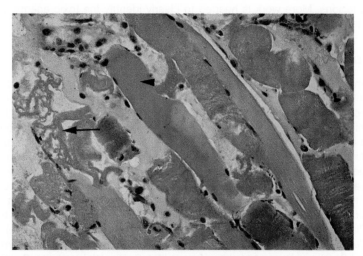

Fig. 2. Photomicrograph of a calf poisoned with *Thrombifolia*. Notice the loss of striation with swelling and hypereosinophilia (*arrowhead*), coagulation, and clumping of sarcomere protein (*arrow*). (Hematoxylin-eosin stain with original magnification of 400X).

considered to be weeds that expand along fences and disturbed areas and they can invade into adjacent fields and pastures. *Cassia* plants generally are erect and lightly branched leguminous trees or shrubs that grow 1.5 m to 2 m tall. The leaves are pinnate, alternate, and often are found in groups of 4 or 5 spaced along the stalk. The flowers generally are yellow and produce a thick, brown seed pod that may be up to 20 cm long and contains many seeds. Poisonings generally occurs when plants invade into corn and soybean fields and the *Cassia* beans contaminate harvested foods and feed, or alternatively, when the whole plant is cut and chopped green with other forages and fed to livestock.

Many species, including cattle, sheep, goats, horses, pigs, rabbits, chickens, and rodents, have been shown to be susceptible to poisoning.[16] Signs of poisoning include diarrhea, colic, tenesmus, weakness, recumbency, myoglobinuria, and wasting. Serum CK and AST activities usually are markedly increased and, with some severe cases, myoglobin-induced nephrosis produce azotemia and other changes of renal failure. Severely poisoned animals develop extensive skeletal muscle and myocardial lesions and the resulting hyperkalemia contributes to altered cardiac contractions, fibrillation, and death. Horses are more likely than some other species to develop liver disease. If high doses are ingested, nearly all species develop hepatic necrosis, and in some cases severely affected animals develop hepatic encephalopathy. Gross lesions include muscle pallor, softening, and secondary changes of nephrosis and occasionally severe hepatic softening and congestion. Histologically, there is skeletal muscle necrosis and degeneration that may be polyphasic making it difficult to differentiate from some nutritional myopathies. *Cassia*-induced liver disease is characterized by extensive centrilobular hepatocyte necrosis that at times can be massive with hemorrhage.

More than 30 potential toxins have been identified in *C occidentalis* but those responsible for producing disease have not been defined clearly. Several other potential toxins have been identified in other *Cassia* spp. Of these toxins, several anthraquinones have been identified in the leaves. The roots contain emodin and the seeds contain chrysarobin (1,8-dihydroxy-3-methyl-9-anthrone) and *N*-methylmorpholine.[17] None of these toxins has definitively proved to be the cause of any or all *Cassia*-induced lesions. More work is needed to clearly identify the toxic agents and their roles in toxicity as well as to determine their mechanism of toxicity.

SELENIFEROUS PLANTS

Selenium (Se) is an essential element and cofactor of approximately 30 biologically important enzymes and proteins. Diseases resulting from Se deficiencies are common and affect livestock in many regions of the world. There is a narrow window between Se deficiency and toxicity, and seleniferous forages or feed misformulations often result in poisoning. Forages containing less than 0.1 parts per million (ppm) Se can cause deficiencies seen as reduced reproductive performance and white muscle disease. On the other hand, chronic Se toxicosis occurs most often when animals consume forages with elevated Se concentrations (10–30 ppm) over a period of weeks to months. Acute Se toxicosis generally is caused by supplementation errors or when animals quickly ingest plants that contain very high Se concentrations (100s to 1000s ppm). Plants that accumulate high Se concentrations (up to 10,000 ppm) include *Astragalus bisulcatus*, *A praelongous*, *Xylorhiza glabriuscula*, *Symphyotrichum ascendens*, and *Stanleya pinnata*, to name a few. In high Se-containing plants, Se is present as selenate, Se-methylselenocysteine and γ–glutamyl-methylselenocysteine, which appear to be more toxic than other selenocompounds, such as selenite and selenomethionine. Other plants, such as *Grindelia* spp or even common forages, such as alfalfa (*Medicago sativa*), when grown in high Se soils, can passively accumulate Se concentrations of 100s ppm to 1500 ppm. These plants are found in seleniferous soils in South Dakota, Wyoming, and other states as well as anywhere Se contaminates soils around mine tailings and pastures and ranges where drainage waters from contaminated sites flow.

Clinical signs of acute poisoning appear within 8 hours to 36 hours postexposure and include depression, dyspnea, pulmonary edema, and death. Chronic exposure of lower doses over several weeks to months may produce heart failure with subsequent edema, thoracic, and abdominal transfusions, and vascular distension that is classically seen as jugular pulse. Damaged animals are crippled and most die. In acutely poisoned sheep, histologic lesions include acute swelling and necrosis of cardiomyocytes (**Fig. 3**) with pulmonary edema and vascular congestion. Animals that survive longer develop more extensive lesions with focally extensive myocardial necrosis and fibrosis with adjacent edema and chronic inflammation (**Fig. 4**). The myocardial Purkinje cells also may be swollen and vacuolated with peripheral edema and infiltrates of lymphocytes and macrophages. The livers from these animals were congested with dilation and congestion of many of the central veins.[18] Chronic Se poisoning in livestock is species-specific. Pigs are uniquely sensitive to chronic Se poisoning and develop characteristic poliomyeloencephalomalcia in addition to the characteristic Se-related hoof lesions and lameness observed in horses and cattle.[19] Horses also are susceptible to chronic Se poisoning and often quickly develop mane and tail alopecia from brittle hair that breaks easily, resulting in a bobtailed and roached mane appearance (**Fig. 5A**). Poisoned horses also develop hoof lesions seen first and horizontal lesions in the hoof wall that may progress to laminar necrosis resulting in sloughing of the entire hoof (**Fig. 5B**). If mane and tail are not lost, then they can be sampled, fragmented, and analyzed. Such sequential sampling can be used to approximate when poisoning occurred.[20]

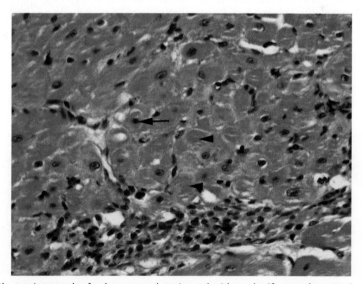

Fig. 3. Photomicrograph of a sheep acutely poisoned with a seleniferous plant. Notice the myocyte swelling and hypereosinophilia (*arrowheads*). There is also nuclear pyknosis (*arrow*) with focal mixed inflammation. (Hematoxylin-eosin stain with original magnification of 200X).

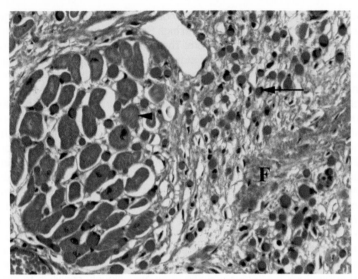

Fig. 4. Photomicrograph of the heart of a cow that survived nearly 2 weeks after ingesting highly seleniferous plants. Notice the extensive loss of myofibers with some small islands of swollen and degenerative myocytes (*arrowhead*) surrounded by extensive fibrosis (F) with clusters of small remnant vessels (*arrow*). (Hematoxylin-eosin stain with original magnification of 200X).

In contrast, sheep are relatively resistant to chronic Se exposure. Often, they do not develop hair loss or hoof lesions when chronically exposed to feeds containing 20 ppm to 30 ppm Se for up to 5 months. These clinically normal ewes had liver Se concentrations of up to 75 ppm (wet weight). Anecdotal reports and 1 recent study suggest that ewes had decreased reproductive performance when fed alfalfa pellets made with Se-rich western aster to obtain a final Se concentration of 25 ppm Se. In a separate study, however, ewes dosed for 72 weeks with feed containing up to 20 ppm Se (as sodium selenite) did not develop clinical or histologic changes suggestive of toxicity and with no detected alterations in gestation or lactation.[21] More work is needed to determine the chronic reproductive effects of high Se exposures in other species.

The mechanism of Se toxicity has not yet been defined clearly. Some have proposed that intermediate substrates, such as glutathione and S-adenosylmethionine,

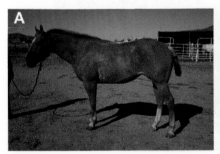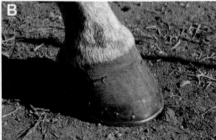

Fig. 5. (*A*) Horse with chronic selenosis. Notice the roached mane and bobtail appearance. (*B*). Hoof of a horse with chronic selenosis. Notice the ring of growth ridges and abnormal growth.

are depleted, thus disturbing their respective enzyme activities and leaving cells susceptible to oxidative damage.[22] Alternatively, free radicals and additional oxidative damage may be produced when Se reacts with various thiols.[23] Se also may be incorporated into amino acids in place of sulfur. These seleno–amino acids are included in proteins that are dysfunctional because they lack key disulfide structures.[24] It is likely that these and possibly other mechanisms all play a role in Se toxicity.

Serum, whole blood, liver, and skeletal muscle Se toxicokinetics have been studied in cattle and sheep. In a classic case of poisoning in cattle, the half-life of Se in the different tissues range from approximately 40 days to 115 days, depending on the tissue.[25]

When diagnosing cases of acute and chronic Se toxicosis, whole-blood and liver Se (either by necropsy or liver biopsies) concentrations should be determined to evaluate the Se status and likelihood of Se exposure. These results can be supported by histologic findings and examination of ranges and feed. In cases of suspected acute selenosis, grazed ranges should be examined for the presence and consumption of Se-accumulating species. Additionally, rumen contents should be analyzed for Se content. If chronic selenosis is suspected, available forages should be analyzed for Se content to determine if Se concentrations are elevated in the forages. Plants containing Se concentrations more than 500 ppm always should be considered extremely toxic because less than 0.5 kg of the plant may be lethal to livestock. Mine reclamation areas are especially dangerous and, if Se contamination is a problem, western aster or Se-accumulating species that are out-competing other forages always should be avoided. In some areas, these plants can contain Se concentrations of several thousand ppm Se and they nearly always are lethal, if ingested. Horses never should be grazed on high Se forages. Intermittent use of ranges with forages containing slightly elevated Se concentrations is possible with sheep and cattle, with caution, allowing detoxification every couple of weeks in pastures with safe forages. Additionally, livestock always should have access to minerals, including Se, and care should be taken to not overgraze available forages and subsequently force livestock to consume vegetation with higher concentrations of Se, because sheep and cattle select forages with lower concentrations of Se, if given a choice with similar feed value.[26]

SUMMARY

There are many plants that cause myoskeletal and myocardial lesions in livestock. Many of the cardioglycoside-containing plants are lethal when ingested in small amounts. When diagnosing cases of plant poisoning, it is necessary to examine clinical signs, serum biochemistries, toxin or metabolite tissue analyses, field studies, and plant toxin chemistry analysis as well as histopathology data from any samples collected. A thorough investigation can provide knowledge to better understand risk and to modify grazing patterns to avoid future poisonings. Additionally, the clinical effects of many of the myoskeletal plants can be reversed with supplemental veterinary care and by eliminating access to the plants.

DISCLOSURE

The authors have nothing to disclose.

REFERENCES

1. Blaustein MP, Robinson SW, Gottlieb SS, et al. Sex, digitalis, and the sodium pump. Mol Interv 2003;3:68–72, 50.

2. Bandara V, Weinstein SA, White J, et al. A review of natural history, toxinology, diagnosis and clinical management of *Nerium oleander* (common oleander) and *Thevetia peruviana* (yellow oleander) poisoning. Toxicon 2010;56:273–81.

3. Bonner WA, DeGraw JI, Bowen DM. Toxic constituents of white snakeroot. Tetrahedron Lett 1961;112:417–20.

4. Beier RC, Norman JO, Reagor JC, et al. Isolation of the major component in white snakeroot that is toxic after microsomal activation: possible explanation of sporadic toxicity of white snakeroot plants and extracts. Nat Toxins 1993;1:286–93.

5. Davis TZ, Stegelmeier BL, Lee ST, et al. White snakeroot poisoning in goats: Variations in toxicity with different plant chemotypes. Res Vet Sci 2016;106:29–36.

6. Lee ST, Cook D, Davis TZ, et al. A Survey of Tremetone, Dehydrotremetone, and structurally related compounds in *Isocoma spp.* (Goldenbush) in the Southwestern United States. J Agric Food Chem 2015;205:872–9.

7. Stegelmeier BL, Davis TZ, Green BT, et al. Experimental rayless goldenrod (*Isocoma pluriflora*) toxicosis in goats. J Vet Diagn Invest 2010;22:570–7.

8. Davis TZ, Green BT, Stegelmeier BL, et al. The comparative toxicity of Isocoma species in calves. Toxicon X 2020;5:100022.

9. Davis TZ, Stegelmeier BL, Lee ST, et al. Experimental rayless goldenrod (*Isocoma pluriflora*) toxicosis in horses. Toxicon 2013;73:88–95.

10. Meyerholtz KA, Burcham GN, Miller MA, et al. Development of a gas chromatography-mass spectrometry technique to diagnose white snakeroot (Ageratina altissima) poisoning in a cow. J Vet Diagn Invest 2011;23:775–9.

11. Smetzer DL, Coppock TW, Ely RW, et al. Cardiac effects of white snakeroot intoxication in horses. Equine Pract 1983;5:26–32.

12. White JL, Shivaprasad HL, Thompson LJ, et al. White snakeroot (Eupatorium rugosum) poisoning clinical effects associated with cardiac and skeletal muscle lesions in experimental equine toxicoses. In: Seawright AA, Hogarty MP, James LF, et al, editors. Plant toxicology. Queensland (Australia): Queensland Poisonous Plant Committee, Department of Primary Industries, Animal Research Institute; 1985. p. 411–22.

13. Baker DC, Keeler RF. *Thermopsis montana*-induced myopathy in calves. J Am Vet Med Assoc 1989;194:1269–72.

14. Keeler RF, Johnson AE, Chase RL. Toxicity of *Thermopsis montana* in cattle. Cornell Vet 1986;76:115–27.

15. Keeler RF, Baker DC. Myopathy in cattle induced by alkaloid extracts from *Thermopsis montana, Laburnum anagyroides* and a *Lupinus* sp. J Comp Pathol 1990; 103:169–82.

16. Vashishtha VM, John TJ, Kumar A. Clinical and pathological features of acute toxicity due to *Cassia occidentalis* in vertebrates. Indian J Med Res 2009;130: 23–30.

17. Yadav JP, Arya V, Yadav S, et al. *Cassia occidentalis* L.: a review on its ethnobotany, phytochemical and pharmacological profile. Fitoterapia 2010;81:223–30.

18. Tiwary AK, Stegelmeier BL, Panter KE, et al. Comparative toxicosis of sodium selenite and selenomethionine in lambs. J Vet Diagn Invest 2006;18:61–70.

19. Panter KE, Hartley WJ, James LF, et al. Comparative toxicity of selenium from seleno-DL-methionine, sodium selenite, and *Astragalus bisulcatus* in pigs. Fundam Appl Toxicol 1996;32:217–23.

20. Davis TZ, Stegelmeier BL, Hall JO. Analysis in Horse Hair as a Means of Evaluating selenium toxicosis and long-term exposures. J Agric Food Chem 2014; 62:7393–7.

21. Davis PA, McDowell LR, Wilkinson NS, et al. Tolerance of inorganic selenium by range-type ewes during gestation and lactation. J Anim Sci 2006;84:660–8.
22. Vernie LN, Ginjaar HB, Wilders IT, et al. Amino acid incorporation in cell-free system derived from rat liver studied with the aid of selenodiglutathione. Biochim Biophys Acta 1978;518:507–17.
23. Kaur R, Sharma S, Rampal S. Effect of sub-chronic selenium toxicosis on lipid peroxidation, glutathione redox cycle and antioxidant enzymes in calves. Vet Hum Toxicol 2003;45:190–2.
24. Raisbeck MF. Selenosis. Vet Clin North Am Food Anim Pract 2000;16:465–80.
25. Davis TZ, Stegelmeier BL, Panter KE, et al. Toxicokinetics and pathology of plant associated acute selenium toxicosis in steers. J Vet Diagn 2012;24:319–27.
26. Pfister JA, Davis TZ, Hall JO. Effect of selenium concentration on feed preferences by cattle and sheep. J Anim Sci 2013;91:5970–80.

Plants Containing Urinary Tract, Gastrointestinal, or Miscellaneous Toxins that Affect Livestock

Bryan L. Stegelmeier, DVM, PhD*, T. Zane Davis, PhD,
Michael J. Clayton, DVM

KEYWORDS

- Poisonous plants - Nephrotoxins - Oak - Oxalates

KEY POINTS

- Plants that affect the urinary tract and kidneys include oxalate-containing plants, oaks, plants that cause hemolysis, calcinogenic plants, pigweed, and others.
- Many plants affect the gastrointestinal tract even though their other prominent lesions result in their inclusion in other systems.
- Buttercup, nightshade, mustard, bindweed, and castor bean are plants that produce gastrointestinal lesions.
- Other miscellaneous plant including cyanogenic plants and bracken fern that commonly poison livestock.

URINARY SYSTEM TOXINS OR NEPHROTOXIC PLANTS

Many commonly used plants are oxalate-containing plants, with soluble or insoluble oxalates. The insoluble oxalates, such as calcium (Ca) oxalate, are present as crystals in plants. These crystals are irritating to mucosal membranes and, when eaten, damage the oral cavity and gastrointestinal tract. Such plants are not palatable and generally are avoided; however, if animals are forced to eat them, they develop oral mucosal hyperemia, swelling, and marked hypersalivation. Plant-soluble oxalates include sodium and potassium oxalate and oxalic acid. These are absorbed quickly and, if plant concentrations are high, they cause systemic poisoning. Although many plants contain some oxalates, only a few species of the *Agave, Beta, Bassia, Chenopodium, Halogeton* (**Fig. 1**), *Oxalis, Rhuem, Rumex, Sarcobatus*, and *Setaria* genera contain enough to be reported as toxic. The type of poisoning depends both on the animal

USDA/ARS Poisonous Plant Research Laboratory, 1150 East 1400 North, Logan, UT 84341, USA
* Corresponding author.
E-mail address: Bryan.Stegelmeier@USDA.GOV

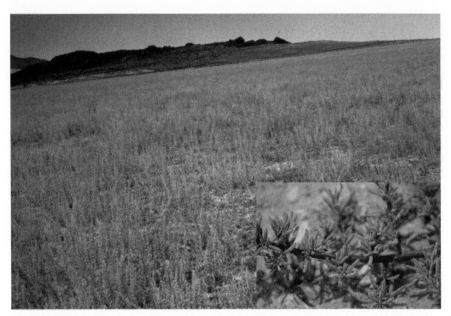

Fig. 1. Halogeton (*Halogeton glomeratus*) is a noxious Eurasian weed. Since its introduction in North America it has spread to cover millions of acres. It tends to grow as a monoculture in disturbed areas along roads, in holding pens and heavily used areas around loading pens, or in watering tanks. Catastrophic poisonings most often occur when hungry sheep are unloaded in such halogeton-infested areas. The inset is a halogeton branch showing the thick tubular or globoid leaves.

species poisoned and plant oxalate concentrations. As ruminants adapt and metabolize oxalates, they are much less susceptible to chronic poisoning. All animals can be fatally poisoned, if they ingest too much too quickly. Horses and other monogastric animals are more likely to develop chronic poisoning (low oxalate doses for extended durations). Plants with greater than 10% soluble oxalates usually are nephrotoxic, causing fatal renal failure. Lower soluble oxalate concentrations can produce secondary hyperparathyroidism, resorption, and loss of bone with secondary osseous proliferation and dysplasia. This is because soluble oxalates effectively bind and sequester Ca and magnesium, which can result in functional deficiencies, including altered neurologic function.[1] Because Ca supplementation does not alter acute poisoning and nephrosis, additional mechanisms of toxicity probably contribute to nephrosis. An oxalate metabolite, Ca oxalate monohydrate (COM), has been shown to damage mitochondrial function-impairing oxidative phosphoralyation.[2] COM crystals also alter membrane structure and function, resulting in physical damage as well as increased reactive oxygen species that further damage cells.[3] Additionally, oxalate poisoning reduces activities of tricarboxylic acid cycle enzymes (succinate dehydrogenase, isocitrate dehydrogenase, malate dehydrogenase, and others). This enzyme inhibition, combined with increased oxygen stress (decreased antioxidant enzymes and glutathione with increased reactive oxygen species and lipid peroxidation), certainly contributes to disease. More work is needed to better define how these different toxic mechanisms contribute to disease.[4,5]

Acute oxalate poisoning is characterized by hypocalcemia, lethargy, anorexia, muscle tremors, weakness, stiffness, diarrhea, ataxia, tachypnea, dyspnea, tetany, recumbency, rumen atony, coma, and death. Animals that are forced to move may develop hyperesthesia and seizures. Animals that survive these early changes develop azotemia and, if severe, they develop clinical renal failure and potentially encephalopathy. Gross lesions in most animals are minimal and characterized by gastritis or rumenitis with serosal edema and hemorrhage. Secondary accumulation of pleural fluids and ascites as well as pulmonary edema also may occur. The kidneys often are pale and swollen. In chronic poisoning, the kidneys often become pale, firm, and shrunken.[5] Histologic lesions are associated with deposition of birefringent COM crystals in the renal tubules, abomasal mucosa, and gastric vasculature. There is degeneration and necrosis of the tubular epithelium of the proximal convoluted tubules. Affected tubules typically are distended with crystalline material and have flattened and degenerative cortical tubular epithelium in acute cases (**Fig. 2**). Animals that survive for several days have gross changes of thinning of the renal cortex with discoloration between the cortex and medulla. The discoloration results from the accumulation of crystalline materials in the tubules.

Chronically poisoned animals, especially horses, show weakness, stiffness, intermittent lameness, inability to work, weight loss, and swelling of the osseous structures of the head. Grossly and histologically, they develop fibrous osteodystrophy with swelling of the nasal bones, maxilla, and mandible (**Fig. 3**). Associated histologic changes include increased osteoclast activity and dystrophic mineralization with proliferation of fibrous connective tissue.[6]

Oxalate poisoning is best diagnosed by associating histologic COM crystals with the clinical signs and field evidence of exposure and consumption of oxalate-containing plants. Treatment largely has been unsuccessful, although oral Ca therapy also may be useful in binding soluble oxalate in the rumen to prevent further absorption. Certainly, allowing ruminants to adapt with limited exposures to produce low-dose exposures to soluble oxalates for 8 days to 25 days decreases the risk of poisoning.[5] Additionally, risk assessment can be facilitated by analyzing the oxalate concentrations of potentially toxic plant populations.

Oaks (*Quercus* spp) are common throughout the world and they include hundreds of species of shrubs and trees. All species are considered toxic, with seedlings, early bud growth, and acorns being highly toxic and the cause of most intoxications. Poisoning generally occurs in early spring or fall, when toxic acorns or early growth are available and alternative forages are limited. Toxicity has been attributed to tannins; however,

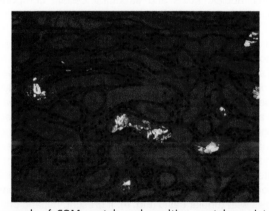

Fig. 2. Photomicrograph of COM crystals and resulting crystal-associated nephrosis in a sheep poisoned with halogeton. This section was stained with hematoxylin-eosin at original magnification of 100X. The photograph was made using polarized filters to identify the prominent intracellular crystals.

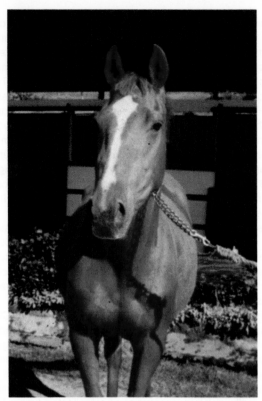

Fig. 3. Horse with oxalate-related fibrous osteodystrophy. This as a case is best appreciated by palpation where the bony proliferations on the lateral surfaces of the maxilla and mandible are apparent.

purified tannins are toxic only at relatively high doses, suggesting there probably is an unidentified toxic component. Tannins are polyphenolic compounds that cross-link proteins, glycoproteins, nucleic acids and structural cellular components resulting in cellular degeneration and necrosis.[7] Poisoning occurs when large doses are ingested over several days to weeks. Primarily a ruminant toxin, calves are highly susceptible and goats seem to be able to metabolize tannins and are less susceptible to poisoning.[8,9] Although oaks predominantly cause gastrointestinal mucosal damage and nephrosis, at some doses and durations, they can cause liver necrosis. Initial signs of poisoning include lethargy, constipation, tenesmus, polydipsia, polyuria, and a brown discoloration to the urine. These are followed by hemorrhagic diarrhea, abdominal pain, rumen atony, and anorexia. Oak-induced renal disease is characterized by isosthenuria, glucosuria, proteinuria, and hematuria, with serum biochemical changes of hyperkalemia, hyperphosphatemia, azotemia, and hypercreatinemia. Gross lesions include oak material/acorns in the rumen contents, subcutaneous edema, perirenal edema, mesenteric edema, ascites, hydrothorax, and ulcerative/hemorrhagic rumenitis, gastritis, and enteritis. Microscopic lesions are characterized by diffuse cortical renal tubular degeneration and necrosis with tubular casts (**Fig. 4**). If present, hepatic changes include hepatocellular degeneration and necrosis with focally extensive hemorrhage.

A most likely diagnosis of poisoning is made by associating the clinical presentation, pathologic findings, and evidence of ingestion. Chemical detection of tannin

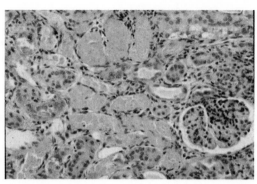

Fig. 4. Kidney of a cow poisoned by oak acorns. Notice the extensive necrosis of the proximal convoluted tubules with eosinophilic granular casts. (hematoxylin-eosin stain original magnificaiton was 100X).

metabolites has limited use because they are readily eliminated and often undetectable in tissues of poisoned animals. Poisoning can be prevented by limiting intake of oak materials to less than 50% of the diet. Treatment of poisoned animals generally is symptomatic and supportive for the gastric and renal damage.

Acer rubrum (red maple) causes severe hemolysis and nephrosis in horses, donkeys and zebras. Toxicity in other livestock has not been reported. Doses of less than 1.5 g leaf/kg body weight, are reported to be poisonous. The wilted and shed leaves are most toxic. Although only red maple has been associated with poisoning, red-maple hybrids should be considered toxic until proved otherwise. Most poisoning occurs in the fall, after storms cause branches to fall into paddocks or when trimmings are fed to animals. Although the cause has not been identified, oxidative hemolysis usually develops within 24 hours of exposure. Clinically, this is seen as anorexia, depression, intravascular and extravascular hemolysis, icterus, anemia, hemoglobinuria, respiratory distress, Heinz body anemia, colic, laminitis, coma, and death. Postmortem findings include icterus and enlarged and swollen spleen, liver, and kidneys and often red urine. Treatment is symptomatic and includes blood transfusions, fluid replacement, and oxygen therapy. Antioxidants, such as ascorbic acid, also may be helpful.

Allium spp (onions) contain an oxidant (N-propyl disulfide) that causes acute hemolytic anemia. Because only large amounts of onion contain enough toxin, it rarely poisons livestock.

The genus *Amaranthus* spp (pigweeds) includes more than 60 species and hybrids that have global distribution. These are annual weeds with prolific seed production that allows them to spread and dominate paddocks, fields, and disturbed areas along fences, ditches, and roads. Although all can accumulate nitrates, only *Amaranthus retroflexus* (red pigweed) and several additional species have been reported to be nephrotoxic and cardiotoxic in livestock.[7,10–12] Clinical poisoning appears to require plant ingestion for several days to several weeks. Additionally, the signs of poisoning can be delayed 5 days to 10 days after exposure, suggesting the elimination of these toxins is slow. The clinical signs of nitrate-associated poisoning include sudden onset of tachypnea, weakness, and recumbency. The syndrome progresses rapidly to death or to a full recovery within 24 hours or less. Pathologic lesions are minimal or absent but can be of darkened, brownish blood in tissues. Pigweed-associated renal disease requires extended ingestion. Once initiated, clinical poisoning quickly progresses in 1 day to 2 days from weakness to muscle tremors, ataxia, knuckling of pasterns, recumbence, paralysis, hemorrhagic diarrhea, hemorrhages, coma, and death. Serum biochemistry changes include increases in potassium, phosphorous, blood urea nitrogen, and creatinine. Gross histologic lesions predominantly are of fluid accumulation with straw-colored fluid in the abdominal and thoracic cavity with pale, potentially swollen kidneys, and prominent perirenal edema. Microscopically, there is marked degeneration and necrosis of the convoluted renal tubular epithelium with interstitial edema. Many renal tubules are dilated and contain proteinaceous debris and casts. The disease in surviving animals often progresses into interstitial renal fibrosis.[7,12–15] Pigweed induced cardiovascular disease usually affect pigs, resulting in sudden death. Histologically, these animals have localized areas of myocardial hemorrhage, necrosis with subsequent fibrosis, and scarring. Many other tissues subsequently may be congested and edematous with occasional effusions.[16,17]

Identifying poisoning is made by linking exposure and ingestion with the clinical signs and lesions. Nitrate poisoning can be confirmed by monitoring serum methemoglobinemia, analyzing serum or ocular fluid for nitrates, analyzing forages for nitrates, and correlating these with the clinical disease. Identifying nephrotoxic or cardiotoxic diseases is more challenging because these lesions are correlated with field studies that verify ingestion and clinical presentation. Because treatment has had no overall effect on survival, prevention by avoiding exposure is recommended. Because animals with pigweed-induced renal disease that survive are likely to have diminished renal function, the prognosis is guarded.

The calcinogenic glycoside-containing plants (*Solanum malacoxylon*, *Solanum verbascifolium*, *Solanum torvum*, *Nierembergia veitchii*, *Trisetum flavescens*, and *Cestrum diurnum*) contain glycosides of 1,25-dihydroxycholecalciferol (calcitriol) or physiologically similar compounds that act as active vitamin D (cholecalciferol), resulting in hypercalcemia and calcification of many tissues and organs. Cholecalciferol increases Ca absorption in the intestinal tract; increases Ca resorption from bone; and decreases renal Ca excretion, resulting in marked hypercalcemia and hyperphosphatemia. These mineral imbalances result in hyperostosis and eventually metastatic calcification.

Clinical poisoning is seen first as depression, weakness, weight loss, infertility, anorexia, cardiac arrhythmias, impaired stilted gait, lameness, recumbence, and death. Biochemically, there is both hypercalcemia and hyperphosphatemia and with progressing renal disease increases in BUN, creatinine, and phosphorus. At necropsy, mineralization, seen as gritty, white deposits, often is seen in kidneys, intestines, stomach, heart, lungs, arteries, bones, tendons, and ligaments. Renal lesions include mineralization of the renal tubular basement membranes, glomerular tufts, and Bowman capsule. Mineralization may involve many other tissues, such as bronchioles, alveoli, endocardium, vessel walls, and walls of the intestine and stomach. Secondary changes include hyperplastic thyroid cells and atrophy of the parathyroid.

Mineralization generally is not reversible and many tissues may remain mineralized for years. Mineralization in the walls of the aorta and tendons are especially persistent.[18–20] Consequently, avoiding exposure is essential. Most of these calcinogenic plants are toxic when grazed and they also are toxic when included in green forage; however, their calcinogenic potential decreases when they are stored for extended periods in dried feeds.

PLANTS THAT CONTAIN GASTROINTESTINAL TOXINS

Mechanical damage results from foxtail, bristle grass, sandbur, cheatgrass, and many other similar plants are poor-quality forages and their awns often are embedded in the mucous membranes of the gums and tongue, causing ulcers and abscesses. Affected animals salivate excessively and they may have difficulty eating. Awns also may migrate deep into tissues, producing infection, abscesses, and loss of function. Because many of these are invasive species, they often displace good forage and also contaminate harvested feeds.

Ranunculaceae (buttercup family) often contain ranunculin that quickly is converted to a potent mucosal irritant, protoanemonin. Clinical signs of poisoning include blistered lips, stomatitis, gastroenteritis, increased salivation, abdominal pain, and diarrhea. Most poisonings occur in sheep because buttercup is not very palatable to other livestock. Dried plants appear to be nontoxic.

The nightshades—*Solanum rostratum* (buffalo bur), *Solanum ptychanthum* (black nightshade), *Solanum dulcamara* (bittersweet), *Solanum elaeagnifolium* (silverleaf nightshade), *Solanum carolinense* (Carolina horse nettle), *Solanum dimidiatum* (western horse nettle), and *Solanum triflorum* (cutleaf nightshade)—are a diverse group of toxic plants, resulting in several poisoning syndromes. Some steroidal glycoalkaloids cause severe gastroenteritis. Others contain cholinesterase inhibitors that cause neurologic disease. The most common toxin is an alkaloid named solanine that is a potent mucosal irritant resulting in severe gastroenteritis (**Fig. 5**). Solanine concentrations are highest in the berries that often poison both livestock and humans. Poisoned animals often develop anorexia, increased salivation and slobbering, abdominal pain, diarrhea, dilation of pupils, dullness, depression, weakness, progressive paralysis, prostration, and rarely death. Treatment generally is symptomatic and most animals quickly recover when exposure is discontinued.[7]

Ricinus communis (castor bean) is an ornamental that in many places has become a weed. The seeds are very toxic and they often contaminate feeds and food. The toxin, ricin, inhibits protein synthesis (by inhibiting ribosomal function) and it can cause severe immunologic disease with anaphylaxis. Poisoning develops within 12 hours to 48 hours after ingestion as animals develop a dull appearance, depression, anorexia, thirst, weakness, colic, trembling, sweating, incoordination, difficult breathing, progressive central nervous system depression, fever, bloody diarrhea, convulsions, and death. Most recognized poisonings are fatal and treatment of those identified early is directed primarily are reducing absorption. Activated charcoal and cathartics may be likely choices for livestock.[21,22]

Convolvulus arvensis (field bindweed or morning glory) is an invasive, noxious weed that invades and often dominates many pastures, paddocks, and disturbed areas.

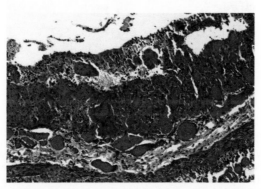

Fig. 5. Intestine of a Syrian hamster treated with ground cutleaf nightshade (*Solanum triflorum*). Notice the extenvise hemorrhagic enteritis with necrosis of enterocyte deep within the intestinal crypts. (hematoxylin-eosin with the original magnificant of 50X).

Poisoning appears to exclusive for horses because there are no reports of toxicity in other species. Horses grazing extensively on bindweed may develop diarrhea, colic, gastrointestinal ulceration, and intestinal thickening and fibrosis. The resinoid convolvulin and several tropane alkaloids have been suggested as the toxins, but this has not been confirmed experimentally.[23] More work is needed to better understand this poisoning, to determine the pathogenesis, and to identify methods to avoid poisoning.

Brassica spp (white mustard, yellow mustard, wild mustard, charlock, black mustard, and Indian mustard). *Erysimum cheiranthoides* (wormseed mustard), *Raphanus raphanastrum* (wild radish), *Thlaspi arvense* (fanweed or field pennycress), *Barbarea vulgari* (yellow rocket or winter cress), and others accumulate nitrates. Though nitrates account for most of their toxicity, several additional toxins have been proposed, and various syndromes have been associated with mustard ingestion. The only proved toxicities, however, are related to nitrates and isothiocyanates. These sporadic diseases such as wooden tongue and hemorrhagic gastroenteritis are poorly characterized.[24,25] Their intermittent occurrence has made identifying the cause and character of poisoning difficult. In most cases, animals recover if they are removed from the source.

MISCELLANEOUS TOXIC PLANTS

Thousands of plants, including those used for food and feeds, contain cyanogenic glycosides. Those associated with poisoning include many types of cherries (*Prunus* spp [**Fig. 6**]); elderberry (*Sambucus* spp); serviceberry (*Amelanchier alnifolia*); various sorghum, Johnson grass, and Sudan grass (*Sorghum* spp); corn (*Zea* spp); vetches (*Vacia sativa*); white clover (*Trifolium repens*); birdsfoot trefoil (*Lotus* spp); and arrowgrass (*Triglochin* spp). Most plant cyanides are sequestered in plants as glycosides, such as amygdalin, prunasin, and lucumin. These glycosides are hydrolyzed, producing toxic cyanide or prussic acid. Hydrolysis primarily occurs when the plant is damaged by crushing, chewing, freezing, or wilting. The cyanide slowly degrades with drying or ensiling. The concentration of cyanogenic glycosides is highest in young rapidly growing plants and often increases with stresses, such as frost, drought, or herbicide treatment.[26,27] Cyanide displaces oxygen by avidly binding with iron in cellular cytochrome oxidase. This inhibits cellular respiration. Unused oxygen accumulates as

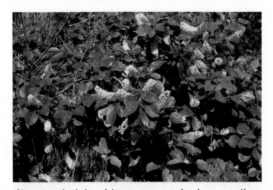

Fig. 6. Chokecherry (*Prunus virginiana)* is a common shrub or small tree that grows along rivers, stream, and cannel banks. All parts contain cyanogenic glycosides except the fleshy part of the berry (the pits are toxic). Ruminants are most susceptible to poisoning and although chokecherry is not very palatable, cattle ingest toxic doses when other forages are scarce.

oxyhemoglobin, making blood and tissues of poisoned animals cherry red. Low, nonlethal doses of cyanide also have been associated with goiter, spinal cord degeneration, and cystitis. It has been suggested these changes are due to neurologic myelin damage.[28]

Clinical poisoning is characterized by hyperventilation, dyspnea, anxiousness, hypotension, and staggering followed by convulsions, paralysis, and death. The blood and tissues may be bright red immediately after death, but darkens between 2 and 6 hours postmortem. Petechial hemorrhages also may be found in the abomasum, endocardium, and epicardium (probably due to stress and agonal struggling). Poisoned animals also may have an almond smell, but this dissipates rapidly postmortem. Diagnosis is made by associating the clinical signs and lesions with evidence of plant consumption. Because cyanide quickly dissipates from tissues after death, tissues such as liver, muscle, and rumen contents, must be collected within a couple of hours, frozen in sealed, airtight containers, and quickly analyzed. Intravenous sodium nitrite and sodium thiosulfate oxidize hemoglobin, forming methemoglobin. Because methemoglobin binds cyanide protecting the cytochrome oxidase system from cyanide, this has been used as a treatment. The best treatment is to avoid harvesting and feeding these plants when they are likely to be toxic. Because some plants are only sporadically toxic, risk assessments can be made by testing potentially toxic feeds for their cyanogenic potential.[26]

Bracken fern (*Pteridium aquilinum* [**Fig. 7**]) has subspecies and varieties throughout the world. They grow in semishaded, well-drained fields and rangelands. They are perennials and, although they are prolific spore producers, they spread primarily through a dense rhizome network. In disturbed areas that have been burned or disturbed, bracken fern expands and dominates the entire plant community. Animals are poisoned when they eat bracken fern while grazing or when it contaminates feeds.[29] Bracken fern toxins include cyanogenic glycosides, thiaminases, steroidal and radiomimetic toxins, and carcinogens. Some have been characterized, but still others have been only suggested. Of these the best described is ptaquiloside, a norsequiterpene glucoside that is mutagenic, clastogenic, and carcinogenic. It damages rapidly dividing cells in the bone marrow and gastrointestinal tract. It also is a potent carcinogen that produces esophageal, gastric, and urinary tract neoplasms.[30] Ptaquiloside

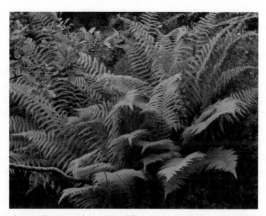

Fig. 7. Bracken fern (*Pteridium* spp) is a prolific perennial that dominates many plant communities. It spreads primarily by an expanding rootstock although it also may produce spores.

concentrations are highest in the vegetative plant parts because the rhizomes, roots, and spores contain very little. Several thiaminases also have been isolated from bracken fern.[31] Thiaminase concentrations are highest in the rhizomes. Prunasin, a cyanogenic glycoside, also has been identified in bracken fern.[32] It has been suggested that chronic cyanide poisoning may account for equine neurologic disease related to bracken fern poisoning. Several syndromes have been associated with bracken fern poisoning. These include acute hemorrhagic disease, bovine enzootic hematuria, bright blindness, upper alimentary carcinomas, and thiamine deficiency. Current evidence suggests these different toxicologic presentations are dependent on dose, duration, and species intoxicated.

Ruminants poisoned with bracken fern generally develop acute hemorrhagic disease and enzootic hematuria though there is a continuum of presentations, varying from hemorrhagic disease to chronic intermittent hematuria with anemia and thrombocytopenia. Hemorrhagic disease occurs most often during late summer when other feed is scarce or when animals are fed hay containing bracken fern. Poisoning livestock must ingest bracken fern for several weeks to years before they become weak and rapidly lose weight. This is followed by fever, dyspnea, and anemia. Hemorrhages develop next ranging from minor mucosal petechia to effusive bleeding that often is seen as large blood clots in the feces. Coagulation times are prolonged and bleeding is extensive even from small wounds, such as small insect bites or other minor scratches. Once animals develop clinical disease, poisoning almost is always fatal. Postmortem examinations usually reveal multiple serosal and soft tissue hemorrhages and bruises, intestinal hemorrhage, and hematuria with hemorrhagic uroepithelium in the bladder and urethra. Later the uroepithelium also may contain numerous vascular, fibrous, or epithelial neoplasms. Although less common, neoplasms in the upper gastrointestinal tract also have been reported. Enzootic hematuria is characterized by intermittent urinary hemorrhage that is due to extensive epithelial and mesenchymal neoplastic transformation of the urinary tract. The neoplastic lesions are of mixed origin because they include vascular, mesenchymal, or epithelial differentiations. The adjacent urinary epithelium often is ulcerated and there are large submucosal hemorrhages. In most cases, mixtures of hemorrhagic and neoplastic lesions are present, making separation of these syndromes artificial. Both the hemorrhagic syndrome and uroepithelial neoplasms have been reproduced experimentally with bracken fern and ptaquiloside.[33] The clinical presentation is dose related because high doses of short duration produce acute poisonings seen as hemorrhagic disease. This is due to ptaquiloside's cytotoxic effects on proliferating bone marrow stem cells. Microscopically, this is seen as depletion of bone marrow megakaryocytes followed by panhypoplasia. The leukogram often has a mixed response. In the initial phase, there is a pronounced monocytosis that is followed by granulocytopenia and thrombocytopenia. Final phases include marked thrombocytopenia with anemia, leukopenia, and hypergammaglobulinemia. Urinalysis generally includes hematuria and proteinuria. Affected animals have both increased susceptibility to infection and a tendency for spontaneous hemorrhage.[34] Ptaquiloside is excreted in the urine and milk of poisoned animals.[35] Ptaquiloside neoplastic transformation may be enhanced by bovine papilloma virus infection; however, this probably is secondary because bracken fern–associated myelodysplasia and subsequent immunosuppression probably promote papilloma virus infection.[36]

Bright blindness is another bracken fern syndrome that may be a less common component of ptaquiloside toxicity characterized by progressive retinal degeneration of sheep. There is marked degeneration and thinning of the retina that is seen as tapetal hyper-reflectivity. Affected sheep may be partially visual and in efforts to see they adopt a characteristic wide-eyed or alert attitude. The pupils respond poorly to light. Ophthalmoscopic findings are those of retinal degeneration characterized by a hyper-reflective fundus with narrowing of arteries and veins and pale tapetum nigrum with patchy spots of gray. Histologically, the lesion is seen as severe atrophy of the retinal rods, cones, and outer nuclear layer that is most pronounced in the tapetal portion of the retina. Affected animals also may have many of the other bracken fern–associated lesions, including bone marrow suppression, hemorrhage, immunosuppression, and urinary tract neoplasia. Retinal degeneration also has been reproduced experimentally in sheep using both powdered bracken fern and purified ptaquiloside.[37,38]

Bracken staggers, or neurologic disease, is the bracken fern poisoning syndrome that is described in monogastric animals. It first was recognized as a neurologic disease when horses consumed contaminated hay. Subsequent studies showed that horses fed diets of 20% to 25% bracken fern for 3 or more months developed the characteristic staggers. The clinical presentation of bracken staggers in horses includes anorexia, weight loss, incoordination, and a crouching stance while arching the back and neck with splayed feet. When forced to move, affected animals tremble and, if they are severely poisoned, horses develop tachycardia and arrhythmias. These signs may progress to convulsions and opisthotonos and such severely affected animals generally die. Because this disease is similar to vitamin B_1 deficiency and most animals respond with thiamine therapy, the pathogenesis of these changes has been attributed to bracken fern thiaminases and antithiamine factors. Perhaps partially due to availability and feeding practices, horses seem particularly susceptible to bracken fern–induced neurologic disease.[29,39] The disease is rare in pigs and the signs are less distinct, including anorexia, weight loss, sudden onset of dyspnea, recumbency, and death. In ruminants, thiamine deficiency generally is associated with polioencephalomalacia ,which is not a common finding in ruminant bracken fern poisoning; however, impaired thiamine metabolism in sheep has been associated with consumption of bracken fern and rock or mulga fern (*Cheilanthes sieberi*) in Australia.[40]

Because bracken fern poisoning, other than thiamine deficiency, essentially is untreatable, poisoning is controlled most easily by preventing exposure. Bracken fern usually is grazed for want of alternative forages. Avoiding exposure by improving pasture management and increasing the production of alternative forage is essential. Recent work has found that some bracken populations contain very low or no ptaquiloside. More work is needed to identify these populations, to determine why they are not toxic and use this information to predict or reduce toxicity. As with most toxic plants, the initial step should be to remove poisoned animals from bracken fern–containing pastures. Treatment of thiamine deficiency in horses is effective if a diagnosis is made early. Thiamine therapy should include animals similarly exposed but not yet showing signs, because they may develop disease days or weeks after removal from the source of bracken. Antibiotics may be useful to prevent secondary infections. Blood transfusions or even platelet transfusions may be appropriate. Most animals that develop hemorrhagic and neoplastic disease do not recover.

SUMMARY

Plants often contain toxins that damage the urinary tract and gastrointestinal systems. These selected plants represent some of the most common toxic plants that affect these systems in livestock in North America. Diagnosis depends on correlating disease and lesions with exposure and chemical analysis of tissues and feeds.

DISCLOSURE

The authors have nothing to disclose.

REFERENCES

1. Naude TW, Naidoo V. Oxalate containing plants. In: Gupta RC, editor. Veterinary toxicology: basic and clinical principles. Boston: Elsevier; 2007. p. 880–91.
2. McMartin KE, Wallace KB. Calcium oxalate monohydrate, a metabolite of ethylene glycol, is toxic for rat renal mitochondrial function. Toxicol Sci 2005;84: 195–200.
3. McMartin K. Are calcium oxalate crystals involved in the mechanism of acute renal failure in ethylene glycol poisoning? Clin Toxicol (Phila) 2009;47:859–69.
4. Van Kampen KR, James LF. Acute halogeton poisoning of sheep: Pathogenesis of lesions. Am J Vet Res 1969;30:1779–83.
5. James LF. Halogeton poisoning in livestock. J Nat Toxins 1999;8:395–403.
6. Walthall JC, McKenzie RA. Osteodystrophia fibrosa in horses at pasture in queensland: Field and laboratory observations. Aust Vet J 1976;52:11–6.
7. Burrows GE, Tyrl RJ. Toxic plants of North America. Second Edition. Ames (Iowa): John Wiley & Sons Inc; 2013.
8. Plumlee KH, Johnson B, Galey FD. Comparison of disease in calves dosed orally with oak or commercial tannic acid. J Vet Diagn Invest 1998;10:263–7.
9. Begovic S, Duzic E, Sacirbegovic A, et al. Examination of variation of tannase activity in ruminal contents and mucosae of goats fed oak leaves and during ruminal application of 3 to 10% annic acid. Veterinaria (Yogoslavia) 1978;27:445–57.
10. Panter KE, Gardner DR, Lee ST, et al. Important poisonous plants of the United States. In: Grupta RC, editor. Veterinary toxicology: basic and clinical principles. New York: Elsevier; 2007. p. 825–72.
11. Stuart BP, Nicholson SS, Smith JB. Perirenal edema and toxic nephrosis in cattle, associated with ingestion of pigweed. J Am Vet Med Assoc 1975;167:949–50.
12. Casteel SW, Johnson GC, Miller MA, et al. *Amaranthus retroflexus* (redroot pigweed) poisoning in cattle. J Am Vet Med Assoc 1994;204:1068–70.
13. Armesto RR, Grande HA, Baroni AC, et al. *Amaranthus quitensis* intoxication in Holando-Argentina heifers. Vet Argen 1989;6:692, 694-692,700.
14. Gonzalez S. Tubular toxic nephrosis in sheep and goats after ingesting plants of the genus *Amaranthus*. Vet Mex 1983;14:247–51.
15. Osweiler GD, Buck WB, Bicknell EJ. Production of perirenal edema in swine with *Amaranthus retroflexus*. Am J Vet Res 1969;30:557–66.
16. Takken A, Connor JK. Some toxicological aspects of grain amaranth for pigs. In: Seawright AA, Hegarty MP, James I, et al, editors. Plant toxicology- proceedings of the Australia-USA poisonous plant symposium. Queensland Department of Primary Industries: Yeerongpilly Australia; 1985. p. 170–7.
17. Sanko RE. Perirenal edema in swine- caused by ingestion of *Amaranthus retroflexus* (pigweed). Vet Med Small Anim Clin 1975;70:42–4.
18. Dirksen G, Plank P, Spiess A, et al. Enzootic calcinosis in cattle. I. Clinical findings and studies. Dtsch Tierarztl Wochenschr 1970;77:321–37.
19. Hanichen T, Hermanns W. The question of reversibility of tissue calcification in enzootic calcinosis of cattle and in experimental hypervitaminosis. Dtsch Tierarztl Wochenschr 1990;97:479–82.
20. Hanichen T, Plank P, Dirksen G. Enzootic calcinosis in cattle. Histomorphological studies of soft tissues. Dtsch Tierarztl Wochenschr 1970;77:338–42.

21. Akande TO, Odunsi AA, Akinfala EO. A review of nutritional and toxicological implications of castor bean (*Ricinus communis* l.) meal in animal feeding systems. J Anim Physiol Anim Nutr (Berl) 2016;100:201–10.
22. Wedin GP, Neal JS, Everson GW, et al. Castor bean poisoning. Am J Emerg Med 1986;4:259–61.
23. Todd FG, Stermitz FR, Schultheis P, et al. Tropane alkaloids and toxicity of *Convolvulus arvensis*. Phytochemistry 1995;39:301–3.
24. Semalulu SS, Rousseaux CG. Suspected oriental mustard seed (brassica juncea) poisoning in cattle. Can Vet J 1989;30:595–6.
25. Staley E. A treatment for tansy mustard poisoning. Bov Pract (Stillwater) 1976; 11:35.
26. Pickrell JA, Oehme F. Cyanogenic glycosides. In: Plumlee KH, editor. Clinical veterinary toxicology. St. Louis (MO): Mosby; 2003. p. 391–2.
27. Vetter J. Plant cyanogenic glycosides. Toxicon 2000;38:11–36.
28. Soto-Blanco B, Stegelmeier BL, Pfister JA, et al. Comparative effects of prolonged administration of cyanide, thiocyanate and chokecherry (*Prunus virginiana*) to goats. J Appl Toxicol 2008;28:356–63.
29. Vetter J. A biological hazard of our age: Bracken fern (*Pteridium aquilinum* Kuhn)- A review. Acta Vet Hung 2009;57:183–96.
30. Castillo UF, Ojika M, Onso-Amelot M, et al. a new toxic unstable sesquiterpene glucoside from the neotropical bracken fern pteridium aquilinum var. Caudatum. Bioorg Med Chem 1998;6:2229–33.
31. Meyer P. Thiaminase activities and thiamine content of pteridium aquilinum, equisetum ramosissimum, malva parviflora, pennisetum clandestinum and medicago sativa. Onderstepoort J Vet Res 1989;56:145–6.
32. Bennett WD. Isolation of the cyanogenetic glucoside prunasin from bracken fern. Phytochemistry 1969;7:151–2.
33. Hirono I, Ogino H, Fujimoto M, et al. Induction of tumors in aci rats given a diet containing ptaquiloside, a bracken carcinogen. J Natl Cancer Inst 1987;79: 1143–9.
34. Pamukcu AM, Price JM, Bryan GT. Naturally occurring and braken-fern-induced bovine urinary bladder tumors. Clinical and morphological characteristics. Vet Pathol 1976;13:110–22.
35. Smith BL, Seawright AA. Bracken fern (pteridium spp.) carcinogenicity and human health–a brief review. Nat Toxins 1995;3:1–5.
36. Leishangthem GD, Somvanshi R, Lauren DR. Pathological studies on bovine papilloma virus-fern interaction in hamsters. Indian J Exp Biol 2008;46:100–7.
37. Watson WA, Barnett KC, Terlecki S. Progressive retinal degeneration (bright blindness) in sheep: A review. Vet Rec 1972;91:665–70.
38. Hirono I, Ito M, Yagyu S, et al. Reproduction of progressive retinal degeneration (bright blindness) in sheep by administration of ptaquiloside contained in bracken. J Vet Med Sci 1993;55:979–83.
39. Kelleway RA, Geovjian L. Acute bracken fern poisoning in a 14-month-old horse. Vet Med Small Anim Clin 1978;73:295–6.
40. Evans WC, Evans IA, Humphreys DJ, et al. Induction of thiamine deficiency in sheep, with lesions similar to those of cerebrocortical necrosis. J Comp Pathol 1975;85:253–67.

Hepatotoxic Plants that Poison Livestock

Michael J. Clayton, DVM, T. Zane Davis, PhD, Edward L. Knoppel, MS,
Bryan L. Stegelmeier, DVM, PhD*

KEYWORDS

- Hepatotoxins • Pyrrolizidine alkaloid • Cocklebur • Saponin • Lantana • Livestock
- Poisoning

KEY POINTS

- The liver is a common target in toxicoses, because many toxicants require metabolic activation to cause cellular injury.
- Plant-derived hepatotoxins largely cause nonspecific clinical, biochemical, and histopathologic changes indicative of hepatic or biliary insult.
- Definitive diagnosis is often challenging and requires field investigation, clinical information, necropsy findings, and detection of the toxic compound.
- Presumptive diagnosis is achieved with clinical information, histopathology, and plant identification in feed or gastrointestinal content.
- Pyrrolizidine alkaloids are likely the most important plant-derived toxins worldwide.

INTRODUCTION

Many toxic plants damage the liver because it is the first organ exposed to intestinal portal blood and has many mixed function oxidases with potential to bioactivate xenotoxins. Enzyme type and activity, and the concentrations of toxins and oxygen, change in hepatocyte populations as portal blood moves down the sinusoid from the portal vessels to the central veins. Toxins are bioactivated by hepatocytes and damage different sections of the hepatic lobule. Some plant toxins are quickly bioactivated and become potent alkylating agents that denature hepatic proteins and nucleic acids in the first hepatocytes they encounter. The result is seen as periportal hepatocellular degeneration and necrosis. Other toxins require more specific bioactivation or lower oxygen tension or oxidative protections as are present in centrilobular hepatocytes. Damage from these toxins results in centrilobular swelling and necrosis.[1,2] Other hepatotoxins may not require bioactivation. These may damage

USDA/ARS Poisonous Plant Research Laboratory, 1150 East 1400 North, Logan, UT 84341, USA
* Corresponding author.
E-mail address: Bryan.Stegelmeier@usda.gov

Vet Clin Food Anim 36 (2020) 715–723
https://doi.org/10.1016/j.cvfa.2020.08.003
0749-0720/20/Published by Elsevier Inc.

all the hepatocytes regardless of their location resulting in massive or panlobular necrosis.

Regardless of the original lesion or its distribution, if the disease is not immediately fatal, the liver is limited in the ways it can respond. This common response is nonspecific fibrosis, biliary hyperplasia, and nodular hepatocellular regeneration and hyperplasia that progresses to overt cirrhosis. Regardless of the inciting cause (toxic, infectious, nutritional, or immunologic), the result (end-stage liver cirrhosis) is similar.[2] This makes identifying specific causes challenging. Field studies documenting exposure, clinical data (hematology, serum biochemistry, and physical examination), gross and histologic evaluation, and laboratory identification of plant parts, toxins, or metabolites must be used in concert to make the best diagnosis. Although some hepatotoxic plants are more likely to produce certain clinical diseases, most are nonspecific.

This brief description of liver disease is applicable to many different etiologies. Nearly all hepatotoxins result in hepatocellular or biliary damage. Clinical signs common to these lesions include inappetence, icterus, hepatic encephalopathy, coagulopathy, edema, ascites, hepatocutaneous syndrome, photosensitization, and polyuria/polydipsia. Hematologic changes include nonregenerative anemia. Changes in serum biochemistry include elevations in alanine aminotransferase, aspartate aminotransferase (AST), alkaline phosphatase (ALP), γ-glutamyltransferase (GGT), and sorbitol dehydrogenase (SDH). There are also increased bilirubin with hyperammonemia, hypoglycemia, and hypoalbuminemia. Chronic liver failure is seen grossly as a shrunken and firm liver with nodules of hyperplasia admixed with fibrosis. Histologic changes include massive fibrosis that often bridges lobules with ovalocyte and biliary epithelial cell proliferation, nodular hepatocyte proliferation with collapse and loss of sinusoidal structure.

DEHYDROPYRROLIZIDINE ALKALOID–CONTAINING PLANTS

Dehydropyrrolizidine alkaloids (PAs) are a large, and diverse group of plant toxins that are found throughout the world in many species of the Boraginaceae, Asteraceae, Orchidaceae, and Fabaceae families (**Figs. 1–3**). It has been estimated that more than 3% of flowering plants worldwide contain PAs and poisoning has been reported

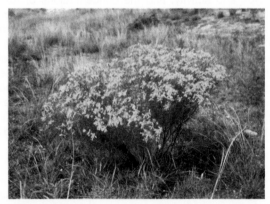

Fig. 1. *Senecio riddellii* is found in the central United States and most commonly poisons cattle. This plant is unique, in that it primarily contains a single dehydropyrrolizidine alkaloid (PA), riddelliine, whereas most PA-containing plants contain mixtures of various PAs. Riddelliine has been proven carcinogenic to rodents and is classified as a potential human carcinogen by the National Toxicology Program.

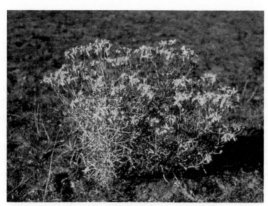

Fig. 2. *Senecio douglasii* var. longilobus (threadleaf or woolly groundsel) is found in several southwestern states. The plant contains four different PAs, and most commonly poisons cattle. Woolly groundsel grows well on abused or arid rangelands.

in livestock, wildlife, and humans. PAs are hepatotoxic, pneumotoxic, and carcinogenic. Many PA-containing plants are invasive, nonnative weeds that often invade and dominate plant populations in fields, pastures, and rangelands. Native PA-containing plants tend to be less invasive, causing problems when they grow or spread when land is disturbed. Most PA-containing plants are not palatable, and poisoning is often associated with contamination of feed and foods. Poisoning caused by grazing and direct consumption is less common and typically occurs when animals are forced to eat the plants because alternative forages are limited. Concentrations of PAs in plant populations is highly variable even in the same plant and location from year to year.[3]

PAs require bioactivation, which occurs primarily in the liver via cytochrome P-450 enzymes. When activated by dehydrogenation or oxidation, PAs form toxic didehydro-pyrrolizidine alkaloids that are potent electrophiles that quickly bind DNA, RNA, proteins, and amino acids. Damage to cellular nucleic acids and proteins results in

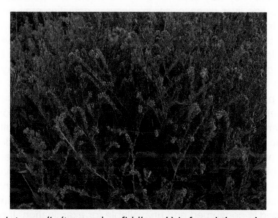

Fig. 3. *Amsinckia intermedia* (tarweed or fiddleneck) is found throughout Canada and the western, midwestern, and northeastern United States, and poisons cattle and horses. This plant has been reported to cause the clinical syndromes "walking disease" in horses and "hard liver disease" in cattle. The plant grows in waste areas and fields.

acute cytotoxicity. Binding to DNA also has an antimitotic effect that can result in megalocytosis, a characteristic histologic finding in which hepatocytes and their nuclei become enlarged because of the inability to divide. There is evidence that protein or DNA adducts persist in tissues for months to years and may be recycled to cause additional damage.

All PAs are not equally toxic. Some are more likely to produce extrahepatic lesions, photosensitivity, or hepatic encephalopathy. There is also significant variation in species susceptibility. Chickens, cattle, pigs, and horses are susceptible, whereas small ruminants and most rodents are resistant. Both susceptibility and resistance to poisoning have been attributed to differences in bioavailability, rumen metabolism, and bioactivation/detoxification mechanisms. Age, sex, and nutritional status also influence susceptibility of individual animals. Young animals are more susceptible than adults. PAs can cross the placenta and they also contaminate milk resulting in fetal and neonatal poisoning. Under some conditions they can poison fetus and nursing neonates, while the less susceptible dam is clinically unaffected. Nutritional stress or excessive hepatic copper concentrations may also increase susceptibility.[3,4]

Most livestock exposure to PAs occurs by ingestion of contaminated hay or prepared feeds. Exposure by grazing may also occur, and plant factors, such as palatability, location, weather, and the availability of other forage, influence the likelihood of exposure, and the amount a grazing animal will ingest. Many PA-containing plants are most toxic in the bud stage; however, there are large variations in PA concentration in the same plant species from year to year and location to location.[5] This variation makes it difficult to predict toxicity and calculate toxic doses when ingestion is suspected.

PA-poisoned animals may display clinical signs of acute liver failure, including anorexia, depression, icterus, visceral edema, and ascites. Clinical signs may develop acutely even in cases of chronic exposure as the threshold of liver dysfunction is reached. High doses result in the acute development of liver failure. Clinical pathology data indicates liver damage and loss of liver function. In most active cases of PA poisoning serum concentrations of AST, SDH, ALP, and GGT are increased. With some time, concentrations of bilirubin, bile acids, and ammonia also increase. In chronic low-dose poisonings, these enzyme elevations may be transient. Enzyme activities and functional indicators may vary depending on the extent of hepatocellular damage and fibrosis. In end-stage liver disease, serum enzyme activities may be normal or even low, whereas indicators of liver function (bilirubin, bile acids, ammonia, albumin, cholesterol, and blood urea nitrogen) may be altered in relation to loss of liver function.[3]

Hepatic histologic lesions of PA poisoning are characteristic, but nonspecific, because other potent alkylating toxins, such as some aflatoxins, may produce similar changes. Acute microscopic changes of PA poisoning include hepatocyte cell swelling, which progresses to degeneration and necrosis. High doses result in acute panlobular hepatocellular degeneration and necrosis, with hemorrhage and low numbers of inflammatory cells. Chronic, low-dose poisonings result in portal, often bridging, hepatic fibrosis with proliferation of bile duct epithelium (ductular reaction). Megalocytosis may also be observed in hepatocytes after chronic exposure.[3,4]

Identification of PA poisoning is often challenging. Clinical signs may be delayed for weeks and even months after ingestion. Because many intoxications are caused by contaminated hay, the clinical disease may not become apparent until after the contaminated feed is consumed and unavailable for examination. If poisoning is suspected, rumen contents and liver samples should be collected and stored frozen. If gross and microscopic findings support PA intoxication these samples can be analyzed for PA and PA metabolites.[6]

Treating PA poisoned animals is generally unrewarding. Some animals do recover, but damage can progress and result in significant loss of hepatic function; such crippled animals often decompensate when stressed. Efforts should be focused on preventing exposure. Because most poisonings are caused by contamination of feed, inspection of fields before harvest is essential. Dry forage should be closely inspected, and contaminated feed discarded. Herbicides are available to control most PA-containing plants.

ALSIKE CLOVER (*TRIFOLIUM HYBRIDUM*)

Alsike clover is a legume forage used for hay, pasture, and soil improvement. The plant resembles red clover, but is distinguished by the absence of crescent-shaped marks on the leaflets. Alsike clover causes poisonings in herbivores characterized by two syndromes. The first syndrome is a primary photosensitization that is seen in cattle, sheep, swine, and horses. The second syndrome, referred to as alsike clover syndrome, is characterized by hepatic dysfunction and photosensitization, and is only reported in horses. The toxic principles have not been completely elucidated, but several phytoestrogen isoflavones and cyanogenic glycosides have been isolated from the plant. These compounds are usually in low enough concentrations that they are probably unimportant and the toxin that is responsible for hepatotoxicity is unknown. Clinical signs and biochemical changes are nonspecific, but include mild colic, anorexia, and serum biochemistry changes of cholestasis and hepatotoxicity. Histopathologic lesions include subacute to chronic biliary hyperplasia and fibrosis. Although the plant is widespread, poisonings are rare.[7]

COCKLEBUR (*XANTHIUM* SPP)

Cocklebur and other xanthium species are widely distributed throughout North America, and other parts of the world (**Fig. 4**). These plants have long been used as part of traditional Chinese medicine to treat headache, sinusitis, urticaria, and arthritis. Xanthium poisoning resulting in hepatotoxicity has been reported in animals and people. The main toxic principles include atractyloside, carboxyatractyloside, and 4'-desulphate-atractyloside. The proposed mechanism of toxicity is inhibition of mitochondrial function and alteration of fatty acid metabolism. Clinical pathology changes include elevations in alanine aminotransferase, AST, ALP, and bilirubin and hypoglycemia. Histologic lesions include dose-dependent hepatocellular vacuolation and centrilobular hepatocellular degeneration and necrosis.[8,9]

SAPONIN-CONTAINING PLANTS

Saponins are glycosides of steroid alcohols known to have antimicrobial and antifungal properties for hundreds of years and are found in numerous plant species. They are present in plants that are nontoxic including soybeans, beans, peas, potatoes, alfalfa, tomatoes, onions, asparagus, spinach, cucumbers, and yams. Other saponin-containing plants that have been reported to cause poisonings in livestock include *Tribulus terrestris*, *Narthecium ossifragum*, *Agave lechuguilla*, and various species of *Brachiaria*, *Panicum*, and *Sesbania* genera. Poisonings from saponin-containing plants in the United States are uncommon, but have been attributed to corn cockle, soapwort, cow cockle, and broomweed. Other reports include Alfombrilla (*Drymaria arenaroides*) in northern Mexico, and *T terrestris*, an annual weed common on semiarid rangelands in Australia, South Africa, North America, and Iran. These poisonings reportedly occur under certain conditions that have not been clearly

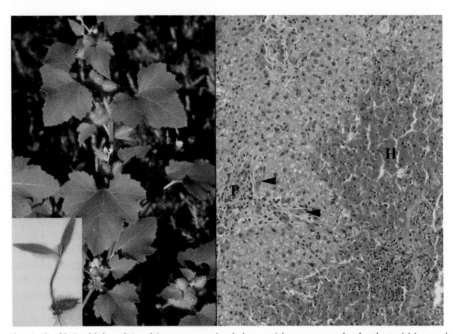

Fig. 4. (*Left*) Cocklebur (*Xanthium strumarium*), burs with numerous barbs that aid in seed dispersal and make the plant unpalatable. The inset is cocklebur in the dicotyledon stage, which is reported to be the most toxic. (*Right*) Bovine liver after acute cocklebur poisoning. Notice the centrilobular to bridging hepatocellular necrosis with massive hemorrhage (H). The hepatic cords have collapsed and there is periportal (P) increased cellularity with infiltrates of lymphocytes and proliferation of ovalocytes (*arrowheads*). (hematoxylin-eosin stain, original magnification 100X).

elucidated. Intoxication causes crystal-associated cholangiohepatopathy in sheep.[10] Grossly, there may be white, crystalline material within the gallbladder, icterus, and facial eczema. Microscopic lesions include cholangitis, and eosinophilic crystalline material within bile ducts, canaliculi, and hepatocytes. The proposed mechanism of action is the formation of free saponins in the gastrointestinal tract, that are then reduced and epimerized to epismilagenin and episarsasapogenin and absorbed into portal circulation.[1] Glucoronidation of these compounds in the liver then results in precipitation as calcium salts in areas of high concentration, such as the hepatocytes and bile canaliculi and ducts.[11]

MISCELLANEOUS AND FUNGAL-ASSOCIATED PLANT HEPATOTOXINS

Several plants were historically important hepatotoxic plants. Horsebrush (*Tetradymia glabrata*) fed exclusively to naive animals often produced liver disease and subsequent photosensitization (**Fig. 5**). Currently livestock handling has changed and poisoning is rarely reported.[12] Both horsebrush and various sage species are important wildlife and livestock winter forages that are safely used.

In other cases, animals are poisoned by ingesting plants that contain toxins that are not synthesized by the plant but are produced by fungal organisms that grow on or within the plant material. There are a variety of mycotoxins that can infect forage or stored grains and hay. These mycotoxins can poison animals and people and can damage many organ systems including the liver. Aflatoxins are an example of a

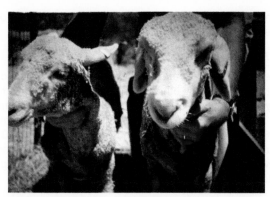

Fig. 5. Photosensitization of sheep with big head (*right*). The left sheep is a normal control animal. This is an acute case with massive edema of the ears and face. This is a historical disease when unconditioned sheep were forced to eat exclusively horsebrush (*Tetradymia* spp) with black sage (*Artemisia nova*). Photosensitization is a nonspecific sign of liver failure with subsequent accumulation of phylloerythrin and increased susceptibility to irradiation-induced dermatitis. Similar dermatitis is seen in sporidesmin-induced liver failure (facial eczema).

mycotoxin that is produced by *Aspergillus* spp and causes poisonings in people and less commonly livestock. Fumonisins are a mycotoxin produced by *Fusarium* spp, and with chronic exposure cause leukoencephalomalacia in horses known as moldy corn poisoning.[13] Lupin toxicosis can occur if lupin stubble becomes infected with the saprophytic fungus, *Diapthoria toxica*. The toxic principles are phomopsins, which inhibit microtubule polymerization, thus hindering mitosis, which results in severe liver disease with secondary photosensitization.[14] Sporidesmin is produced by the saprophytic fungus *Pithomyces chartarum*, which infects different *Lolium* spp including perennial rye and other plants. Poisoning results in diarrhea, inappetence, followed by icterus and photosensitization (facial eczema; see **Fig. 5**). Acute bovine liver disease is an emerging disease associated with the ingestion of *Cynosurus echinatus* resulting in hepatocellular degeneration and necrosis. The toxic principle has not been identified, but a mycotoxin is suspected.[15]

Lantana camara and other *Lantana* species are ornamental shrubs that can act as invasive noxious weeds, replacing nutritious forage. Toxicity is caused by lantadene A and B, pentacyclic triterpenoid toxins present in the leaves, stems, roots, and unripe fruit. They are potent hepatotoxins causing hepatocellular necrosis and fibrosis that often results in photosensitization. Acutely poisoned animals may develop constipation and inappetence as quickly as 2 hours after ingestion. This is followed by photosensitization, dull mentation, and icterus 24 to 48 hours after ingestion. Poisonings have been reported in cattle, small ruminants, and wildlife. Ingestion of 60 mg/kg of dried leaf powder causes hepatotoxicity and cholestasis. Ruminal stasis also occurs 4 to 6 hours after ingestion. As is true with many toxins, hepatic metabolism or bioactivation is required before toxic injury. Differences in metabolism are responsible for differences in species susceptibility. *Lantana* toxins cause intrahepatic cholestasis in addition to hepatocellular damage. Grossly, the liver and kidneys are swollen and pale yellow. Histologic lesions include periportal hepatocellular degeneration and necrosis. In chronic cases, fibrosis with cholestasis and variable biliary proliferation are observed. Clinical pathology changes include elevations in GGT, ALP, and bilirubin. Treatment with surgical rumenotomy and transfaunation has been successful, but is cost prohibitive in a large-scale poisoning event. Oral administration of activated charcoal has also been successfully used for treatment.[16]

Other Emerging Hepatotoxic Plants

It has been suggested that *Salvia reflexa* is hepatotoxic and when included in hay can fatally poison cattle and possibly other species. *S reflexa* is native to North America and is commonly called lance-leaf sage, wild mint, mint weed, narrow-leafed sage, blue sage, sage mint, and Rocky Mountain sage. The plant has blue-green leaves covered in soft hair, with a mintlike odor, and can grow to 30 to 60 cm. Originally it was reported to accumulate nitrates, but until recently it was not known to be hepatotoxic.[17] More work is needed to better characterize this poisoning and identify the toxic components.

SUMMARY

Plants often contain hepatotoxins resulting in liver degeneration, necrosis, and failure. Nonspecific end-stage liver failure or cirrhosis is often the result of poisoning and because this also results from various toxic, infectious, and nutritional disease, identification of the underlying cause is difficult. Diagnosis depends on documenting exposure with clinical signs and lesions. Correlating clinical signs, lesions, and a history of exposure with chemical identification of toxins or their metabolites is required to make a likely diagnosis. This is often complicated because disease is often delayed weeks or months after exposure.

DISCLOSURE

The authors have nothing to disclose.

REFERENCES

1. Burrows GE, Tyrl RJ. Toxic plants of North America, Second Edition. Ames (Iowa): John Wiley & Sons Inc; 2013.
2. Kelly WR. The liver and biliary system. In: Jubb KVF, editor. Pathology of domestic animals. New York: Academic Press Inc.; 1993. p. 319–406.
3. Stegelmeier BL, Edgar JA, Colegate SM, et al. Pyrrolizidine alkaloid plants, metabolism and toxicity. J Nat Toxins 1999;8:95–116.
4. Stegelmeier BL. Pyrrolizidine alkaloid-containing toxic plants (*Senecio, Crotalaria, Cynoglossum, Amsinckia, Heliotropium,* and *Echium* spp.). Vet Clin North Am Food Anim Pract 2011;27:419–28, ix.
5. Molyneux RJ, Johnson AE. Extraordinary levels of production of pyrrolizidine alkaloids in *Senecio riddellii.* J Nat Prod 1984;47:1030–2.
6. Brown AW, Stegelmeier BL, Colegate SM, et al. The comparative toxicity of a reduced, crude comfrey (*Symphytum officinale*) alkaloid extract and the pure, comfrey-derived pyrrolizidine alkaloids, lycopsamine and intermedine in chicks (*Gallus Gallus domesticus*). J Appl Toxicol 2016;36:716–25.
7. Colon JL, Jackson CA, Piero FD. Hepatic dysfunction and photodermatitis secondary to alsike clover poisoning. Comp Cont Edu Pract Vet 1996;18:1022–6.
8. Witte ST, Osweiler GD, Stahr HM, et al. Cocklebur toxicosis in cattle associated with the consumption of mature *Xanthium strumarium.* J Vet Diagn Invest 1990; 2:263–7.

9. Stuart BP, Cole RJ, Gosser HS. Cocklebur (*Xanthium strumarium*, L. var. strumarium) intoxication in swine: review and redefinition of the toxic principle. Vet Pathol 1981;18:368–83.

10. Wina E, Muetzel S, Becker K. The impact of saponins or saponin-containing plant materials on ruminant production: a review. J Agric Food Chem 2005;53: 8093–105.

11. Francis G, Kerem Z, Makkar HP, et al. The biological action of saponins in animal systems: a review. Br J Nutr 2002;88:587–605.

12. Johnson AE. Experimental photosensitization and toxicity in sheep produced by *Tetradymia glabrata*. Can J Comp Med 1974;38:406–10.

13. Ross PF, Nelson PE, Owens DL, et al. Fumonisin B2 in cultured *Fusarium proliferatum*, M-6104, causes equine leukoencephalomalacia. J Vet Diagn Invest 1994;6:263–5.

14. Edgar JA. Phomopsins: antimicrotubule mycotoxins. Handbook of Natural Toxins Volume 6: Toxicology of plant and fungal compounds. Marcel Dekker Inc. 1991. pp 371-395.

15. Read E, Edwards J, Deseo M, et al. Current understanding of acute bovine liver disease in Australia. Toxins 2017;9:8.

16. Sharma OP, Sharma S, Pattabhi V, et al. A review of the hepatotoxic plant, *Lantana camara*. Crit Rev Toxicol 2007;37:313–52.

17. Williams C, Hines H. The toxic properties of *Salvia reflexa*. Aust Vet J 1940;16: 14–20.

Plant-Induced Photosensitivity and Dermatitis in Livestock

Bryan L. Stegelmeier, DVM, PhD*, T. Zane Davis, PhD,
Michael J. Clayton, DVM

KEYWORDS

- Poisonous plants • Photosensitivity • Dermatitis • Hypericin • Furanocoumarins
- Phylloerythrin

KEY POINTS

- Plant-induced photosensitivity is increased sensitivity to radiation-induced dermatitis. Plant-induced photosensitivity and dermatitis in livestock
- Primary photosensitization occurs when livestock ingest plants that contain photodynamic compounds or chromophores.
- Secondary or hepatogenous photosensitization occurs when photodynamic chlorophyll metabolites (phylloerythrin) accumulate in tissues due to liver disease.
- Other plants that cause dermatitis include hairy vetch, various allergenic plants, and dermatitis secondary to systemic disease.

PHOTOSENSITIZATION

Photosensitization is light-induced dermatitis caused by heightened sensitivity of the skin to sunlight, and this is generally due to the presence of photodynamic agents or chromophores in the skin. These chromophores absorb light energy transforming into a high-energy state that damages adjacent proteins, nucleic acids, and membranes. This energy can directly damage molecules or generate reactive molecules that continue or initiate chemical reactions in dermal components. Perhaps the largest contributor to dermal damage is the production of reactive oxygen intermediates and free radicals. The result of all this is epithelial cell damage, degeneration, and necrosis. Because most chromophores are not cytotoxic until they are photoactivated, clinical dermatitis requires solar irradiation and generally only develops after exposure to sunlight. Both hair and dermal pigments absorb light energy and protect the underlying skin. Consequently, radiation-induced dermatitis generally occurs on the muzzle,

USDA/ARS Poisonous Plant Research Laboratory, 1150 East 1400 North, Logan, UT 84341, USA
* Corresponding author.
E-mail address: Bryan.Stegelmeier@USDA.GOV

Vet Clin Food Anim 36 (2020) 725–733
https://doi.org/10.1016/j.cvfa.2020.08.008
0749-0720/20/Published by Elsevier Inc.

ears, eyelids, face, tail, vulva, udder, and coronary bands. However, with severe exposures even black, heavily haired animals can develop photosensitivity. Clinical signs include photophobia and discomfort seen as scratching and rubbing of the ears, eyelids, and muzzle. Affected areas develop erythema followed by edema, serous exudation, scab formation, and skin necrosis. The resulting inflammation may be extensive resulting in epidermal necrosis, sloughing of necrotic layers, and extensive suppurative exudate (**Fig. 1**). Clinically the effect of dermatitis depends on animal function. Lactating cattle that develop dermatitis of the udder and teats often wean immature calves. Horses with white skin and hair on the face, back, shoulders, or girth skin develop dermatitis that impairs using tack and may preclude their use for riding or work for the rest of the season. Sheep and goats often develop big head (marked swelling and dermatitis of the face, ears, and lips) that impairs both growth and production. All of these lesions will recover with appropriate therapy and housing of animals in shaded areas to prevent further damage.[1]

Dermal photodynamic chromophores that cause photosensitization are generally xenobiotics (plant or fungal toxins, drugs, chlorophyll metabolites, or other chemicals). Cattle, swine, and cats have a congenital form of photosensitivity termed porphyria, osteohemochromatosis, or pink tooth that is caused by defective uroporphyrinogen III cosynthetase, an enzyme of hemoglobin synthesis.[2]

Photosensitization is divided into primary and secondary or hepatogenous photosensitization. Primary photosensitization is caused directly by chromophores from plants, drugs, or abnormal metabolites. Secondary photosensitization is caused by defective liver function with subsequent accumulation of photodynamic phylloerythrin, a chlorophyll metabolite. By definition, primary photosensitization does not include hepatic damage, but some poisonings are mixed and the effects are cumulative. Most agents are ingested where the chromophore is absorbed from the digestive tract and reaches the skin unchanged.[1,3] Other plants cause topical dermatitis when the chromophore is absorbed into the superficial epidermis.[4]

Primary Photosensitization

Hypericum perforatum (St. John's wort, goat weed, Tipton weed, amber, or Klamath weed) (**Fig. 2**) is a perennial that grows along roadsides and in meadows, pastures, rangelands, and waste places. It is found in the North American Pacific coast states

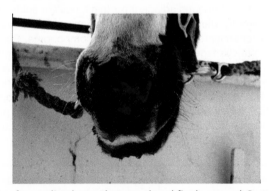

Fig. 1. The muzzle of a yearling horse that was dosed finely ground *Cynoglossum officinale* to obtain a dose of 15 mg total pyrrolizidine alkaloid/kg BW/for 10 days. This filly developed severe liver disease and failure, resulting in severe necrosis of the thinly haired skin over her muzzle. Notice the necrotic crust-covered scabs with central zones of ulceration and hemorrhage.

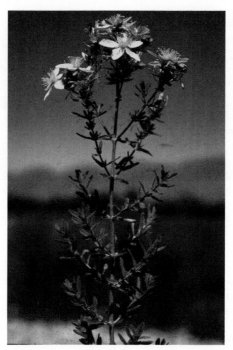

Fig. 2. St. John's wort (*Hypericum perforatum*) is a smooth-branched, erect plant that may reach a height of 2 m. The leaves are covered with clear, small dots that contain the toxic substance (hypericin). The flowers have 5 petals that grow in clusters; they are orange-yellow with small black dots along the edges.

as well as in Europe, Australia, New Zealand, and South America. It typically grows on dry, gravelly, or sandy soils in full sunshine. It may grow in dense patches or mixed among other plants. It is considered a noxious weed in many states. St. John's wort is dangerous at all stages of growth. Young tender shoots may attract animals and are more palatable in the spring. Normally, livestock will not eat mature St. John's wort if other forage is available. However, if included in stored feeds it is readily eaten, and contaminated hay and feeds also cause photosensitization. Signs of clinical poisoning usually appear 2 to 21 days after animals have access to St. John's wort. The principle photodynamic toxin has been identified as hypericin.[5]

St. John's wort has traditionally been used as a herbal medicine, and hypericin is thought to have antidepressant, antiviral, antiangiogenic, and antineoplastic activity.[6,7]

Fagopyrum esculentum and *Fagopyrum tataricum* (North American buckwheat) are upright perennial subshrubs or vines with simple, alternate leaves and perfect flowers. They grow up to 0.6 m tall and are commonly found in disturbed soils along field margins and fences. Native to Asia, they were initially used in many countries as a cover crop. As they have been replaced by better, less-toxic plants, poisoning is uncommon. The buckwheats contain hypericin-like toxins (fagopyrin, photofagopyrin, and pseudohypericin). Poisoning was most common in sheep and cattle.[8]

Furanocoumarin-containing plants

Cymopterus watsonii (spring parsley) (**Fig. 3**) often poisons livestock in early spring when they quickly grow due to spring moisture and they are the only green forage

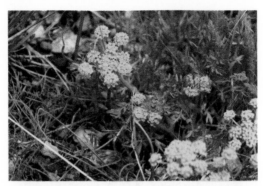

Fig. 3. *Cymopterus watsonii* (spring parsley) and several other similar *Cymopterus* spp. are relatively short perennials that grow 8 to 12 cm tall. All have parsley-like, finely divided leaves, small white or cream flowers, and a long taproot. All are also members of the carrot family.

available. Later in the spring and early summer they mature, produce seeds, senesce, and dry up. Spring parsley grows in pastures and rangelands on well-drained soils, rolling foothills with sagebrush, piñon pines, and junipers at elevations of 1500 to 3500 m.[9]

Pastinaca sativa (wild parsnip) has been associated with livestock and human photosensitization. Wild parsnip is a biennial or perennial Eurasian plant that can grow from 1 to 2 m tall. It has alternate, compound and branched leaves with jagged teeth. It flowers in early summer with hundreds of yellow flowers that form an umbel. Because it has a deep tap root, it is somewhat drought tolerant and can spread and dominate heavily grazed pastures and ranges. Chemically, wild parsnip contains several furanocoumarins—xanthotoxin, bergapten, isopimpinellin, imperatorin, and a putative methoxyimperatorin. Although some incidents have been attributed to livestock ingesting wild parsnip, most lesions may be attributed to contact dermatitis. Ruminants may be less susceptible to poisoning, and wild parsnip furanocoumarins are quickly metabolized (**Fig. 4**). Cutaneous application of wild parsnip extracts produced severe photodermatitis similar to those observed in clinical poisoning.[4] As with other

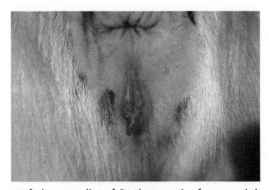

Fig. 4. Vulva of a goat fed a pure diet of *Pastinaca sativa* for several days. Notice the focal necrotizing dermatitis on the exposed unpigmented skin.

causes of primary photosensitization, wild parsnip–induced dermal lesions quickly resolve when exposure to both plant and irradiation is discontinued.

Ammi majus (bishop's weed) is a carrotlike weed found in central and southern states. It grows 20 to 80 cm tall with 3 pinnately compound or dissected leaves with terminal leaflets that are linear to lanceolate. The flowers are compound with small, white petals. Originally from Eurasia, they can be found growing on waste areas and along roadways and fence lines. Most poisonings are reported in lambs and calves.[10]

Thamnosma texana and *Thamnosma montana* (Dutchman's breeches) are perennial weeds of the southwest United States. These are erect plants, 10 to 60 cm high with simple alternate leaves. The flowers are blue to yellow. They are native to dry rocky slopes, and most poisonings are reported in sheep and cattle.[11]

Celery and parsnip when rotting, often are infected with fungi that can produce phytoalexins (commonly xanthotoxin and tripsoralen). These cause photosensitization, which is often topical or contact dermatitis. Phytoalexin-induced photodermatitis is most common in pigs although there are rare reports in other livestock.[12]

Secondary or Hepatogenous Photosensitization

Phylloerythrin is a chlorophyll metabolite that is primarily formed by enteric microorganisms. Secondary or hepatogenous photosensitization can be caused by increased circulating and dermal phylloerythrin concentrations.[1,13] Phylloerythrin is absorbed from the gastrointestinal tract and carried to the liver via the portal circulation. Within the normal liver, the hepatocytes conjugate phylloerythrin and excrete it in the bile. However, if the liver is damaged or if bile excretion is impaired, phylloerythrin accumulates in the liver, blood, and subsequently the skin causing photosensitivity. In most areas this secondary photosensitization is the most common cause in livestock.

Clinical photosensitization develops when serum phylloerythrin concentrations are greater than 8.0 μg/dL. Serum bile acid concentrations are generally greater than 10.0 μmol/L.[14] Development of clinical photosensitivity requires the concert of 3 independent variables. First, liver damage and biliary excretion is impaired such that phylloerythrin accumulates. Second, adequate green forage must be ingested, resulting in intestinal chlorophyll metabolism producing abundant phylloerythrin. And lastly animals must be exposed to enough sunlight to photoactivate dermal phylloerythrin and damage dermal tissues. Scenarios in which these variables are increased results in clinical photosensitization. A good example of this is the historical disease of big head in sheep. This disease occurred when sheep were driven all day, and while hungry they were bedded in monocultures of *Tetradymia* spp. (horsebrush). Horsebrush contains hepatotoxic furanoeremophilanes (furanosesquiterpenes), including tetradymol. Poisoned animals developed fatal liver failure and many that also ingested chlorophyll-rich black sage (*Artemisia nova*) developed photosensitization that was identified as "big head".[15] When one or more components are massively increased, normal excretion may be overwhelmed. The result is often seen as periodic or seasonal photosensitization. For example, increased dermal phylloerythrin concentrations may occur in animals with normal liver function and no exposure to photodynamic xenotoxins when they eat large amounts of green leafy feeds with abundant chlorophyll. It has been suggested that phylloerythrin production may be enhanced by individual animal microbiomes. More work is needed to better determine if and how this metabolism is controlled. Increased phylloerythrin production that overwhelms juvenile excretion pathways is probably the cause of photosensitization seen in many young horses.[14]

The most common cause of hepatogenous photosensitization is hepatocellular dysfunction and cholestasis that occurs with hepatocellular necrosis and subsequent fibrosis. This nonspecific change can be caused by infectious, nutritional, or toxic causes. Hepatotoxic plants that cause such necrosis and fibrosis are presented in the accompanying review in this section. Briefly these include dehydropyrrolizidine alkaloid (DHPA)-containing plants, cockleburs, *Lantana* species, certain clovers etc.[16] Cholestasis can be caused by bile duct obstruction such as cholangitis due to enteric bacterial disease, parasite migrations, or cholelithiasis. In addition, some crystalline cholangitis can also be caused by plant steroidal saponins. The following are select plants that are associated with crystalline cholangitis and secondary photosensitization. *Panicum* spp. associated with toxicity in North America include *Panicum antidotale* (blue *Panicum*), *Panicum coloratum* (Kleingrass), *Panicum dichotomiflorum* (smooth switchgrass), *Panicum maximum* (guinea grass), *Panicum miliaceum* (millet), and *Panicum virgatum* (switchgrass).[17] *Tribulus* spp. such as goathead or puncture vine is found throughout North America and in many parts of the world. It also causes crystalline cholangitis and photosensitization that is known as geeldikkop or yellow head in Africa.[18] *Brachiaria* spp. can contain saponins and other toxins when infected with *Pithomyces cartarum*.[19] *Brachiaria* spp. are warm season grasses that rarely cause problems, as they are seldom grown in North America. Several native saponin-containing North American plants include *Agave lecheguilla* and *Nolina texana* (beargrass or sacahuiste) of the southwest, but these plant are rarely eaten so poisoning is infrequent.[20] In Norway and Europe *Narthecium ossifragum* (bog asphodel) commonly poisons sheep producing crystalline hepatopathy and photosensitivity that has been called alveld or "elf fire."[21]

The diagnosis of secondary photosensitivity is made by correlating the characteristic changes of photoinduced dermatitis with hepatic disease; however, determining the inciting cause is often difficult or even impossible. Hepatogenous photosensitivity will have additional clinical signs and pathologic lesions of hepatic disease including jaundice, hepatic encephalopathy, hyperbilirubinemia, and increased serum bile acids and enzyme activities (sorbitol dehydrogenase, glutamate dehydrogenase, aspartate dehydrogenase, alkaline phosphatase).[14] The challenge is determining the cause of hepatic disease. Many animals do not develop photosensitivity until months or even years after initial hepatic damage. A common scenario would be that contaminated hay is fed and the liver is damaged, but because of reduced exposure to sunlight during the winter months photosensitivity or overt clinical signs of liver disease are not noticed.[22,23] Later in the spring, exposure to sunlight increases and green pastures with abundant chlorophyll results in massive phylloerythrin production. In addition, in early spring many animals may be stressed by poor nutrition, late pregnancy, parturition, and lactation. Animals with hepatic insufficiency cannot excrete the increased amounts of phylloerythrin and subsequently they develop photosensitivity. Identifying the inciting cause of hepatic damage is often difficult. The contaminated feed was fed several months earlier and none is left for inspection or analysis. The source of the feed may not even be available. Serum markers of hepatic disease may have also returned to normal. Because normal hepatocytes are replaced with fibrous connective tissue, there are fewer damaged cells to elevate serum enzymes. Percutaneous liver biopsies often provide the best chance of identifying and diagnosing these cases. Plant-induced hepatopathy generally results in characteristic histologic lesions. For example, pyrrolizidine alkaloids generally cause bridging portal fibrosis with hepatocellular necrosis, biliary proliferation, and megalocytosis (**Fig. 5**). Hepatic biopsy can also be useful for developing a prognosis, as the degree of hepatic damage often correlates to the animal's ability to compensate, recover, and be productive. For some

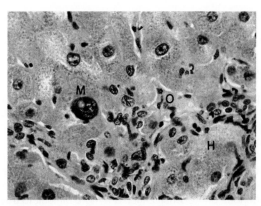

Fig. 5. Liver biopsy taken 14 days after a yearling horse was treated with ground hound-stongue (*Cynoglossum officinale*) to obtain total dehydropyrrolizidine alkaloids dose of 5 mg/kg per day for 10 days. Although this early section lacks the characteristic fibrosis there is evidence of hepatocellular degeneration and biliary proliferation. Notice the marked swelling of hepatocytes (H) that are entrapped by proliferating ovalocytes and biliary epithelia (O). A single megalocyte is also present (M). (Hemotoxylin-eosin stain, original magnification was 400X).

toxins, chemical detection is possible. In PA poisoning, tissue bound metabolites can be extracted from liver and identified chemically confirming exposure.[24] A most likely diagnosis depends on correlating exposure with clinical disease.

OTHER PLANT-INDUCED DERMATITIS

Endophyte-infected fescue (*Festuca arundinacea*) and ergot-infected seed grains can result in ischemic dermal necrosis with damage most severe in the extremities. Other plants such as poison ivy, oak, and sumac (*Toxicodendron radicans, Toxicodendron diversilobum,* and *Toxicodendron vernix*) or stinging nettle (*Urtica* spp.) commonly cause contact dermatitis in people, but they do not seem to affect livestock. Still other plants induce generalized disease that includes many tissues in addition to the skin. Locoweeds cause prominent dermal changes with rough hair coats that fail to shed seasonally. Another example is plants that contain 1,25-dihydroxycholecalciferol (vitamin D) such as *Cestrum diurnum (*a tropical plant in southeastern states) that result in dystrophic and metastatic mineralization of many tissues including the skin.

Finally, hairy vetch (*Vicia villosa* Roth) poisons cattle and rarely horses. Poisoning is characterized by multisystemic disease that most often includes clinically obvious dermatitis. Hairy vetch is a leafy legume that is used in many parts of North America as pasture forage, hay, silage, or as a cover crop. Various toxic syndromes have been reported including fatal neurologic disease; ulcerative mucosal disease with subcutaneous swelling and edema; and granulomatous inflammatory disease of skin, conjunctiva, intestinal tract, and other organs (liver, kidney, spleen, heart, and various glands). It has been suggested this inflammatory reaction is similar to a type IV hypersensitivity reaction. Although an immunoreactive lectin has been suggested, none have been definitively identified.[25] Hairy vetch dermatitis is characterized by alopecia with thickened pleated skin. Microscopically there is extensive dermal edema with perivascular and periadnexal infiltrates of lymphocytes, plasma cells, macrophages, and multinucleated giant cells. Morbidity is low, affecting 10% to 20% of animals, but affected animals rarely recover. The focally extensive inflammation causes organ failure resulting in cardiovascular failure, renal disease, or permanent loss of condition and emaciation.[26]

TREATMENT AND SUMMARY

Managing clinical photosensitivity should be directed at eliminating the photodynamic agent, decreasing exposure to sunlight, and treating the dermal and possible hepatic lesions. Changing the diet and providing housing in the shade is a responsible first step. Both photodermatitis and chemical dermatitis are generally best treated with topical antimicrobial ointments and lotions. If severe, animals may need fluid therapy and systemic antibiotics. Sunscreens, dermal tattooing, and protective hoods have been useful for photosensitized animals that cannot be removed from sunlight. Liver failure and hepatogenous photosensitization are more difficult to treat. Hepatic biopsy helps to identify the most likely cause of hepatic disease and determine the extent of damage. Many inflammatory diseases such as cholangiohepatitis respond well to therapy. Animals with severe lesions generally do not respond to treatment and may have to be euthanized.

DISCLOSURE

The authors have nothing to disclose.

REFERENCES

1. Collett MG. Photosensitisation diseases of animals: Classification and a weight of evidence approach to primary cause. Toxicon 2019;X3:1–12.
2. Elder GH. The cutaneous porphyrias. Semin Dermatol 1990;9:63–9.
3. Hussain SM, Herling VR, Rodrigues PH, et al. Mini review on photosensitization by plants in grazing herbivores. Trop Anim Health Prod 2018;50:925–35.
4. Stegelmeier BL, Colegate SM, Knoppel EL, et al. Wild parsnip (*Pastinaca sativa*)-induced photosensitization. Toxicon 2019;167:60–6.
5. Araya OS, Ford EJ. An investigation of the type of photosensitization caused by the ingestion of St John's Wort (*Hypericum perforatum*) by calves. J Comp Pathol 1981;91:135–41.
6. Jendzelovska Z, Jendzelovsky R, Kucharova B, et al. Hypericin in the Light and in the Dark: Two Sides of the Same Coin. Front Plant Sci 2016;7:560.
7. Miskovsky P. Hypericin–a new antiviral and antitumor photosensitizer: mechanism of action and interaction with biological macromolecules. Curr Drug Targets 2002; 3:55–84.
8. Burrows GE, Tyrl RJ. Toxic plants of North America- 2nd Edition. John Wiley & Sons Inc. Ames Iowa; 2013.
9. Binns W, James LF, Brooksby W. Cymopterus watsoni: a photosensitizing plant for sheep. Vet Med 1964;59:375–9.
10. Dollahite JW, Younger RL, Hoffman GO. Photosensitization in cattle and sheep caused by feeding *Ammi majus* (greater Ammi; Bishop's-Weed). Am J Vet Res 1978;39:193–7.
11. Oertli EH, Beier RC, Ivie GW, et al. Linear furocoumarins and other constituents from *Thamnosma texana*. Phytochem 1984;23:439–41.
12. Beier RC. Natural pesticides and bioactive components in foods. Rev Environ Contam Toxicol 1990;113:47–137.

13. Collett MG. Bile duct lesions associated with turnip (Brassica rapa) photosensitization compared with those due to sporidesmin toxicosis in dairy cows. Vet Pathol 2014;51:986–91.
14. Stegelmeier BL. Equine Photosensitization. Clin Tech Equine Pract 2002;1:81–8.
15. Johnson AE. Experimental photosensitization and toxicity in sheep produced by *Tetradymia glabrata*. Can J Comp Med 1974;38:406–10.
16. Stegelmeier BL. Pyrrolizidine alkaloid-containing toxic plants (*Senecio, Crotalaria, Cynoglossum, Amsinckia, Heliotropium,* and *Echium* spp.). Vet Clin North Am Food Anim Pract 2011;27:419–28, ix.
17. Wina E, Muetzel S, Becker K. The impact of saponins or saponin-containing plant materials on ruminant production–a review. J Agric Food Chem 2005;53: 8093–105.
18. Kellerman TS, Erasmus GL, Coetzer JA, et al. Photosensitivity in South Africa. VI. The experimental induction of geeldikkop in sheep with crude steroidal saponins from *Tribulus terrestris*. Onderstepoort J Vet Res 1991;58:47–53.
19. Graydon RJ, Hamid H, Zahari P, et al. Photosensitisation and crystal-associated cholangiohepatopathy in sheep grazing *Brachiaria decumbens*. Aust Vet J 1991; 68:234–6.
20. Rankins DL Jr, Smith GS, Ross TT, et al. Characterization of toxicosis in sheep dosed with blossoms of sacahuiste (*Nolina microcarpa*). J Anim Sci 1993;71: 2489–98.
21. Flaoyen A, Wilkins AL. Metabolism of saponins from *Narthecium ossifragum*–a plant implicated in the aetiology of alveld, a hepatogenous photosensitization of sheep. Vet Res Commun 1997;21:335–45.
22. Synge BA, Stephen FB. Delayed ragwort poisoning associated with lactation stress in cows. Vet Rec 1993;132:327.
23. Molyneux RJ, Johnson AE, Stuart LD. Delayed manifestation of *Senecio* -induced pyrrolizidine alkaloidosis in cattle: case reports. Vet Hum Toxicol 1988;30:201–5.
24. Brown AW, Stegelmeier BL, Colegate SM, et al. The comparative toxicity of a reduced, crude comfrey (*Symphytum officinale*) alkaloid extract and the pure, comfrey-derived pyrrolizidine alkaloids, lycopsamine and intermedine in chicks (*Gallus gallus domesticus*). J Appl Toxicol 2016;36:716–25.
25. Panciera RJ, Mosier DA, Ritchey JW. Hairy vetch (*Vicia villosa* Roth) poisoning in cattle: update and experimental induction of disease. J Vet Diagn Invest 1992;4: 318–25.
26. Knight AP, Walter RG. A guide to plant poisoning. Jackson (WY): Teton Newmedia; 2001.

Plant-Induced Reproductive Disease, Abortion, and Teratology in Livestock

Bryan L. Stegelmeier, DVM, PhD*, T. Zane Davis, PhD,
Michael J. Clayton, DVM

KEYWORDS

- Poisonous plants • Teratogenic • Abortifacient • Reproductive toxins • Diagnosis

KEY POINTS

- Many plants that affect reproductive function also cause other significant lesions and diseases for which they are better known.
- Plant toxins that affect the reproductive system may not cause maternal fatality, but reproductive failure can be equally costly to herd and economic health.
- Identification of plant toxin–induced teratogenesis is difficult, as resulting birth defects occur months after exposure.
- Pine needle toxins and metabolites detected in fetal and maternal samples indicate maternal exposure and must be correlated with clinical signs and pathophysiologic sequelae of abortion to formulate a likely diagnosis.

REPRODUCTIVE TOXINS

Often toxic plants affect reproductive function, but these reproductive changes are lost in the shadows of more impressive disease and lesions. For example, locoweeds are primarily considered neurotoxins, as they often produce spectacular neurologic disease; however, under some conditions (dose, duration, and poisoning frequency) reproductive failure may be the initial sign of locoweed poisoning. Locoweeds are potent endocrine disrupters, and poisoning quickly alters spermatogenesis, spermatic maturation. They also impair libido resulting in male reproductive failure.[1] Female reproduction is similarly affected, as poisoning quickly produces cystic ovaries with altered estrus. Locoweed also is fetotoxic resulting in placental resorption, abortion, fetal myocardial dysfunction with placental damage, and hydrops amnii. Locoweed poisoned neonates are slow to stand and ambulate and some are unable to nurse. Locoweed-induced birth defects include small calves or lambs with phocomelia.

USDA/ARS Poisonous Plant Research Laboratory, 1150 East 1400 North, Logan, UT 84341, USA
* Corresponding author.
E-mail address: Bryan.Stegelmeier@USDA.GOV

Chronic selenium poisoning has also been associated with reproductive failure. Poisoning occurs as a result of feed mixing errors or when animals graze or eat contaminated feeds containing seleniferous plants. Acute selenium poisoning is generally characterized by sudden death with vascular damage and acute myocardial necrosis. Chronic poisoning is different and characterized by loss of condition, hair and hoof lesions, and anecdotal reports of infertility. Recent work has documented altered spermatic maturation, resulting in marked motility deficits in chronically poisoned rams.[2] Initial studies suggest bulls are not similarly affected at similar dosages and durations. Chronically poisoned ewes may develop early embryonic death and reduced conception rates. Additional studies are needed to better characterize these changes and to determine if cattle are similarly affected.

Many other toxic plants damage specific organ systems that can secondarily affect reproduction. For example, plant-induced liver failure also alters reproductive capability. Similarly, severe plant-induced photosensitivity will impair affected animals' ability to maintain body condition, breed, and conceive at regular intervals.

TERATOGENIC PLANTS

Lupines: in North America the *Lupinus* genus includes more than 150 species that are similar and difficult to taxonomically classify. Although fatal lupine poisoning has historically killed hundreds of sheep, currently the more common effect of lupines is cattle teratogenesis known as crooked calf disease. Lupines are considered highly nutritious legumes and, in many ranges, they are an important component of livestock and wildlife nutrition. However, they are also rich in many different toxic and teratogenic alkaloids. As both the plant identification and potential toxicity are difficult to predict, sampling with professional identification and chemical analysis is essential for both diagnosis and predicting risk.

Crooked calf disease is a congenital condition in calves that are born with skeletal contracture–type malformations, and /or cleft palate. The musculoskeletal contractures include axial lesions such as scoliosis, lordosis, torticollis, and kyphosis. It also produces appendicular contractures that most often involve the front legs and include permanent contractures, rotational defects, massive joint deformation and ankyloses and bony deformation (**Fig. 1**). Specific lupine populations and later specific lupine alkaloids have been identified as the cause of crooked calf disease. Exposure time and duration are critical, as disease depends on pregnant cows grazing toxic lupines during days 40 to 100 of gestation.[3,4] The extent of lupine-induced birth defects depends on both dose and duration of poisoning. Some calf deformities are so severe that they produce dystocia and may preclude vaginal delivery. Other minimally affected calves may not be able to stand and nurse. Still others may only have benign lesions that with time resolve so that affected calves grow normally and finish normally. Cleft palate is a common change that can be overlooked, nevertheless, it is a serious lesion, as it decreases the ability to nurse and increases incidence of inhalation pneumonia. Although clinical lupine-induced teratogenesis is most common in cattle, similar birth defects have been reproduced in various other rodent and livestock species, suggesting that many species are susceptible.[3]

Lupines generally expand in disturbed areas and are common in ranges and pastures that are overgrazed or drought stressed. Although many lupines seem similar and may even be classified as the same species, there are large population differences with unique alkaloids and concentrations that may produce birth defects. For example, *Lupinus sulphureus*, a yellow lupine from Oregon, Washington, and British Columbia, has 7 distinct populations and all 7 have unique alkaloid profiles with

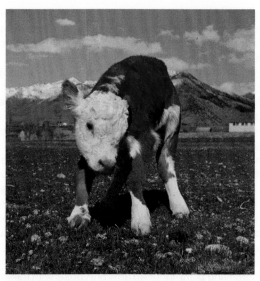

Fig. 1. A newborn calf with "crooked calf disease." Notice the angular limb deformities in both front legs; both knees are partially fused (ankylosis), and there is marked lateral rotation of the right front leg. There is also mild kyphosis involving the thoracic vertebrae, and the cranial vertebrae have mild ankylosis with left rotation.

varying teratogen concentrations resulting in distinct incidence of disease and the relative risk.[5]

Lupine teratogens include anagyrine[6] and ammodendrine.[7] Physiologic studies have shown that the mechanism of toxicity is due to alkaloid-induced reduction in fetal movement during the critical stages of gestation.[8] This is due to desensitization of skeletal muscle nicotinic acetylcholine receptors (nAchR).[9] Similar mechanisms have been identified in other plants that produce similar contracture defects including poison hemlock (*Conium maculatum*) and wild tree tobacco (*Nicotiana glauca*). All of these toxins have also been shown *in vitro* to inhibit human fetal-muscle nAChR and human autonomic nAChR.[10] Lupine alkaloids are most concentrated in new early growth and and they gradually decrease as the plant biomass increases; however, they often are highest in the seeds making the pods dangerous. As the pods age they shatter, dispersing the seeds, and alkaloid concentrations decline until the dried senescent plant becomes relatively nontoxic. The incidence of lupine-induced crooked calf disease is variable geographically and from year to year. This is directly attributed to expanding lupine populations as a result of certain environmental conditions. This and the lack of alternative forages force susceptible animals to eat lupines.

Lupine teratogens can be detected in serum and urine of grazing animals; however, their elimination is rapid with a half-life of 6 to 7 hours.[11] As crooked calf disease is often not clinically apparent until months after exposure when the affected calf is born, plant teratogens will not be present in fetal or maternal fluid or tissues. Documenting exposure is generally made by identifying toxic lupines in pastures or ranges the cattle used when they were susceptible. Sampling suspect lupines that cattle may have eaten during susceptible times is recommended, as chemical analysis can support the diagnosis of lupine-induced crooked calf disease. In many cases lupine-infested ranges can be safely used if grazed at the appropriate time. Management strategies to avoid critical exposure include changing calving season, intermittent grazing with short clearance times in lupine-free pastures, and limiting use of lupine ranges with nonpregnant or stocker animals.[11] Once affected calves are born, there is no treatment of the malformations. Euthanasia is recommended for calves with serious skeletal defects and cleft palate.

Other plants that cause contracture type birth defects: as suggested there are several additional plants that cause contracture-type skeletal defects and cleft palate. Poison hemlock (*C maculatum*), wild tobacco (*N glauca*), and tobacco stalks (*Nicotiana tabacum*) have been documented to cause birth defects in cattle and swine, albeit less commonly than lupine-induced teratogenesis. These birth defects have been experimentally induced in cattle, swine, sheep, and goats.[3] The birth defects include angular limb deformities, arthrogryposis, scoliosis, torticollis, and cleft palate. The teratogenic effects have also been shown to be due to plant toxin neuromuscular effects, resulting in inhibition of fetal movement during critical gestation developmental times.[3,12] In cattle, the susceptible period of pregnancy is 40 to 100 days, the same as lupine-induced crooked calf syndrome. In swine, sheep, and goats the susceptible period of gestation is 30 to 60 days.[3] Cleft palate has been induced in fetal goats when pregnant goats were treated with plant or purified toxins on days 32 to 41 of gestation with incidence of nearly 100%.[3]

As with lupine, identifying plant-induced arthrogryposis with these plants is made by associating these terata with exposure during susceptible gestation times. In acute poisoning, alkaloids from all of these plants can be detected in liver, urine, blood, gastric contents, and other samples.[13] However, when birth defects are clinically apparent, the abortifacient toxins have been excreted. Preventing poisoning is based on recognizing the plants and avoiding livestock exposure when hungry, and pregnant animals may be at susceptible stages of gestation.

Veratrum californicum (false hellebore or corn lily): *V californicum* was first found to cause craniofacial birth defects in pregnant ewes that grazed *V californicum*. Often morbidity was high affecting nearly 25% of pregnant ewes in the flock. These malformations ranged from mild superior brachygnathism to severe cyclopia with anencephaly (**Fig. 2**).[14] These spectacular malformations resulted in producers referring to the syndrome as monkey faced lamb disease.[15] Since these first observations, the susceptible gestation time has been identified in various species; the teratogenic *Veratrum* toxins have been identified; experimental toxicity has been reproduced and described in a variety of experimental models; and the mechanism of toxicity defined.

V californicum grows primarily in moist, open meadows and marshes or along edges of waterways, ponds, or lakes in the high mountain ranges of the western North America. *V californicum* is an erect plant growing up to 2.5 m tall with smooth, parallel veined, oval to lanceolate leaves that are about 30 cm long.[16] More than 50 complex steroidal alkaloids have been identified, including several neurologic toxins; several toxins that bind to sodium channels resulting in cardiotoxic and respiratory effects; and the teratogens cyclopamine and jervine that both induced congenital cyclopia.[15] These teratogenic effects are gestation age specific, as the cyclopic defect only occurs when pregnant ewes ingests the plant during the 14th day of gestation. Exposure before the 19th day of gestation may cause embryonic death. Exposure between 28 and 33 days of gestation often produces phocomelia and tracheal stenosis.[17,18] Both cyclopamine and jervine disrupt the sonic hedgehog signaling pathway, which is critical in craniofacial embryonic development.[19]

Although livestock frequently graze *Veratrum*, neurologic disease is uncommon. The clinical presentation of the monkey faced lamb disease is distinct and characterized by extended gestation, dystocia, or lack of parturition. Most monkey faced lambs must be delivered by cesarean section, which is not cost-effective in sheep, so most

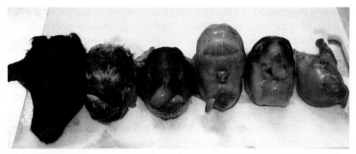

Fig. 2. A series of lambs with "monkey faced lamb disease." Notice the spectrum of cranio-facial defects that range from mild superior brachygnathism (first lamb on the left) to anencephaly (sixth lamb on far right). The second lamb has severe superior brachygnathism with microphthalmia. The third lamb also has microphthalmia and maxillary agenesis with subsequent proboscis formation. The fourth lamb has prominent synophthalmia with maxillary agenesis and no nasal development. The fifth lamb has cyclopia with nasal development forming a proboscis-like growth that extends from the forehead and maxillary agenesis. The ewes from these lambs were hand bred and dosed with ground *Veratrum californicum* on the 14th day of gestation. It has been suggested that the variation in teratogenesis is probably due to differences in gestation age. In this study the ewes were synchronized using intravaginal pessaries; however, the ewes probably ovulated at different times. This suggests that hours and possibly even minutes in gestation age may affect the type and extent of teratogenesis.[14]

affected ewes are euthanized. Diagnosis is made by correlating exposure during susceptible gestation age and production of lambs with craniofacial defects. Breeding ewes should be excluded from *Veratrum*-containing pastures and ranges in order to avoid teratogenesis.

ABORTIFACIENT PLANTS

Pine needle–induced abortion: when pregnant cattle eat needles or bark from ponderosa pine (*Pinus ponderosa*) or several other related pine trees they may abort, resulting in dead or premature calves, retained placentas, and uterine infections. Most poisoning occurs during the winter when cattle are in late gestation and weather forces animals into the trees for cover and the snow further reduces availability of alternative forages. Other pine trees associated with abortions in cattle include lodgepole pine (*Pinus contorta*) and Monterey cypress (*Cupressus macrocarpa*). Additional trees have been reported to contain isocupressic acid, the pine needle toxin, but these have not been associated with clinical abortions. Both fresh green and old dry ponderosa pine needles can cause abortions, suggesting any needles, dry duff around the tree, or dried trimmings could cause abortions. Cattle and bison are uniquely susceptible to abortion, as other species have not been shown to abort when exposed or treated with pine needles or their toxins.[20]

Although the exact physiologic mechanism of abortion has not been identified, the abortifacient pine needle compound has been identified as isocupressic acid. Isocupressic acid is quickly metabolized and the resulting agathic acid, imbricatoloic acid, and dihydroagathic acid are also abortifacient.[21] Tetrahydroagathic acid is a unique metabolite that can be detected in the serum of poisoned animals for longer than 72 hours, making it an excellent biomarker of exposure.[20] It is speculated that pine needles affect the fetal/placental blood flow resulting in fetal hypoxia, stress, and subsequent early parturition.[22] More research is needed to identify the exact mechanism of abortion and develop antidotes or methods to reduce abortion.

Factors that affect abortion incidence include gestation stage, dose, duration, animal condition, environmental stress, and nutritional status. There is variation in response, as some cows abort within a few days of exposure and others may abort several weeks after a single exposure. Other cows require daily doses of nearly 2 weeks duration to produce abortions. Late gestation cows are the most susceptible.[23] The initial signs of poisoning include weak uterine contractions, incomplete cervical dilation, dystocia, and placental retention (**Fig. 3**). Aborted calves are often stillborn or may be small weak calves that require assistance to stand and nurse. Complications of abortion include endometritis, agalactia, rumen stasis, and death.[24]

Pine needle abortion should be a differential in abortions with a retained placenta in late-term gestation with exposure. Fetal tissues and fluids as well as maternal serum can be analyzed for pine needle metabolites; however, positive results indicate only exposure, and other causes of late term abortion should be excluded. Currently, the best method to prevent abortions is to deny pregnant cattle access to pine needles. Providing adequate food and shelter can also help reduce losses. If cows abort from ingesting pine needles, veterinary care is essential to prevent postpartum complications, and the survival of premature calves depends on fetal maturity and the quality of available neonatal care.

Nitrate-accumulating plants: another relatively common plant toxicity occurs when certain pasture and cultivated forages accumulate nitrates. A common presentation of nitrate poisoning in pregnant cattle is abortion that may have a high enough incidence to be described as an abortion storm. In the rumen and possibly in other portions of the gastrointestinal tract, nitrates are reduced to nitrite. Nitrites are quickly absorbed and when in circulation bind and oxidize hemoglobin producing methemoglobin. Methemoglobin is nonfunctional, as it will not bind oxygen. Poisoning is most common in cattle, but there are also reports of nitrate poisoning in horses, cats, and dogs.[25,26] Infrequent poisoning in sheep and goats has been attributed to their quick elimination

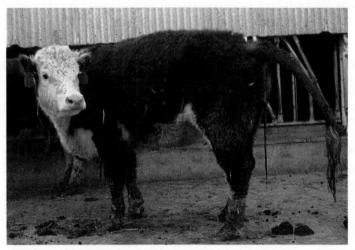

Fig. 3. Cow that recently aborted a near-term calf after she was treated with freshly ground ponderosa pine needles. Notice the retained placenta, swollen vulva, and minimal mammary gland development.

of nitrate in the urine (nitrate half-life in sheep is about 4 hours compared with 9 hours in cattle). Nitrate clearance in bovine fetuses is even longer with a half-life of more than 24 hours. Some have suggested that fetal hemoglobin has high nitrite affinity, which may contribute to abortion.[27] Poisoning is cumulative and all other potential sources, such as water or feed additives, should be considered. Nitrates accumulate in all plant parts but may be especially high in stalks and leaves. Seeds or grains are generally safe. Crops that commonly accumulate toxic nitrate concentrations (>0.5%) include oats, beets, rape, turnips, soybeans, barley, flax, alfalfa, millet, rye, sorghum, Sudan grass, Johnson grass, wheat, and corn. Common nitrate-accumulating weeds include ragweed, pigweed, wild oats, musk thistle, lambsquarter, Canadian thistle, field bind-weed, jimson weed, barnyard grass, cudweeds, sunflowers, fireweed, skeleton plant, cheese weed, sweet clover, smart weed, dock, Russian thistle, milk thistle, night-shades, and golden eye. Many of these weeds invade fields where they can contam-inate forages especially in newly planted hay fields. Dried and stored forages retain their toxicity. Nitrate accumulation is also provoked or enhanced by nitrogen fertiliza-tion, drought or frost stress, and some herbicide treatments.[26,28]

Initial signs of poisoning include exercise intolerance, weakness, trembling, brown or cyanotic mucous membranes, dyspnea, brown discolored blood, abortion, and death. Abortions occur 3 to 7 days postexposure and are frequently associated with sublethal nitrate poisoning. Some clinical nitrate-associated abortion storms have been attributed to plants with nitrate concentrations as low as 0.5%, a concentration that may be considered safe for nonpregnant animals. The lesions of nitrate poisoning can be minimal and easily overlooked, especially if the postmortem examination is delayed. Acutely poisoned animals may have chocolate-colored blood and many tis-sues may appear brown. As methemoglobin is quickly reduced post mortem, this co-lor diminishes quickly. If promptly measured, blood methemoglobin concentrations will be elevated. Feed nitrate analysis is essential for documenting exposure. Tissue and blood nitrate concentrations quickly degrade postmortem; however, both clini-cally poisoned animals and aborted fetuses have elevated ocular fluid nitrates that persist post mortem. Consequently, submission of the entire eye is the optimal sample for analysis. Fetal ocular nitrate concentrations higher than 20 μg NO_3/mL (20 ppm) highly suggest maternal nitrate poisoning.

Poisoned animals may be treated with intravenous methylene blue (8 mg/kg in cat-tle). As methylene blue is rapidly cleared, treatment may need to be repeated every 2 hours. In most cases the animals die quickly, precluding treatment. Poisoning is best prevented by recognizing crops, weeds, and forages that are likely to accumulate nitrates; testing potentially toxic feed; and avoiding contact with susceptible species. Forage nitrate concentration of greater than 0.5% and water concentrations greater than 200 ppm should be considered dangerous. Contaminated forages can still be used if they are mixed and diluted with good feed or fed to less susceptible species.

SUMMARY

Plants often contain reproductive toxins that alter fertility, produce birth defects, or cause abortion. Diagnosis depends on documenting exposure with clinical signs and lesions. Although serum or tissue analysis for plant toxins or their metabolites is useful in cases of abortion, this is not the case with birth defects, as the problem does not become clinically apparent until months after early gestation exposure.

DISCLOSURE

The authors have nothing to disclose.

REFERENCES

1. Panter KE, James LF, Stegelmeier BL, et al. Locoweeds: Effects on reproduction in livestock. J Nat Toxins 1999;8:53–62.
2. Davis TZ, Stegelmeier BL. Characterization of the effects of high selenium feed on spermatogenesis in rams. J Anim Sci 2019;97:449–50.
3. Panter KE, James LF, Gardner DR. Lupines, poison-hemlock and Nicotiana spp: toxicity and teratogenicity in livestock. J Nat Toxins 1999;8:117–34.
4. Shupe JL, Binns W, James LF, et al. Lupine, a cause of crooked calf disease. J Am Vet Med Assoc 1967;151:198–203.
5. Cook D, Lee ST, Gardner DR, et al. The alkaloid profiles of Lupinus sulphureus. J Agric Food Chem 2009;57:1646–53.
6. Keeler RF. Lupin alkaloids from teratogenic and nonteratogenic lupins. II. Identification of the major alkaloids by tandem gas chromatography-mass spectrometry in plants producing crooked calf disease. Teratology 1973;7:31–5.
7. Keeler RF, Panter KE. Piperidine alkaloid composition and relation to crooked calf disease- inducing potential of Lupinus formosus. Teratology 1989;40:423–32.
8. Panter KE, Keeler RF, Bunch TD, et al. Congenital skeletal malformations and cleft palate induced in goats by ingestion of Lupinus, Conium and Nicotiana species. Toxicon 1990;28:1377–85.
9. Lee ST, Wildeboer K, Panter KE, et al. Relative toxicities and neuromuscular nicotinic receptor agonistic potencies of anabasine enantiomers and anabaseine. Neurotoxicol Teratol 2006;28:220–8.
10. Green BT, Lee ST, Panter KE, et al. Actions of piperidine alkaloid teratogens at fetal nicotinic acetylcholine receptors. Neurotoxicol Teratol 2010;32:383–90.
11. Lopez-Ortiz S, Panter KE, Pfister JA, et al. The effect of body condition on disposition of alkaloids from silvery lupine (Lupinus argenteus pursh) in sheep. J Anim Sci 2004;82:2798–805.
12. Panter KE, Bunch TD, Keeler RF, et al. Multiple congenital contractures (MCC) and cleft palate induced in goats by ingestion of piperidine alkaloid-containing plants: reduction in fetal movement as the probable cause. J Toxicol Clin Toxicol 1990;28:69–83.
13. Lee ST, Stonecipher CA, Dos Santos FC, et al. An evaluation of hair, oral fluid, earwax, and nasal mucus as noninvasive specimens to determine livestock exposure to teratogenic lupine species. J Agric Food Chem 2019;67:43–9.
14. Welch KD, Panter KE, Lee ST, et al. Cyclopamine-induced synophthalmia in sheep: defining a critical window and toxicokinetic evaluation. J Appl Toxicol 2009;29:414–21.
15. Binns W, Shupe JL, Keeler RF, et al. Chronologic evaluation of teratogenicity in sheep fed Veratrum californicum. J Am Vet Med Assoc 1965;147:839–42.
16. Kingsbury JM. Poisonous plants of the United States and Canada. Englewood Cliffs (NY): Prentice-Hall, Inc.; 1964.
17. Keeler RF, Young S, Smart R. Congenital tracheal stenosis induced by maternal ingestion of Veratrum californicum. Teratology 1985;31:83-8.
18. Keeler RF, Stuart LD, Young S. When ewes ingest poisonous plants: the teratogenetic effects [Veratrum californicum]. Vet Med 1986;81:449.
19. Gaffield W, Keeler RF. Structure and stereochemistry of steroidal amine teratogens. Adv Exp Med Biol 1984;177:241–51.
20. Gardner DR, James LF, Panter KE, et al. Ponderosa Pine and Broom Snakeweed: Poisonous plants that affect livestock. J Nat Toxins 1999;8:27–34.

21. Gardner DR, Panter KE, Stegelmeier BL. Implication of agathic acid from Utah juniper bark as an abortifacient compound in cattle. J Appl Toxicol 2010;30:115–9.
22. Ford SP, Christenson LK, Rosazza JP, et al. Effects of Ponderosa pine needle ingestion on uterine vascular function in late-gestation beef cows. J Anim Sci 1992;70:1609–14.
23. Short RE, Staigmiller RB, Bellows RA, et al. Endocrine responses in cows fed ponderosa pine needles and the effects of stress, corpus luteum regression, progestin, and ketoprofen. J Anim Sci 1995;73:198–205.
24. Stegelmeier BL, Gardner DR, James LF, et al. The toxic and abortifacient effects of ponderosa pine. Vet Pathol 1996;33:22–8.
25. Worth AJ, Ainsworth SJ, Brocklehurst PJ, et al. Nitrite poisoning in cats and dogs fed a commercial pet food. N Z Vet J 1997;45:193–5.
26. Hintz HF, Thompson LJ. Nitrate toxicosis in horses. Equ Pract 1999;20:5–6.
27. Casteel SW, Evans TJ. Nitrate. In: Plumlee KH, editor. Clin vet toxicol. St Louis (MO): Mosby; 2003. p. 127–30.
28. Burrows GE, Tyrl RJ. Plants causing sudden death in livestock. Vet Clin North Am Food Anim Pract 1989;5:263–89.

Ruminant Mycotoxicosis
An Update

Michelle S. Mostrom, DVM, PhD*, Barry J. Jacobsen, PhD

KEYWORDS

- Molds • Fusarium • Mycotoxins • Ruminants • Toxicosis • Review

KEY POINTS

- Crop mold damage occurs in field and storage. Fungi associated with damage before harvest or field molds include *Fusarium*, *Alternaria*, *Aspergillus*, and *Penicillium* and with damage in storage include *Aspergillus* and *Penicillium*.
- Moisture and temperature are primary factors determining the ability of molds to grow and their rate of growth, and the rate at which molds produce mycotoxins.
- It is vital to establish and sustain a functional rumen flora with adequate diet and sufficient roughage to maintain ruminal capacity to inactivate certain mycotoxins.
- Commonly recognized mycotoxins and associated adverse effects in affected ruminants are discussed.
- Exposure to multiple mycotoxins and potentially emerging mycotoxins in ruminant feed is increasingly frequent with climatic changes, and mycotoxin interactions are relatively unknown in ruminants, especially in small ruminants.

INTRODUCTION

Recent trends in weather patterns are for higher climatic variation in temperatures and precipitation. Often the result is warmer and wetter seasons with more opportunities for mold invasion of crops and multiple mycotoxins, secondary mold metabolites, produced at significant concentrations in those crops and forages contaminating animal rations. Mycotoxins are naturally occurring low-molecular-weight compounds produced by fungi growing on plants in the field or during storage periods on feed commodities. The source of toxigenic fungi or mold in both cases is the field. *Fusarium* species and *Claviceps purpurea* can act as plant pathogens on cereal crops or grasses in the field. *Fusarium verticillioides* and *Aspergillus flavus* can produce mycotoxins on water stressed or senescent plants, particularly corn. Fungi that occur on developing kernels in the field or delayed harvest grains can later proliferate in storage,

The authors have nothing to disclose.
North Dakota State University, Veterinary Diagnostic Laboratory, 4035 19th Avenue North, Dept. 7691, PO Box 6050, Fargo, ND 58108-6050, USA
* Corresponding author.
E-mail address: Michelle.mostrom@ndsu.edu

especially on ensiled cereals or baled forages, are typically the *Fusarium*, *Penicillium*, and *Aspergillus* species. Additional fungi have been associated with grasses, endophytes, such as *Neotyphodium lolii* in perennial ryegrass and *N coenophialum* in tall fescue. Numerous, coexisting mycotoxins can be produced by fungi invading plant material; however, only a relative few mycotoxins have been recognized as toxic to animals and are regulated worldwide. Not only environmental changes associated with climate change, but also greatly decreased crop diversity on a global basis has resulted in the reappearance of some fungal toxins (ergot alkaloids, citreoviridin, T-2 toxin) that were infrequently detected in the past.[1] This article focuses on mycotoxins affecting ruminants in North America. Briefly discussed are emerging mycotoxins, which are not well-defined fungal metabolites nor is their toxicity determined in ruminants.[2] Ruminants are often considered less sensitive to mycotoxins owing to rumen microflora metabolism conversion to less toxic compounds. However, ruminants occupy wide agricultural niches from forage pastures to dry lots using localized feed sources or feedlots using numerous commercial sources of grains or byproducts, which expose animals to diverse toxins under widely different conditions. Often the more moldy and potentially highly contaminated feeds end up at a feedlot, and in poor crop years, beef cows can be fed contaminated screenings, straw and cereal byproducts, poorly preserved silages or baled forages, or be turned out onto moldy fields for crop salvage. Less than optimal feedstuffs creating suboptimal rumen microbial flora could result in reduced ruminal capacity to detoxify certain mycotoxins and adverse effects. This review covers factors associated with mold production in feedstuffs and major mycotoxins affecting ruminants.

CROP MOLDS AND POTENTIAL MYCOTOXINS

Frequently in cases of ill-thrift in livestock, veterinarians need to evaluate the sources and quality of feedstuffs and, if is testing warranted, obtain a representative sample of suspect feed or feeds that livestock have been consuming. Feeds can be cultured by mycologists and plant pathologists for mold identification, providing a record or biological indicator of storage conditions and suggesting potential mycotoxins. Mold cultures can provide direction in analytical testing for mycotoxins. Stored grains and seeds can be damaged by insects and fungi if not properly conditioned and protected. Damage from field and storage molds can include reduced germination, heating, a decrease in market grade and grain value, loss of feed and oil quality, mycotoxin contamination, fires, explosions, and worker health hazards associated with dust and mycotoxin inhalation and falling through crusted grain. Mold damage occurs both before and after harvest. Those fungi associated with damage before harvest are termed field molds and these fungi grow in equilibrium with relative humidities of greater than 90% to 95% (**Table 1**). Fungi associated with damage in storage can grow in equilibrium with relative humidity between 65% and 85% (**Table 2**). Grains and seeds readily absorb or lose moisture and will achieve moisture in equilibrium with the moisture vapor available in the air between seeds or grains. Moisture and temperature are the primary factors determining the ability of molds to grow and their rate of growth. The growth of storage fungi results in increased temperatures and increased moisture owing to the metabolism of these fungi. Thus, once these molds begin growth, grains and seeds will gain in moisture and allow growth of storage fungi that require higher equilibrium moistures. For example, *Aspergillus glaucus* can grow at 15% moisture in starchy grains, but as it grows it produces heat and moisture that allows the growth of *Aspergillus candidus* or even *A flavus* or *Penicillium* species that require 16% to 18% moisture. Growth of *A glaucus* and *A candidus* can be quite

Table 1
Field mold problems that can cause predisposition to storage mold damage and reduce germination

Crop	Disease Name/Pathogen Genus	Favored by
Cereal grains	Fusarium head blight, scab Several *Fusarium* spp Black head molds *Alternaria* and *Cladosporium* spp Head molds *Fusarium* and *Penicillium* spp Black point *Helminthosporium* spp	Warm, wet weather at anthesis and shortly after Plants killed prematurely (eg, by diseases, frost) Wet weather-delayed harvest, snow cover Wet weather during grain maturation
Corn	Ear and kernel rots *Fusarium* spp, *Gibberella*, *Diplodia*, *Helminthosporium*, *Bipolaris* *Aspergillus*, *Penicillium*	Warm, wet weather in 21 d after pollination, delayed harvest, hail, bird, or insect damage. *Fusarium verticillioides* and *F proliferatrum*; droughty conditions, insect damage to ear; Fusarium; hail damage *Aspergillus*; droughty conditions, insect damage to ear. *Penicillium*; hail damage milk stage or later, insect damage, cool, wet weather-delayed harvest
Soybeans	Pod and stem blight; *Phomopsis*, *Diaporthe* spp, Anthracnose; *Colletotrichum*	Wet weather during pod-fill, weather-delayed harvest Wet weather during pod-fill
Peas, lentils, chickpea, dry bean	*Ascochyta* blight, *Asochyta*, gray mold; *Botrytis*, Anthracnose; *Colletotrichum*	Wet weather during pod-fill
Safflower	*Alternaria* blight, *Alternaria*	Warm temperatures and high humidity from flower to seed set, wet weather-delayed harvest
Hay	*Fusarium* spp, *Cladosporium*, *Alternaria*	These fungi cannot grow at moisture <20%

rapid and will generate temperatures as high as 140°F. A good management practice is to avoid blending low and high moisture grains; grain moisture in a blending process will progress to the high moisture levels.

Grain and seeds are at highest quality and have the lowest storage risk when they are fully mature before harvest, free of field mold damage, have no mechanical damage to the seed coat, and where the harvest is not delayed by weather or other factors. The intact seed coat is a formidable barrier to seed infection by storage molds and extra care in preventing mechanical damage during harvest and handling is critical to managing storage mold damage. Grain or seeds infected by field molds such as *Fusarium*, *Helminthosporium*, *Penicillium*, *Sclerotinia*, *Botrytis*, *Ascochyta*, *Alternaria*, and *Cladosporium* are at higher risk for damage by storage molds than intact seeds and will likely have lower germination rates. **Table 1** lists diseases caused by field molds that may predispose grains and seeds to damage by storage molds. **Table 3** lists selected molds and associated mycotoxicoses in ruminants. Even though toxigenic molds may grow under a given set of conditions, they do not necessarily produce mycotoxins. The mold can undergo additional stress conditions, leading to mycotoxin

Table 2
Percentage relative humidity (%RH), equilibrium moisture (%) for various grains and seeds and storage fungi that can grow at these moistures

% RH	Starchy Grains, Corn, Wheat, Barley (% Equilibrium Moisture)	Soybean, Pea, Bean, Lentils (% Equilibrium Moisture)	Peanut, Canola, Camelina, Safflower (% Equilibrium Moisture)	Fungi
65–70	12.5	12.0	5.0	*Aspergillus halophilus* *Aspergillus restrictus*
70–75	14.0	13.0	6.0	*Aspergillus glaucus*
75–80	15.0	14.0	7.0	*Aspergillus candidus*
80–85	16.0	15.0	8.0	*Aspergillus flavus* *Penicillium* sp
85–90	18.0	18.0	10.0	As above + *Penicillium*
>95	22.0	20.0	13.0	Yeasts/bacteria/most field molds

production, which can be generated fairly rapidly in the field or storage conditions. More than 1000 μg/kg (ppb or parts per billion) of aflatoxins can be produced on *A flavus* inoculated corn within 4 days and *Fusarium* mycotoxins (zearalenone, deoxynivalenol [DON], and HT-2 toxin) can be found in >1 mg/kg (ppm or parts per million) levels within 4 to 7 days after hail damage on maturing corn. The use of mold spore counts is limited; it provides an indication of mold presence (mold spores can deteriorate) and whether the feedstuff has "gone bad," but does not equate to the presence or identification of a mycotoxin(s). Spore counts will often indicate fungi that are highly prolific in spore production (*Cladosporoium, Penicillium, Aspergillus, Alternaria, Mucor* spp., etc), while not revealing the presence of mycotoxigenic species that produce fewer spores such as *Claviceps* or *Fusarium*. Most mycotoxins can remain stable for years in feeds, and many survive ensiling and food processing. Mycotoxins (eg, aflatoxins and fumonisins) can be concentrated several-fold in cereal byproducts.

AFLATOXINS

Aflatoxins are an important group of structurally related difuranocoumarin compounds produced primarily by *A flavus, Aspergillus parasiticus,* and *Aspergillus nomius*. These mycotoxins are found worldwide, but more commonly are produced in warm, subtropical and tropical climates. Aflatoxins can occur before harvest on starchy cereal crops, cottonseeds, and peanuts or after harvest on stored commodities (see **Table 3**). Aflatoxins are potent hepatotoxins, immunosuppressants, carcinogens, and mutagens and can be important public health problems. Clinical signs of aflatoxicosis include poor weight gains and feed conversion, liver disease with elevated hepatic enzymes and bilirubin, prolonged clotting times, and decreased immune competence (ie, vaccine failure or poor antibiotic response). Aflatoxins affect cell-mediated immunity, cytokine production, and nonspecific humoral factors, such as complement, interferon, and some bactericidal serum components.[3] Governments regulate the allowable concentrations of aflatoxins in animal feeds, human foods, and fluid milk (**Table 4**).

Strains of *A flavus* typically invade damaged or senescent plant tissue and mainly produce aflatoxin B_1. Aflatoxin B_1 is generally found in the highest concentration

Table 3
Summary table of fungi, mycotoxins, environmental conditions of fungi growth and clinical disease in ruminants

Mycotoxin	Fungi	Feed Affected	Environmental Conditions	Clinical Signs	Lesions	References
Aflatoxins B1, B2, G1, G2	Aspergillus flavus, A Parasiticus, A nomius	Cereal grains Peanuts Cottonseed Dried fruits (dairy products) Others	13–42°C (54–108°F) Optimum: 25–30°C (81–86°F), 75% relative humidity, grain moisture >18%; peanut moisture >8%9%; oxygen >0.5%	Hepatotoxic, reduced feed conversion and weight gains, rough hair coats, lethargy, immunosuppression, hemorrhage, abortions, death, increased liver enzymes (especially γ-glutamyltransferase), increased bilirubin, increase prothrombin time	Hepatic fatty degeneration, megalocytosis and necrosis, fibrosis, biliary hyperplasia, possible veno-occlusive lesions, hemorrhages	3,9,15,91
Sterigmatocystin	Aspergillus glaucus, A versicolor, A nidulellus	Wheat Cereals Hay, forages	Stored cereals at 14%–15% moisture Wet weather	Hepatotoxin, kidney damage Carcinogen Lower milk production Diarrhea		4,92
Deoxynivalenol (DON) vomitoxin	Fusarium graminearum, F culmorum	Cereal grains Cereal byproducts, Silages, Straws, hay	Optimum growth at about 21–28°C water activity >0.87	Lower feed intake, low weight gains, diarrhea Lower milk production Immune alterations Hepatotoxicity (young preruminant)		3,15,30,93
Zearalenone	F graminearum, F culmorum, F equisetti	Cereals Silages, hay	Warm days, cool nights High oxygen Moisture >30%– 40% Hail damage	Swelling vulva Mammary gland hyperplasia and secretion Abnormal estrus Rectal and vaginal prolapses Infertility		3,41

(continued on next page)

Table 3
(continued)

Mycotoxin	Fungi	Feed Affected	Environmental Conditions	Clinical Signs	Lesions	References
Tricothecenes (T-2 toxin HT-2 toxin Diacetoxyscirpenol)	*Fusarium poae, F sporotrichioides, F equiseti, F acuminatum*	Cereal grains (overwintered under snow) Straw, hay	Moderate to low temperature Sharp fluctuations in temperatures, hail, Wet, high humidity	Anorexia, inflammation and hemorrhage of mouth throughout gastrointestinal tract, bloody diarrhea, poor growth, abortions, cytotoxicity, immune suppression, death	Hemorrhage Dermonecrosis	3,36,93
Fumonisins B1 and B2	*Fusarium verticillioides, F proliferatum, Aspergillus niger*	Corn in the field Dried grapes	Drought followed by cool, wet weather during pollination	Inappetence Decreased feed intake Decreased milk production Increased hepatic enzymes	Milk hepatopathy Possible tubular nephrosis (lambs)	18,56,59
Roridin E Satratoxins G and H Verrucarin J	*Stachybotrys atra (syn. S alternans and S chatarum)*	Wet forage Silage Grain	Temperature 0–40°C Relative humidity 90% Moisture content of 15% in substrates	Anorexia, fever Salivation, oral necrosis Bloody diarrhea Skin necrosis Abortions, death	Hemorrhage and necrosis of gastrointestinal tract	93,94
Ochratoxin A	*Aspergillus alutaceus var alutaceus (ochraceus), Penicillium viridicatum*	Wheat Cereal grains	Grain moisture of 16%–18% and equilibrium relative humidity >85%, Temperatures 12–25°C (54–77°F)	Hepatotoxic and nephrotoxic Poor feed conversion and weight gains Ill thrift Polyuria and polydipsia Immunosuppressive	Enlarge kidneys Renal interstitial fibrosis Dilated renal tubules Thickened basement membranes	18,60–62
Citrinin	*Penicillium citrinum, P viridicatum, Monascus ruber*	Wheat Barley Oats Rye	Grain moisture of 16%–18% and equilibrium relative humidity >85%, Temperature 12–25°C (54–77°F)	Uremia	Degeneration and necrosis of proximal convoluted tubules	3,62

Toxin	Fungi	Substrate	Conditions	Clinical signs	Lesions	References
Unknown toxicant? (patulin?)	Aspergillus clavatus	Hydroponically grown sprouted barley or wheat, Sprouted grains, Beer residues (malting byproducts)		Posterior ataxia, Knuckling of fetlocks, Tremors, recumbency, Salivation, Paralysis, Death	Degenerative and necrotic neuronal changes of the brainstem and neurons of ventral horn of spinal cord, Vacuolation and myelin depletion in spinal cord	66–70
Tremorgen toxins, Lolitrem B, Paspalitrem A and B, Paxilline	Neothyphodium lolii, Claviceps paspali	Perennial ryegrass (Lolium perenne), Dallis grass (Paspalum dilatatum)		Staggers, Tremors, Seizures		3,15,64,65
Diplonine, Others?	Stenocarpella maydis (Diplodia maydis)	Ear corn	Wet weather and moderate temperatures 7–14 d near mid-silk in (50% plants with silks)	Ataxia, Incoordination, High-stepping gait, Salivation, Paresis/paralysis, Perinatal death	Neonatal deaths—spongiform degeneration in myelin, Adults—rare laminar brain spongiosis	84,86
Patulin	Penicillium, Aspergillus, Byssochlamys	Silages, Apple juice	0–25°C	Impaired cellulose digestion, Decreased feed intake, Decrease milk production, Liver damage, Neurotoxicosis?		3,32,95,96
Roquefortine, Mycophenolic acid, Andrastin A, PR toxin, Marcfortines A,B,C	Penicillium roqueforti (P paneum Frisvad, P caneum Frisvad)	Corn and grass silage	Low oxygen, High levels or organic acid	Ill thrift, Poor milk production, Poor reproduction, Immunosuppression, Inappetence, ketosis		72,73

(continued on next page)

Table 3
(continued)

Mycotoxin	Fungi	Feed Affected	Environmental Conditions	Clinical Signs	Lesions	References
Sporidesmin	*Pithomyces chartarum* (facial eczema)	Dead plant material and pasture litter	Warm, humid weather during late summer and fall	Photosensitization Skin edema and necrosis Sheep—hepatic lesions and urinary cystitis	Marked lobular liver pattern and later on atrophy and marked fibrosis, regeneration tissue, distorted liver capsule	3,82
Cyclopiazonic Acid	*Aspergillus, Penicillium*	Stored grains Sunflowers	Hot weather, can co-occur with aflatoxins from *A flavus*	Anorexia, dehydration Weight loss Muscle spasms	Necrosis of liver, spleen, kidneys, myocardium	3,74
Slaframine (can co-occur with swainsonine that can produce locoism)	*Slafractonia leguminicola* (formerly *Rhizoctonia leguminicola*)	Clover (*Trifolium sp.*) Alfalfa Black patch disease	Wet weather and cool temperatures during regrowth of forages (mid- to late summer)	Excessive salivation Lacrimation Watery diarrhea Bloat Dyspnea	Severe cases—dilated fluid-filled intestines	18,105
Ergot alkaloids	*Claviceps purpurea, C Africana, C cyperi*	Rye Triticale Cereal grains Sorghum Nut sedges	Cool, damp spring weather delaying pollination increases infection and warm weather favors growth of sclerotia	Vasoconstriction with loss of extremities (ears, feet, tail) Hyperthermia Decreased milk production Reproductive failure Open-mouth breathing	Thickening of blood vessel walls of extremities Tissue necrosis and sloughing	3,97
Dicoumarol	*Aspergillus fumigatus, Penicillium, Mucor*	Sweet clover hay (*Melilotus*) Sweet vernal grass	Damp weather Baled wet hay	Prolonged clotting time inhibiting vitamin K epoxide reductase Hemorrhages	Hemorrhages	18
Citreoviridin	*Penicillium citreonigrum* (*P citreoviride*)	Rice	High humidity High temperatures	Human—cardiac beriberi Respiratory failure Heart palpitations and failure		1

Data from Refs. 1,3,4,9,15,18,30,32,36,41,56,59–62,64–70,72–74,84,86,91–97,105

Table 4
Guidelines for maximum mycotoxins in total rations for animal feeds (mg/kg = ppm; ug/kg = ppb)

Mycotoxins	Dairy Cattle		Beef Cattle		Other	Reference
DON (Vomitoxin) Grain and grain byproducts at 10 ppm	5 ppm	>4 mo of age— ruminating dairy	10 ppm	>4 mo of age—ruminating beef and feedlot cattle	2 ppm	Calves (<4 mo), lambs and kids	US FDA, advisory limits[98]
Distillers grains, brewers grains, gluten feed, gluten meals derived from grains at 30 ppm	5 ppm	Complementary and complete feedstuffs	5 ppm	Complementary and complete feedstuffs	2 ppm	Calves (<4 mo) lambs and kids	EC[99]
	1 ppm	Lactating dairy and young calves	5 ppm	Cattle			Canada—RG-8[100]
Aflatoxins Total of: B1 + B2 + G1 + G2	20 ppb	Corn, peanut products, cottonseed meal, and other animal feeds and feed ingredients	300 ppb 300 ppb 100 ppb 20 ppb	Feedlot beef using corn, peanut products · Beef regardless of age or breeding status using cottonseed meal · Breeding beef using corn, peanut products · Immature animal using corn, peanut products and other feed ingredients, excluding cottonseed meal	20 ppb	Corn, peanut products, cottonseed meal, and other animal feeds for other ruminants	FDA action level[101]
Aflatoxin M1	0.5 ppb 0.05 ppb				Fluid milk Raw milk, heat-treated milk	FDA action level[102] EC[103]

(continued on next page)

Table 4
(continued)

Mycotoxins	Dairy Cattle		Beef Cattle		Other	Reference
Fumonisin Total of: FB1 + FB2 + FB3	15 ppm [30 ppm in corn, ≤50% of diet]c	Lactating dairy cattle	30 ppm [60 ppm in corn, ≤50% diet] 15 ppm [30 ppm in corn, ≤50% diet]	Ruminants ≥3 mo old raised for slaughter Breeding ruminants	5 ppm [10 ppm in corn, ≤50% of diet]	Others and Ruminants <3 mo old	US FDA guidance levels 2001[104]
Zearalenone			10 ppm	Cows (1.5 ppm if other toxins present)	0.5 ppm	Calves, sheep, lambs, goats	EC[99] Canada—RG8[100]
HT-2 toxin	0.025 ppm	Dairy	0.1 ppm				Canada—RG8[100]
Ochratoxin A	0.25 ppm	Cereals and cereal products					EC[99]

Data from Refs.[98–104]

and considered the most toxic and carcinogenic of the aflatoxins. Strains of *A parasiticus* can produce aflatoxins B_1 and B_2, and G_1 and G_2 that fluoresce blue or green, respectively, under ultraviolet light. Aflatoxins M_1 and M_2 are 4-hydroxylated metabolites of aflatoxin B_1 and B_2, respectively, and can occur in aflatoxin-contaminated feed and in tissues, milk, and dairy products. Aflatoxin B_1 has been associated with hepatocellular carcinoma in humans and is included in group 1 as a human carcinogen by the International Agency for Research on Cancer. Aflatoxin M1 is less toxic and classified by International Agency for Research on Cancer as a human carcinogen in group 2B. Sterigmatocystin, a mycotoxin produced by *Aspergillus versicolor* and other molds, is a precursor in the synthesis of aflatoxins, a hepatotoxin and carcinogen, and capable of toxicosis similar to, but less toxic than aflatoxins.[4] Concentrations of sterigmatocystin (<500 ppb) have been detected more frequently in forages, as compared with grains, during wet years (M. S. Mostrom, DVM, unpublished data, 2017–2019).

Aflatoxins are low-molecular-weight, lipophilic compounds that are passively absorbed from the gastrointestinal tract. Absorption of aflatoxin may occur in the mouth or esophagus before the entering the rumen, based on detection of aflatoxin M_1 in the plasma within 5 minutes after dosing dairy cows.[5] Aflatoxins are absorbed from the intestinal tract into the hepatic portal system. Young animals absorb aflatoxins more efficiently than older animals. Rumen microbial degradation of aflatoxins has been studied and findings are inconsistent. Aflatoxins can be degraded slightly in the rumen, but type of ration, feeding time, animal species, individual animal, and incubation time in rumen influence degradation of aflatoxins.[6–8] Aflatoxin B_1 can bind reversibly to albumin, with unbound aflatoxin B_1 passing from the circulation into tissues. Aflatoxins do not readily accumulate in tissues, although repeated exposures can generate toxic effects in tissues. Aflatoxins may cross the placenta and damage fetal tissue; however, little work has focused on reproductive effects. Aflatoxin elimination is through the bile, feces, urine, and into milk and eggs. Most species eliminate the toxin within 24 hours after exposure.[9]

The liver and, to a lesser extent, the kidney, intestinal tract, and other organs biotransform aflatoxin B_1 into several products, with the most important activation by cytochrome P450 into an 8,9-epoxide. The covalent binding of aflatoxin 8,9-epoxide to DNA, RNA, and proteins results in tissue adducts and reduced synthesis of these products, disruption of cellular processes, and organ function.[3] The outcome results in cellular necrosis, immune suppression (both humoral and cell-mediated immunity), mutagenesis, and neoplasms. Additional biotransformation products (eg, AFM_1, AFM_2, AFQ_1, aflatoxicol) are less toxic; conjugation of these products with glucuronide and sulfate are detoxification reactions. The metabolite aflatoxicol, which is a carcinogen to animals and possibly a carcinogen to human, can be oxidized back to aflatoxin B_1 and serve as a source for AFB_1 in the body. Aflatoxicol has been detected in milk, eggs, fermented dairy products, and tissues. Pasteurization and ultrapasteurization of milk with various level of fat content did not destroy aflatoxicol.[10] Aflatoxin M_1 is the major excretion product in urine and milk and can be monitored for exposure. Aflatoxin M_1 appears quickly in milk; goats in mid lactation given a single oral dose of 0.8 mg aflatoxin B_1 per head had detectable concentrations of aflatoxin M_1 in milk 1 hour after administration, maximum concentrations in milk 3 to 6 hours after administration, and concentrations of less than 50 ng/L (0.05 ppb, the European Union maximum allowed level) 36 hours after aflatoxin B1 administration.[11] Excretion of M_1 in milk varies with animal species and individual, lactation status, and milkings after exposure. Feeding practices impact potential aflatoxin M_1 contamination of milk. For example, when concentrates were fed predominately at night, aflatoxin M_1

contamination was higher in morning milk compared with evening milk, and aflatoxin M_1 in milk was higher during the winter season when animals, including cows, buffalos, goats, sheep, and camels, were fed more concentrates than during the summer when fed on grass.[12] Aflatoxin M_1 excretion in milk approaches a steady-state condition about 3 to 6 days after daily ingestion of aflatoxins.[9] The dietary threshold for cows to excrete aflatoxin in milk is about 15 μg aflatoxins/kg ration (ppb); lactating cows consuming a diet with or 20 μg or less of aflatoxins/kg (ppb) will excrete less than 0.1 μg aflatoxin M_1/kg (ppb) in milk (US Food and Drug Administration [FDA] action limit is 0.5 ug/L or ppb in milk). The ratio of aflatoxin M_1 excreted in milk to the amount of aflatoxin B_1 ingested is generally between nondetectable and 4% in cows, between 1% and 3% in dairy ewes,[13] and approximately 0.26% in dairy goats.[11] After removal from the contaminated ration, aflatoxin M_1 becomes undetectable in milk after 2 to 4 days.

All animals are susceptible to aflatoxins, but the sensitivity varies between species. Young animals and monogastrics are more at risk for toxicosis. The major impact in dairy herds is decreased milk production and milk residue violations, with recent questions focused on possible immune suppression. Aflatoxins in the total ration of immature ruminants and dairy cows should not exceed 20 ppb. **Table 4** lists the FDA action levels set for aflatoxins in animal feeds. Ruminants fed rations of aflatoxins over several hundred parts per billion aflatoxins may exhibit some decreased feed intake and growth. Chronic aflatoxicosis in cattle is associated with clinical signs of reduced appetite, feed efficiency, milk production, and icterus.[14] Hepatic enzymes are typically elevated and prothrombin time can be prolonged. The sensitive indicator of aflatoxicosis is decreased performance, the cause of which is multifactorial, involving nutritional interactions, anorexia, altered hepatic protein and lipid metabolism, and disruptions of hormonal metabolism.[15] Sheep are considered the most resistant domesticated species to toxic effects of aflatoxins. Lambs fed elevated concentrations of aflatoxins (1.00–1.75 ppm) in concentrate for more than 5 years were slower to grow, had decreased fertility, and developed hepatic cell carcinoma and nasal tumors, but did not develop liver pathology consistent with aflatoxicosis.[16]

High concentrations of aflatoxins can occur in field crops with insect damage and hot weather, such as a case of moldy, unharvested sweet corn containing more than 2300 ng aflatoxin/g (ppb) of corn that caused death in a cow grazing the field[17]; sweet corn is considered more hazardous than field corn because of its higher sugar content. Veterinarians need to consider multiple sources of aflatoxins in rations and commodity storage conditions on a farm.

A diagnosis of aflatoxicosis is based on typical clinical signs, lesions, and demonstrating toxic (not trace) concentrations in the ration. Positive fluorescence of grain under a black light (blue-green color at 365 nm) suggests *Aspergillus* metabolites, but not aflatoxins. Various analytical methods can be used to determine aflatoxins in feedstuffs; the most important aspect of analysis is to acquire a representative sample of the suspect feed or feeds. When sampling for aflatoxins in feed, the more random and larger the sampling, the better the chances will be to detect aflatoxins. In a small sample, even 1 contaminated kernel can dramatically alter analytical results. Uneven distribution of mold and mycotoxins in a storage facility requires multiple samples at both the perimeter and center of the bin.[18,19] A more representative sample is obtained by periodic sampling from a flowing or moving stream of suspect feed to generate a large sample volume (5–10 kg), mixing the sample, and subsampling for analysis. To avoid inadequate or insufficient sampling, retain a minimum of 5 kg from each batch of feed or grain purchased or used.[19] No specific treatment is available for aflatoxicosis beyond quickly removing the contaminated ration and replacing with an uncontaminated feed. Providing optimum dietary protein, vitamins, and trace elements may aid recovery, although some affected animals may not recover. To prevent aflatoxin production after harvest, storage moisture of less than 12% is recommended for cereals grains and less than 8% to 9% moisture for oilseeds over a wide range of temperatures. Store grains and oil seeds in clean, weatherproof structures; cleaning grain to remove light weight or broken grain can decrease mycotoxins. Several measures have been taken to reduce aflatoxin contamination of feeds, including mold inhibitors, fermentation, physical separation, thermal treatment (roasting), irradiation, ammoniation, ozonation, and using mycotoxin adsorbents. No method is without drawbacks, including cost, large-scale application, and only partial success. Treating grain with anhydrous ammonia may decrease aflatoxin concentrations by about 30%. Numerous products are marketed to sequester or bind mycotoxins and decrease absorption from an animal's gastrointestinal tract, although in the United States these agents are typically sold as anticaking or free-flow agents. Agents tested include sodium calcium aluminosilicates, activated charcoal, bentonite, various clays, yeast cultures, and esterified glucomannan. Several of these compounds show potential in partially binding aflatoxin B_1 and decreasing aflatoxin M_1 contamination in milk.[20–22] Positive responses in reducing aflatoxin M_1 in milk are not consistent for all of these binders; refereed publications indicate that some clay products only partially bind aflatoxins in ruminants with unknown rumen compounds competing for binding sites on clay. Incorporating sodium calcium aluminosilicates or clay products at low concentrations in the diet is a reasonable investment to partially sequester aflatoxin, decreasing potential toxicosis and milk residues in lactating cows. The use of yeast products may stimulate some immune responses and partially offset some adverse effects, but do not seem to substantially decrease toxicosis or milk residues. To date, the US FDA has not licensed any product for use as a mycotoxin binder in animal feeds.

TRICHOTHECENES

Fusarium molds are the most economically important source of trichothecene mycotoxins. Trichothecenes are sesquiterpenoid compounds with an epoxy group at C12-13 that is considered essential for toxicity. Although more than 100 trichothecene mycotoxins have been identified, veterinary medicine is focused on a relatively few trichothecenes. Type A trichothecenes include some of the most toxic trichothecenes, T-2 toxin, its deacetylated metabolite HT-2 toxin, and diacetoxyscirpenol (anguidine). Type B trichothecenes are common field contaminants of grains and include DON (or vomitoxin) and its acetylated derivatives 15- and 3-acetyl DON (15- and 3-AcDON), nivalenol, and fusarenon-X (4-acetylnivalenol). In North America, *Fusarium graminearum* characteristically produces DON and 15-AcDON; during cooler, wet conditions the production of 3-AcDON and nivalenol can be detected in cereals. The relative cytotoxicity of the type B trichothecenes has been evaluated in vitro using bioassays. Generally, the toxicity of DON, 15-AcDON, fusarenon-X, and nivalenol were similar, and 3-AcDON is considered slightly less toxic.[23] Another study of DON and 3- and 15-AcDON on cell proliferation, intestinal barrier function and in vivo intestinal structure showed that 15-AcDON had higher toxicity owing to its ability to activate mitogen-activated protein kinase.[24] Trichothecenes are stable compounds and can remain present at toxic concentrations in feed for years. Field reports of trichothecene toxicity in livestock in North America typically involve DON contamination. Most trichothecene exposures are of a chronic to subchronic nature with low dietary DON concentrations associated with nutritional impairment, reduced production, and possible diminished immune responses. Swine and monogastrics (including preruminant animals) are more sensitive to trichothecenes.

Fusarium is most common in temperate climates, but contamination of grains is reported worldwide. Although not a trichothecene, the estrogenic mycotoxin zearalenone is produced by several *Fusarium* species and often found together with DON in North America. *Fusarium* infection of immature corn can result in higher trichothecene and zearalenone concentrations in the cob, as compared with kernel mycotoxin concentrations. In unusually wet, cool periods, *Fusarium* mycotoxins not only occur in the grain, but also in the vegetative part of the plant (hay and straw). *Fusarium* contamination can occur in hay baled wet or stored in higher moisture conditions (>20%) and in silage inadequately packed or where aerobic conditions exist. Wheat straw contamination with DON in scabby years may be as high as 50 to 100 mg DON/kg (ppm, dry weight basis).[25] These extremely high levels of contamination are relevant when contaminated forages are used for fiber in dairy feeds or bedding for swine.

Trichothecenes have multiple effects on eukaryotic cells, including inhibition of protein, RNA, and DNA synthesis; alteration of membrane structure and mitochondrial function; stimulation of lipid peroxidation; hypoxia and oxidative stress; induction of programmed cell death or apoptosis; and activation of cytokines and chemokines.[3,26] The hallmark clinical sign of trichothecene toxicosis in animals is feed refusal, which has led to speculation that animals may not voluntarily consume enough contaminated ration to cause marked poisoning. However, when the only available feedstuffs are contaminated with trichothecenes, poisoning can result. Diarrhea is common after trichothecene ingestion. Altered intestinal absorption of compounds and impaired permeability are caused by morphologic and functional damage to intestinal mucosa.[27] Significant metabolism of trichothecenes can occur both in the rumen and gastrointestinal tract before absorption. The rumen metabolite of oral DON is de-epoxy DON. De-epoxidation of DON to de-epoxy DON is considered a deactivation step resulting in a much less toxic compound.[28] Rumen microbes, in particular protozoa, seem to be active in the deacetylation of the trichothecenes.[7] Liver metabolism of trichothecenes occurs and in a study of fusarenon-X (a B trichothecene) in goats, the parent compound was rapidly absorbed and metabolized to nivalenol in liver microsomes, with an oral bioavailability of 15.8% reported in goats.[29]

It is vital to establish and sustain a functional rumen flora with an adequate diet and sufficient roughage to maintain the ruminal capacity to inactivate certain mycotoxins, including DON and its acetylated derivatives. Intensive feeding practices of calves raised in the veal and beef industry that feed milk replacer and cereal grains for up to 6 months with limited intake of roughage lead to nonoptimal ruminal development and, with the shortage of roughage in a diet, predisposes these calves to DON toxicity.[30] In a recent study by these authors, the absolute oral bioavailability of DON was greater in nonruminating calves at 50.7 ± 33.0% compared with ruminating calves at 4.1 ± 4.5%, with the higher oral bioavailability in the nonruminating calves similar to that in pigs (54%–100%). In a related case, a group of 1- to 3-month-old calves fed milk replacer and feed concentrate contaminated with 1.13 mg DON/kg feed, with little roughage in the ration, developed liver failure that resolved by replacing the contaminated corn and by stimulating ruminal development with a higher roughage diet.[30] These data suggest that the DON concentration in a preruminant diet, especially if lacking roughage, should be less than the US FDA advisory level of 2 ppm in the total ration (see **Table 4**).

Low concentrations of DON do not seem to adversely affect ruminating beef growth or reproduction. In 1 study, cross-bred steers fed up to 9.2 mg DON/kg diet (ppm) for 84 days during the growing period and up to 12.6 mg DON/kg diet (ppm) for 100 days during the finishing period had no significant differences in beef performance, including feed intake, feed efficiency, rate of gain, or carcass quality.[31] The FDA advisory level for DON in the final ration for beef cattle more than 4 months of age is 10 mg/kg or ppm (see **Table 4**). Pregnant yearling heifers consumed DON contaminated barley at 10.2 mg DON/kg diet or 13 mg DON/kg diet from midgestation through the first 45 days of lactation.[31] No significant changes were noted in feed intake, heifer weight gain, or calf body weights; calf weight gains were slightly higher for calves nursing heifers fed the DON-contaminated barley during calving and lactation. Ovine responses to trichothecene exposure are similar to beef cattle. In general, beef cattle and sheep are more tolerant of higher DON concentrations in their rations than dairy cattle. The different susceptibilities could be associated with greater stress for dairy cows and increased dry matter intake, faster rumen turnover, and decreased rumen microbial degradation time for dairy cows.[32] When feeding dairy cows, questions arise about possible impact of DON on milk production and milk residues with data from several controlled studies are available. Primparous Holstein cows fed DON-contaminated grains up to 12.09 mg DON/kg of dry matter concentrate (maximum daily intake 104 mg DON) for 10 weeks in a lactation study had no changes in total milk output, feed intake, and no detectable residues (<1 ng/mL or ppb) of DON or de-epoxy DON in milk.[33] High-producing dairy cows provided DON-contaminated barley diets up to 14.6 mg DON/kg concentrate (approximately 8.5 ppm in diet, 0.31 mg DON/kg body weight) for 3 weeks showed no significant changes in milk production or feed intake.[34] The FDA advisory level for DON in the final ration for dairy cattle more than 4 months of age is 5 mg/kg or ppm (see **Table 4**). Lactating cows dosed orally with 920 mg of DON had only trace DON levels in serum (<2 ng DON/mL) detected at 24 hours after administration.[35] Free and conjugated DON were detected in cow's milk at low levels (<4 ng/mL) with an estimated 0.0001% of the administered dose excreted in milk.

Clinical signs of the more toxic trichothecenes include emesis, feed refusal and weight loss, diarrhea, immunomodulation, coagulopathy and hemorrhage, and cellular necrosis of mitotically active tissues such as the intestinal mucosa, skin, bone marrow, spleen, testis, and ovary.[3,15] T-2 and HT-2 toxin, often found together in plants, are some of the most toxic trichothecenes detected in feeds. Ruminants can rapidly deacetylate T-2 toxin to HT-2 toxin. It is often difficult to distinguish the effects of T-2 toxin from HT-2 in vivo; therefore, it is reasonable to sum the concentrations of these toxins together to evaluate clinical effects. Decreased feed consumption was reported in beef calves (85–200 kg) orally dosed with T-2 toxin at 0.3 mg/kg (approximately 10 mg T-2/kg diet or ppm) for 6 weeks.[36] Calves dosed with 0.6 mg/kg (approximately 20 mg T-2/kg diet) developed marked anorexia, weight loss, rough hair coats, and intermittent diarrhea. In a field case, clinical signs of anorexia, periodic elevated temperatures, abortions in midgestation, and a 20% death loss were associated with feeding moldy, high moisture corn to lactating Holstein dairy cows during a 5-month period in late winter.[37] Among the fungi cultured from corn were F tricinctum, F roseum, and F moniliforme and various Penicillium spp. A sample of feed from this field investigation contained 2 mg T-2 toxin/kg, which was considered a low value because of analytical methodology (low recovery). Additional mycotoxins could have been present in the feed and contributed to the clinical toxicity in the dairy cows, but were not analyzed. **Table 5** lists several Fusarium species and their associated production of mycotoxins.

Wet, cooler conditions in the northern United States and in Canada during the fall have been associated with significant concentrations of T-2 and HT-2 toxins in grass hay bales (approximately 9 ppm) and in corn (up to 6 ppm) (M. Mostrom, DVM,

Table 5
Fusarium species and related mycotoxins produced by the molds

Fusarium	Mycotoxins
F graminearum	DON, 15-AcDON, 3-AcDON, nivalenol, zearalenone
F culmorum	DON, 3-AcDON, nivalenol, zearalenone
F equiseti	Nivalenol, zearalenone, diacetoxyscirpenol
F poae	Nivalenol, diacetoxyscirpenol, T-2, HT-2
F acuminatum	Diacetoxyscirpenol, T-2, HT-2
F sporotrichioides	Diacetoxyscirpenol, T-2, HT-2
F verticillioides (moniliforme) F proliferatum	Fumonisins

unpublished data, 2009–2019). Dramatic weather patterns including hurricanes, tornadoes, and heavy thunderstorms have created wet and cooler conditions in central and southern United States, leading to *Fusarium* growth on wet pasture grasses and production of T-2 toxin, HT-2 toxin, and other mycotoxins in pastures used for livestock grazing and in stored feeds from flood waters. Feeder calves have been fed contaminated corn silage in a ration with almost 5 ppm (T-2 + HT-2 toxins) with no adverse effects, supporting earlier research (M. Mostrom, DVM PhD, unpublished data, 2010). However, higher concentrations of type A trichothecenes in rations should be avoided in pregnant animals and dairy. T-2 toxin can cross the placenta. Because T-2 toxins are rapidly metabolized in animals and excreted, no public health concerns have been associated with residues in edible tissues, milk, and eggs.[38]

Owing to the vague nature of toxic effects attributed to low concentrations of trichothecenes, a solid link between a low level of exposure and a specific trichothecene(s) is difficult to establish. Mycotoxins may play a role in some subtle animal diseases, but diagnostic consideration needs to move beyond just testing the feed for toxins and evaluate nutrition, disease, management, and environmental conditions. Storage of grains at less than 13% to 14% moisture (<0.70 α_w) and hay/straw at less than 20% moisture are important in preventing trichothecenes production. After the contaminated feed is removed from the diet and exposure stopped, animals generally have a good prognosis for recovery. The use of mycotoxin adsorbents (bentonites, aluminosilicates, and some zeolites) to bind trichothecenes in dietary rations, decreasing the clinical effects in ruminants, is problematic, with some of the β-glucans and mannans showing potential.[39] Few in vivo studies for multiple mycotoxin binding have been reported in ruminants, although the combination of different adsorbents (mineral and organic) seems to be more effective to counteract adverse effects of several mycotoxins in feed. A potential cost-effective process to reduce DON contamination of wet, stored cereal grains (15%–20% moisture) is through the incorporation of sodium metabisulfite, with or without propionic acid, into grain.[40] A decrease in DON concentrations was paralleled by an increase in DON sulfonate, which was considered biologically less active in pigs. The stability of DON sulfonate in the rumen is unknown.

ZEARALENONE

Zearalenone, chemically described as 6-(10-hydroxy-6-oxo-*trans*-1-undecenyl)-β-resorcyclic acid lactone, is a nonsteroidal estrogenic mycotoxin produced by several species of *Fusarium* fungi. The primary producer of zearalenone is *F graminearum* (teleomorph *Gibberella zeae*). Additional *Fusarium* fungi capable of producing zearalenone include *F culmorum*, *verticillioides* (*moniliforme*), *sporotrichioides*, *semitectum*, *equiseti*, and *oxysporum*. Zearalenone can occur not only in the parent form, but also in decreased metabolites of α- and β-zearalenol, α- and β-zearalanol, zearalanone and conjugated metabolites of zeralenone-14-O-β-glucoside, zearalenone-16-O-β glucoside and zeralenone-14-sulfate.[38,41] Contamination of cereal grains by zearalenone has been reported worldwide, primarily in temperate climates. Typically, zearalenone concentrations are low in grain contaminated in the field, but increase under storage conditions with moisture greater than 30% to 40% and adequate oxygen. Very high concentrations of zearalenone, which can occur naturally in some field samples, generally resulted from improper storage at high moisture rather than production in the field. Ear corn stored in a crib and exposed to winter weather is particularly prone to fungal invasion and production of zearalenone.

After oral exposure, zearalenone is generally well-absorbed with a relatively low bioavailability owing to extensive presystemic metabolism taking place in the rumen, enteric cells, and the liver.[41] One study in pigs reported the oral absorption of zearalenone at approximately 80% to 85%.[42] After zearalenone administration, zearalenone can be localized in reproductive tissues (ovary and uterus), adipose tissue, and interstitial cells of the testes.[43,44] Zearalenone can undergo reduction of the keto group on C-8 into diastereoisomeric zearalenols (α and β). The α-zearalenol metabolite, which is about 3 times more estrogenic than zeraralenone, is the main metabolite formed in pigs and humans. Species differences in zearalenone susceptibility might be related to hepatic biotransformation, with the highest amount of α-zearalenol produced by pig hepatic microsomes, whereas cattle rumen microbes produce α- and β-zearalanol, with the latter metabolite less toxic.[41] After a single intravenous injection of zearalenone at 1.2 mg/kg body weight in goats (24–28 kg), the elimination half-life was 28.58 hours and β-zearalenol was the predominant metabolite.[45] Although the liver plays a major role in glucuronidation, the intestinal mucosa is also active. Zearalenone metabolites are excreted into the urine and bile and can undergo enterohepatic recirculation with eventual excretion in the feces. Zearalenone and metabolites can interact directly with the cytoplasmic receptor that binds 17β-estradiol and translocate receptor sites to the nucleus.[46] In the nucleus, stimulation of RNA leads to protein synthesis and clinical signs of estrogenism. The transfer of zearalenone into edible tissues is not expected; cattle consuming 0.1 mg zearalenone kg/d of feed had no detectable concentration of the parent compound or metabolites in muscle, kidneys, liver, and dorsal fat.[47] Dairy cows fed rations with purified zearalenone at 50 mg zearalenone per day and 165 mg zearalenone per day for 21 days had no detectable concentrations of zearalenone or α and β-zearalenol in the milk or plasma.[48] One cow dosed with 544.5 mg zearalenone per day for 21 days had maximum concentrations of 2.5 ng zearalenone/mL and 3.0 ng α-zearalenol in the milk. Cows dosed orally with a 1-day dose of 1.8 or 6.0 g zearalenone had maximum milk levels on day 2 of 4.0 and 6.1 ng zearalenone/mL, respectively. In dairy milk, the transfer rates for forms of zearalenone varied between 0.008% and 0.050%, with β-zearalenol (of low estrogenic potency) detected as the main metabolite.[38] Zearalenone has major effects on reproduction that can lead to hyperestrogenism. Typical clinical signs are swelling of the vulva, increase in uterine size and secretions, mammary gland hyperplasia and secretion, prolonged estrus, anestrus, increased incidence of pseudopregnancy, infertility, decreased libido, and secondary complications of rectal and vaginal prolapses, and possibly abortions.

Zearalenone has low acute toxicity in most species. In most natural conditions, the concentrations of zearalenone in feed are less than 20 mg/kg (ppm) and generally less than 5 mg zearalenone/kg feed.[49] Prepubertal swine are the most sensitive, cattle may exhibit some adverse effects, and chickens seem to be the least sensitive species. Females are more sensitive than males and cycling females may be more sensitive than pregnant sows. Abortions have been associated in field cases with natural *Fusarium* mold exposure, but have not been reproduced with purified zearalenone.[50] In an experimental study, 18 cycling heifers were dosed with 0 or 250 mg of purified zearalenone daily through 1 nonbreeding estrous cycle and the next 2 consecutive estrous cycles during which the heifers were bred.[51] The authors calculated that treated heifers were given an average of 250 mg zearalenone/364 kg body weight/d or 0.69 mg zearalenone/kg body weight/d. The control and treated heifers had conception rates of 87% and 62%, respectively, at a statistical probability of $P<.065$.

In an ovine study, zearalenone was administered orally at concentrations or greater than 3 mg/animal/d to ewes before mating, depressing ovulation rates and reduced lambing percentages.[52] Ewes administered a similar range of oral doses of zearalenone (0, 1.5, 3, 6, 12, and 24 mg/ewe/d) for 10 days, starting 5 days after mating, showed no effect of zearalenone exposure after mating on pregnancy rate or embryonic loss. Breeding rams fed a diet containing 12 mg zearalenone/kg feed for 8 weeks had no significant adverse effects on semen volume, concentration, motility, or morphology during the trial. Following zearalenone exposure to livestock and occurrence of clinical signs, the contaminated feed must be removed, and animals will generally return to normal reproductive status after 3 to 7 weeks.

The US FDA has not established guidelines for zearalenone in animal feeds. The European Union has promulgated maximum zearalenone in complete feedstuffs for calves, dairy cattle, sheep and goats at 500 μg/kg (ppb), with no guidelines for adult beef cattle.[53] Based on anecdotal evidence from field cases, a suggested maximum zearalenone concentration in the final ration for adult beef cattle should be less than 2000 μg/kg (ppb or <2 ppm), and zearalenone concentrations need to be lower in feed with the occurrence of phytoestrogens from alfalfa, red and white clovers in the diet, and when fed to cattle during pregnancy and early postnatal period (M.S. Mostrom, DVM, unpublished data, 2009–2019). When naturally contaminated feed must be used, incorporation into rations for less susceptible species, such as feedlot animals or poultry, should be considered.

FUMONISINS

Fumonisins are a group of heat stable, water soluble mycotoxins generally produced in white and yellow corn in the field by *Fuarsium verticillioides* (syn. *F moniliforme*) and *F proliferatum*. A period of water stress during the growing season followed by insect damage and wet, cooler conditions during pollination of corn favors development of fumonisins. Toxicity is associated with fumonisins B1 and B2, with fumonisin B2 usually occurring at about 30% of fumonisin B1. Although recently concentrations of fumonisin B2 are occurring in corn with little detection of fumonisin B1. Additional fungi have been identified as producers of fumonisins including *Aspergillus niger*, an industrially used fungi, discovered to produce fumonisins B2 and B4 on raisins and grapes.[54] Fumonisins can be concentrated in corn screenings, because infected kernels are highly friable, thus avoid feeding corn screenings in drought years to horses that are the sensitive species to fumonisins. Fumonisins are chemically characterized as an aliphatic hydrocarbon with a terminal amine group and tricarboxylic acid side chains, and are structurally similar to sphingolipids in cellular membranes.[55] Fumonisins inhibit enzymes involved with the conversion of sphinganine to sphingosine, which can interfere with cellular growth, differentiation, and cell communication, resulting in toxicity and carcinogenicity. Ruminants are fairly resistant to fumonisins.

Feed containing 148 μg fumonisins/g (ppm) was less palatable to feeder calves (approximately 230 kg) and the calves developed elevated liver enzymes and mild liver lesions (see **Table 3**).[56] In a chronic study of feeder steers (86–127 kg) fed *F monili-forme* culture material with 417 ppm fumonisins B1 and B2 in the final corn mixture, a few days of feed refusal were observed in the calves.[57] The liver sphinganine:sphingosine ratios in the fumonisin fed calves were greater than 1; normal ratios are considered to be less than 0.5. Renal and hepatic damage were reported in lambs fed high concentrations of fumonisins (approximately 470 ppm).[58] Dairy cows seem to be more susceptible to fumonisins and FDA guidelines recommend lower fumonisin concentration in their rations, as compared with ruminants fed for slaughter (see **Table 4**). Dairy cows provided a naturally contaminated ration with 100 μg fumonisin/g (ppm) for 7 days prepartum and 70 days post partum developed reduced feed intake and milk production.[59]

OCRHRATOXIN A AND CITRININ

Ochratoxins are phenylalanine-dihydroisocoumarin compounds produced primarily by *Aspergillus alutaceus var. alutaceus* (*A ochraceus*) and *Penicillium viridicatum*, with toxin production generally occurring in storage but also can occur before harvest. Ochratoxins can occur in small grains, such as rye, barley, wheat, and in corn, millet, sorghum, rice, oil seeds, and a wide variety of foods. Ochratoxins are potent nephrotoxins, immunosuppressants, and possible human carcinogens. They cause oxidative stress and inhibit protein synthesis and deplete humoral factors, especially immunoglobulins, and decrease natural killer cell activity.[3,38] The most toxic of the ochratoxins is ochratoxin A. Another nephrotoxic mycotoxin often found with ochratoxins is citrinin. Citrinin is produced by *Penicillium* molds under similar conditions of ochratoxins (see **Table 3**). Ruminants are more resistant to ochratoxin, as compared with monogastrics, because rumen protozoal metabolism can quickly inactivate ochratoxin A to the less toxic ochratoxin α. The elimination half-life in ruminants is short, about 17.3 hours as compared with 100 hours in pigs.[32] However, rapid changes in rations and an increased percentage of protein-rich concentrates can decrease ruminant metabolism of ochratoxin A to less toxic compounds. Regulatory concerns for ochratoxin A in ruminants involve chronic exposure, and unlike swine and poultry, the likelihood for residues in edible tissues or milk of ruminants is low to negligible.[38]

Ochratoxin A and citrinin target the renal proximal tubule. Adult cattle given a single oral dose of ochratoxin A at 13 mg/kg body weight developed anorexia, reduced milk production, diarrhea, and incoordination, with eventual recovery.[60] The toxic effects of ochratoxin are more likely at chronic low-level exposures, and repeated feeding of goats at 3 mg/kg body weight was lethal after 6 days.[61] In several suspect field cases in cattle, the repeated feeding of ochratoxin A at 3 mg/kg ochratoxin (up to 6 ppm) and citrinin (up to 4 ppm) that was detected in feeds caused clinical signs in cattle of uremia, including depression, anorexia, profuse diarrhea, dehydration, hypothermia, and death.[62] Histologic lesions included nephrosis with proximal tubule damage, hyaline casts, dilated tubules and fibrosis in the kidneys, and fatty changes in the liver.

TREMORGENS

The term "staggers" refers to a group of nervous disorders, of different fungal origins, that are characterized by similar clinical signs, including muscle tremors, incoordination, and generalized weakness exacerbated by stress.[15] Perennial ryegrass (*Lolium perenne*) is a common pasture grass in New Zealand, Australia, Europe, and northwestern United States. Cases of staggers predominantly occur on intensively grazed pastures. Disease outbreaks generally occut in the summer and fall and are character-ized by high morbidity, low mortality, and no lesions nor biochemical changes in recovered animals. A group of indole terpenoids, including lolitrem A and B, paxilline and related compounds are produced by an endophyte, *Neothyphodium lolii*, and are thought to act on GABA receptors disrupting neuromuscular control. Lolitrem B is the predominant tremorgen responsible for clinical signs, which start as head tremors and muscle fasciculations of the neck and shoulders and later involve extremities. With disease progression, animal tend to sway, lie down, and convulse when stressed. The maximum tolerable dose is about 2 mg toxin (lolitrem B)/kg dry matter in sheep and cattle.[63] Deaths rarely occur, and animals can recover completely within 7 days when removed from infected grasses and kept in a quiet, secure location.

Paspalum staggers or Dallis grass staggers are associated with infection of dallis and bahia (*Paspalum spp.*) grasses by *Claviceps paspali* and formation of indole-diterpene tremorgens or paspalitrems, such as paspalinine and paspalitrem A and B. Animals can be at risk with ingestion of sclerotia and perhaps honeydew formed in the grasses. Paspalitrem B is the most abundant mycotoxin associated with tremors in cattle and sheep. Sporadic outbreaks of tremors in cattle, similar to paspalum stag-gers, have been associated with grazing Bermuda grass (*Cynodon dactylon*) infected with *Claviceps cynodontis*.[64] Infected seedheads of Bermuda grass contained scle-rotia and paspalitrems and paspaline-like indole-diterpenes and low concentrations of ergonovine and ergine. Prevention of tremorgenic mycotoxins in forages is aimed at pasture improvement programs and maintenance of beneficial endophyte infection, in perennial ryegrass, for example, while decreasing the negative effect of the indole-diterpene compounds on health.[65]

ASPERGILLUS CLAVATUS

Numerous field outbreaks of tremors, posterior ataxia with knuckling of fetlocks, paresis, recumbency, and death have been reported in sheep and beef and dairy cat-tle.[66–68] The animals generally maintain a good appetite. A common denominator is feeding sprouted cereals, hydroponically grown sprouts, or malted byproducts contaminated with *Aspergillus clavatus*. Pathology includes degeneration of large neu-rons in the brain stem and neuronal chromatolysis in the spinal cord gray matter.[69,70] Although *A clavatus* can produce patulin, no specific mycotoxin was associated with these outbreaks. Several field outbreaks of neurotoxicosis in Belgium cattle, accom-panied by lesions involving neuronal degeneration in the central nervous system and axonal degeneration in the peripheral nervous system, were associated with *A clava-tus*–contaminated malting residues and traces of patulin in the compacted fodder.[71]

SILAGE AND FORAGE MOLDS

Ruminant diets contain a significant amount of fiber, usually grass, hay, straw, and si-lages. These feedstuffs can be contaminated in the field with *Fusarium*, *Alternaria*, *Claviceps*, and *Cladosporium* molds. Under poor growth, production, or storage con-ditions, additional fungal spoilage and mycotoxin contamination continue in forages. Generally, when oxygen is excluded from acidic silages or tight forage bales, further mold growth and mycotoxin production is unlikely; however, if air gains access to these feedstuffs, they are at risk for storage molds. Corn and grass silages are often contaminated with molds, including *Aspergillus*, *Penicillium*, *Mucor*, *Geotrichium*, and *Monascus*.[63,72–74] *Fusarium* spp. require oxygen for growth, are pH sensitive, and generally vanish in days following routine silage methods. However in wet years, significant concentrations of *Fusarium* mycotoxins (DON, 15-AcDON, and zearalenone) can routinely be detected in corn silages, and occasionally lower amounts of T-2 and HT-2 toxins can be found in hays and straws in the Midwest. *Geotrichum candidum* occurs in silages and gives off a rancid odor that tends to repel animals, decreasing feed consumption.[75] In Europe, *Penicillium* molds, particularly *Penicillium roqueforti*, contaminate corn silage, grass, and sugar beet products and can produce numerous mycotoxins, including roquefortines, andrastin A, mucophenolic acid, and PR toxin. In a field case, *P roqueforti* was identified on barley kernels stored in a bunk silo for 1.5 months before feeding dairy cows.[76] Adverse effects noted in the cows were inappetence, ketosis, mastitis, paralysis, and abortions; roquefortine C, an indole alkaloid, was identified at approximately 25.6 mg/kg (ppm) in feed grain. No additional *Penicillium* mycotoxins including patulin, PR toxin, or penicillic acid were found, and clinical signs disappeared after feeding the moldy grain stopped. The toxicity of roquefortine in ruminants has not been established. Oral administration of roquefortine to ewes by stomach tube of equivalent amounts of 0 to 25 mg roquefortine/kg silage through 1 estrous cycle (16–18 days) resulted in no clinical illness or changes in serum chemistry or hematology parameters.[77] The only apparent effect was a decrease in rumen pH by 0.5 units, perhaps owing to a shift to gram-positive bacteria.

Stored straw and hay can also be invaded by *Stachybotrys atra*, a mold that likes growing on cellulose in cool, damp conditions. Stachybotryotoxicosis, a historic disease in the 1930s and 1940s, has been reported in ruminants and horses in Eastern Europe (see **Table 3**). Sporadic cases in animals have been reported elsewhere. Intense interest in *Stachybotrys* stems from black mold growth on drywalls in flooded buildings or in wet, poorly ventilated areas and has been associated with pulmonary hemorrhage and respiratory difficulties in humans. *Stachybotrys* can be occasionally cultured from silages and improperly stored grains.

Several recent reviews on mycotoxins occurring in silage have focused on prevention and mitigation strategies to minimize mycotoxins.[74,78–80] The use of silage additives can include homofermentative lactic acid bacteria, heterofermentative lactic acid bacteria, a combination of inoculants, non–lactic acid bacteria species, yeast, enzymes, and chemical additives to provide aerobic stability, assist with fermentation efficiency and animal productivity, inhibit molds and detrimental silage microorganisms, and improve nutrition quality for cattle use.[78] Several detoxification strategies for mycotoxins in silage are feed dilution, which can decrease the ingestion of a mycotoxin but increase the feed-out rate and result in more silage mold, adsorption by a sequestering agent to decrease bioavailability of toxins in the gut, mycotoxin detoxification by exogenous microorganisms (bacteria, yeast, fungi, and enzymes) and exogenous natural or recombinant enzymes.[79] Mycotoxin adsorbents can comprise a large and complicated class of silicate minerals with unique structures and physical, chemical, and mineralogical characteristics, varying capacities in cation exchange, distribution of particles, and surface areas.[80] The complex interactions and factors that affect adsorption of toxins by binders make it difficult to define and predict, and the reader is referred to these reviews for further information. Further research is needed to evaluate in vivo effectiveness to detoxify mycotoxins in ruminants and the stability of toxins through the whole food chain, the field to fork approach is required for the reduction of adverse contaminants and to avoid recontamination.[80] Some studies also indicate that these mineral adsorbents or binders can also cause undesirable effects in livestock, including interaction with veterinary substances and binding nutrients such as vitamin A, zinc, copper, and manganese in feed; causing oxidative stress and reduced cell viability, and apoptosis; and adding possible contaminants if mineral adsorbents contain variable concentrations of accessory mineral and heavy metals that could alter animal health.[81] Also note that some laboratories providing mycotoxin analysis for toxins and concentrations in feed commodities are selling mycotoxin binders to clients, which is a concern for conflict of interest.

PHOTOSENSITIZATION

Photosensitization is clinically characterized as skin (without protection of hair, wool, or pigmentation) hyper-reactivity to sunlight because of photodynamic compounds. The condition may be primary or secondary. Primary photosensitization occurs when photodynamic compounds are absorbed through the skin or gastrointestinal tract and reach the skin to interact with light. Secondary photosensitization is the most common form of photosensitization and occurs when a breakdown product of chlorophyll in the gut or phylloerythrin accumulates in the plasma and skin because of hepatic injury. Phylloerythrin can absorb and release energy, creating a phytotoxic reaction in skin. Facial eczema or pithomycotoxicosis is reported in ruminants grazing intensive pasture systems containing dead plant material contaminated with *Pithomyces chartarum*. Toxicoses generally occur in late summer and fall when hot, dry weather and occasional rain and high humidity promote the growth and sporulation of *P chatarum* and production of sporidesmin mycotoxins. The most predominant mycotoxin is sporidesmin A.[82] Clinical signs usually occur 10 to 14 days after ingestion of sporidesmin and reflect cholestatic liver disease and dermal photosensitization. Edema and erythema of the ears, eyelids, face, and lips are visible in sheep. Animals can develop secondary bacterial infection and become icteric. Dairy cows may develop a sudden decrease in milk production and ill thrift followed by dermal photosensitization several weeks later.

   The term lupinosis applies to a hepatic disease in sheep and cattle resulting from ingestion of phomopsins produced by *Diaporthe toxica* and *D wooddii* on dead lupin plants. The hepatotoxicosis is prevalent in Western Australia, where dead lupin plants are used for fodder in the summer and autumn.[83] Phomopsins are cytotoxic and antimitotic agents. The course of the disease may be acute, subacute, or chronic, depending on the dose and exposure time. Clinical signs are severe liver damage, inappetance, lethargy, icterus, and death. Abortions occur in late pregnant sheep and cattle. Photosensitization is seen in cattle, but rarely in sheep.

DIPLODIA

Another fungus contaminating corn or maize worldwide is *Stenocarpella maydis* (syn. *Diplodia maydis*). Ear corn is most susceptible to *Diplodia* infection within 1 or 2 weeks of midsilk (50% of plants with silks), with wet weather and moderate temperatures allowing spores to splash onto the plant and infect the stalk or ear. The *Diplodia* spores germinate and penetrate the ear shank, starting at the base of the ear and growing toward the tip; ear rot appears as white–grey–brownish mycelia. *Diploidia* is not considered a mycotoxin producer in the United States; however, in southern Africa, diplodiosis is an important mycotoxicosis in harvested maize fields used for winter forage. *Diplodia* can cause a neuromuscular paretic syndrome (eg, high-stepping gait, ataxia, incoordination, constipation, salivation, paresis, and paralysis) in sheep and cattle and stillbirths and neonatal deaths associated with spongiform degeneration in white matter of the brain in offspring of exposed sheep or cattle.[84] The toxin diplonine, isolated from *S maydis* cultures, induced neurologic signs in guinea pigs.[85] A report of diplodiosis in Argentina involved beef heifers grazing a harvested maize field for about 2 weeks and developing incoordination of hindquarters, stiffness, ataxia, recumbency, and paralysis.[86]

EMERGING MYCOTOXINS

The term "emerging mycotoxins," although not well-defined, refers to a group of "mycotoxins, which are neither routinely determined, nor legislatively regulated; however, the evidence of their incidence is rapidly increasing."[87] Emerging mycotoxins include some of the *Fusarium* toxins, enniatins, beauvericin, fusaproliferin, moniliformon, culmorin, butanolide, *Aspergillus*-produced toxins, sterigmatocystin, emodin and cyclopiazonic acid, *Penicillium* produced mycophenolic acid, and *Alternaria* toxins including alternariol and alternariol monomethyl ether, tenuazonic acid, and others.[2] Some of these mycotoxins have been recognized but are not commonly tested for in animal feeds and others are recently detected. Knowledge of the occurrence in animal feed and acute and chronic toxicity of these compounds in animals, particularly ruminants, is being developed but sparse.[88] The reader is referred to recent articles by Gruber-Dorniger and colleagues,[2] Panasiuk and colleagues,[88] Khoshal and colleagues,[89] and Internet sources such as the US National Institutes of Health's National Library of Medicine or Pubmed Central.

DISCUSSION

Mycotoxins occurring on grains and in grasses can adversely affect ruminants. The detection and characterization of mycotoxins occurring in silages, forages, and some of the cereal byproducts that are routinely fed to dairy and beef is increasing with recognition of emerging mycotoxins, but toxicity data are often lacking in ruminants, particularly small ruminants and impacts on the fetus. Multiple mycotoxins can be detected in moldy feed (eg, aflatoxins, fumonisins, DON, zearalenone in grains, grain byproducts, and silages) and our knowledge of interaction(s) of effects in ruminants is sparse. Some mycotoxins can exist in conjugated form, either soluble (masked mycotoxins) or incorporated into, associated with, or attached to macromoleucules in plants (insoluble or bound mycotoxins).[90] The significance of conjugated mycotoxins is being discovered, particularly data regarding the toxicity or bioavailability of these mycotoxins. Dose–response relationships often have not been established for reproductive or immune effects of mycotoxins in ruminants. In general, ruminants tend to be less susceptible to mycotoxins as compared with monogastrics and young animals; however, the preruminant or young animal can be as susceptible as monogastrics. Developing and maintaining adequate rumen flora and function is critical for metabolism and/or deactivation of some of the mycotoxins (ie, DON and ochratoxin).

The more mycotoxins discovered and characterized, the more livestock producers want to test those toxins in feed for possible explanation of health effects. Mycotoxin analyses for multiple toxins, especially emerging mycotoxins, in more complex matrices (eg, silages, haylages) can require expensive instrumentation such as liquid chromatography and tandem mass spectroscopy, pure standards, and if available, stable isotope standards that can minimize matrix effects. Testing feed for mycotoxins is not the quick, easy answer to oftentimes difficult problems involving adequate nutrition, environment, animal physiology, genetics, other toxins, and disease. More research is needed for effective, cost-efficient inactivation of mycotoxins (esp. trichothecenes) in ruminants.

Government regulations for maximum mycotoxins in commodities are typically established to protect the consumer from harmful effects of these compounds, and regulations for mycotoxins in food and feed will probably expand with better analytical methods. Recent history indicates that growing food and feed commodities will be challenged with climactic changes and sustained moisture conditions for both the field and storage, with a trend for increasing mold and mycotoxin contamination in animal feeds.

A major question from livestock producers when submitting animal feeds for mycotoxin testing is to determine if feed is "safe to feed." No feed sample submitted for mycotoxin analysis can ever be labeled by the laboratory as "safe to feed to animals" because laboratories do not have the analytical capability or mycotoxin standards to test for all possible mycotoxins produced by molds and toxicity data in ruminants, particularly pregnant ruminants, are lacking for many mycotoxins. Laboratories are typically testing for common mycotoxins, not all toxins. Based on mold cultures, analytical findings, and knowledge of mycotoxin concentrations associated with clinical effects, feed can be channeled for use in various animals under specified conditions. Often the moldy and more contaminated feeds are used in feedlots, where the physiologic demands of pregnancy and lactation are avoided and a more frequent turnover in sources or batches of feed decrease the duration of exposure. This approach is not foolproof to avoiding mycotoxicosis. Common sense is "do not feed moldy feed"; a practical approach is to test suspect feeds in a ration, avoid moldy feed if possible, and dilute out with clean feed to minimize the effects or channel feed to animals that are more tolerant of mycotoxin feed contamination.

REFERENCES

1. Pitt JI, Miller MD. A concise history of mycotoxin research. J Agric Food Chem 2017;65(33):7021–33.
2. Gruber-Dorninger C, Novak B, Nagl V, et al. Emerging mycotoxins: beyond traditionally determined food contaminants. J Agric Food Chem 2017;65(33): 7052–70.
3. CAST (Council for Agricultural Science and Technology). Mycotoxins: risks in plant, animal and human systems, Task Force Report No. 139, Ames (IA): CAST; 2003.
4. EFSA CONTAM panel (European Food Safety Authority Panel on Contaminants in the Food Chain). Scientific opinion on the risk for public and animal health related to the presence of sterigmatocystin in food and feed. EFSA J 2013; 11(6):3254, 81.
5. Gallo A, Moschini M, Masoero F. Aflatoxins absorption in the gastro-intestinal tract and in the vaginal mucosa in lactating dairy cows. Ital J Anim Sci 2008; 7:53–63.
6. Kiessling KH, Pettersson H, Sandholm K, et al. Metabolism of aflatoxin, ochratoxin, zearalenone and three trichothecenes by intact rumen fluid, rumen protozoa and rumen bacteria. Appl Environ Microbiol 1984;47:1070–3.
7. Westlake K, Mackie RI, Dutton MF. *In vitro* metabolism of mycotoxins by bacterial, protozoal and ovine ruminal fluid preparations. Anim Feed Sci Tech 1989; 25:169–78.
8. Upadhaya SD, Sung HG, Lee CH, et al. Comparative study on the aflatoxin B1 degradation ability of rumen fluid from Holstein steers and Korean native goats. J Vet Sci 2009;10:29–34.
9. Meerdink GL. Aflatoxins. In: Plumlee KH, editor. Clinical veterinary toxicology. St Louis (MO): Mosby; 2004. p. 231–5.
10. Carvajal M, Rojo F, Méndez I, et al. Aflatoxin B_1 and its interconverting metabolite aflatoxicol in milk: the situation in Mexico. Food Addit Contam 2003;20: 1077–86.

11. Mazzette A, Decandia M, Acciaro M, et al. Excretion of aflatoxin M_1 in milk of goats fed diets contaminated by aflatoxin B_1. Ital J Anim Sci 2009;8(Suppl 2): 631-3.

12. Asi MR, Iqbal SZ, Arino A, et al. Effect of seasonal variations and lactation times on aflatoxin M_1 contamination in milk of different species from Punjab, Pakistan. Food Control 2012;25:34-8.

13. Battacone G, Nudda A, Cannas A, et al. Excretion of aflatoxin M_1 in milk of dairy ewes treated with different doses of aflatoxin B_1. J Dairy Sci 2003;86(8): 2667-75.

14. Newberne PM. Chronic aflatoxicosis. J Am Vet Med Assoc 1973;163:1262-7.

15. Raisbeck MF, Rottinghaus GE, Kendall JD. Effects of naturally occurring mycotoxins on ruminants. In: Smith JE, Henderson RS, editors. Mycotoxins and animal foods. Boca Raton (FL): CRC Press; 1991. p. 647-77.

16. Lewis F, Markson LM, Allcroft R. The effect of feeding toxic groundnut meal to sheep over a period of five years. Vet Rec 1967;80:312-4.

17. Hall RF, Harrison LR, Colvin BM. Aflatoxicosis in cattle pastured in a field of sweet corn. J Am Vet Med Assoc 1989;194:938.

18. Osweiler GD. Mycotoxins. In: Kluge JP, editor. Toxicology (the national veterinary medical series). Philadelphia: Williams & Wilkins; 1996. p. 409-36.

19. Osweiler GD. Mycotoxins. Contemporary issues of food animal health and productivity. Vet Clin North Am Food Anim Pract 2000;16:511-30.

20. Smith EE, Phillips TD, Ellis JA, et al. Dietary hydrated sodium calcium aluminosilicate reduction of aflatoxin M1 residue in dairy goat milk and effects on milk production and components. J Anim Sci 1994;72:677-82.

21. Diaz DE, Hagler WM, Blackwelder JT, et al. Aflatoxin binders II: reduction of aflatoxin M1 in milk by sequestering agents of cows consuming aflatoxin in feed. Mycopathologia 2004;157:233-41.

22. Kutz RE, Sampson JD, Pompeu LB, et al. Efficacy of Solis, NovasilPlus and MTB-100 to reduce aflatoxin M1 levels in milk of early to mid lactation dairy cows fed aflatoxin B1. J Dairy Sci 2009;92:3959-63.

23. Sundstøl Eriksen G, Pettersson H, Lundh T. Comparative cytotoxicity of deoxynivalenol, nivalenol, their acetylated derivatives and de-epoxy metabolites. Food Chem Toxicol 2004;42:619-24.

24. Pinton P, Tsybulskyy D, Lucioli J, et al. Toxicity of deoxynivalenol and its acetylated derivatives on the intestine: differential effects on morphology, barrier function, tight junction proteins, and mitogen-activated protein kinases. Toxicol Sci 2012;30(1):180-90.

25. Mostrom M, Tacke B, Lardy G. Field corn, hail, and mycotoxins. In: Proceedings, North Central Conference of the American Association of Veterinary Laboratory Diagnosticians, Fargo, North Dakota. North Dakota State University, Fargo (ND). 2005.

26. Wu Q, Wu W, Kuca K. From hypoxia and hypoxia-inducible factors (HIF) to oxidative stress: a new understanding of the toxic mechanism of mycotoxins. Food Chem Toxicol 2020;135:110968. Available at: https://doi.org/10.1016/j.fct.2019.110968. Accessed January 7, 2020.

27. Ueno Y. General toxicology. In: Ueno Y, editor. Trichothecenes - chemical, biological, and toxicological aspects. New York: Elsevier; 1983. p. 135-46.

28. Valenta H, Danicke S, Doll S. Analysis of deoxynivalenol and de-epoxy-deoxynivalenol in animal tissues by liquid chromatography after clean-up with an immunoaffinity column. Mycotoxin Res 2003;19:51-5.

29. Phruksawan W, Poapolathep S, Giorgi M, et al. Toxicokinetic profile of fusarenon-X and its metabolite nivalenol in the goat (*Capra hircus*). Toxicon 2018;153:78–84.

30. Valgaeren B, Theron L, Croubels S, et al. The role of roughage provision on the absorption and disposition of the mycotoxin deoxynivalenol and its acetylated derivatives in calves: from field observations to toxicokinetics. Arch Toxicol 2019;93:293–310.

31. Anderson VL, Boland EW, Casper HH. Effects of vomitoxin (deoxynivalenol) from scab infested barley on performance of feedlot and breeding cattle. J Anim Sci 1966;74:208.

32. Jouany J-P, Diaz DE. Effects of mycotoxins in ruminants. In: Diaz DE, editor. The mycotoxin blue Book. Nottingham (England): Nottingham University Press; 2005. p. 295–321.

33. Charmley E, Trenholm HL, Thompson BK, et al. Influence of level of deoxynivalenol in the diet of dairy cows on feed intake, milk production, and its composition. J Dairy Sci 1993;76:3580–7.

34. Ingalls JR. Influence of deoxynivalenol on feed consumption by dairy cows. Anim Feed Sci Technol 1996;60:297–300.

35. Prelusky DB, Trenholm HL, Lawrence GA, et al. Nontransmission of deoxynivalenol (vomitoxin) to milk following oral administration to dairy cows. J Environ Sci Health 1984;B19:593–609.

36. Osweiler GD, Hook BS, Mann DD, et al. Effects of T-2 toxin in cattle. In: Proceedings United States Animal Health Association, 85th Annual Meeting, St Louis, MO. Richmond, VA: US Animal Health Association. October 11-16, 1981; p. 214–31.

37. Hsu IC, Smalley EB, Strong FM, et al. Identification of T-2 toxin in moldy corn associated with a lethal toxicosis in dairy cattle. Appl Microbiol 1972;24:684–90.

38. Fink-Gremmels J, van der Merwe D. Mycotoxins in the food chain: contamination of foods of animal origin. In: Frans JM, Smulders I, Rietjens MCM, et al, editors. *Chemical Hazards in food of animal origin. Food safety assurance and veterinary public heath No. 7*. The Netherlands: Wageningen Academic Publishers; 2019. p. 241–61. Available at: http://doi.10.3920/978-90-8686-877-3_10. Accessed January 15, 2020.

39. Vila-Donat P, Martin S, Sanchis V, et al. A review of the mycotoxin absorbing agents, with an emphasis on their multi-binding capacity, for animal feed decontamination. Food Chem Toxicol 2018;114:246–59.

40. Dänicke S, Pahlow G, Beyer M, et al. Investigations on the kinetics of the concentration of deoxynivalenol (DON) and on spoilage by moulds and yeasts of wheat grain preserved with sodium metabisulfite (Na2S2O5, SBS) and propionic acid at various moisture contents. Arch Anim Nutr 2010;64:190–203.

41. European Food Safety Authority CONTAM Panel (EFSA panel on contaminants in the food chain), Knutsen HK, Alexander J, et al. Scientific opinion on the risks for animal health related to the presence of zearalenone and its modified forms in feed. EFSA J 2017;15(7):4851, 123.

42. Biehl ML, Prelusky DB, Koritz GD, et al. Biliary excretion and enterohepatic cycling of zearalenone in immature pigs. Toxicol Appl Pharmacol 1993;121:152–9.

43. Kuiper-Goodman T, Scott PM, Watanabe H. Risk assessment of the mycotoxin zearalenone. Regul Toxicol Pharmacol 1987;7:253–306.

44. Ueno Y, Ayaki S, Sato N, et al. Fate and mode of action of zearalenone. Ann Nutr Aliment 1977;31(4–6):935–48.

45. Dong J, He ZJ, Tulayakul P, et al. The toxic effects and fate of intravenously administer zearalenone in goats. Toxicon 2010;55:523–30.
46. Katzenellenbogen BS, Katzenellenbogen JA, Mordecai D. Zearalenones: characterization of the estrogenic potencies and receptor interactions of a series of fungal β-resorcylic acid lactones. Endocrinology 1979;105:33–40.
47. Danicke S, Gadeken D, Ueberschar KH, et al. Effects of *Fusarium* toxin contaminated wheat and of a detoxifying agent on performance of growing bulls, on nutrient digestibility and on the carryover of zearalenone. Arch Tierernahr 2002;56(4):245–61.
48. Prelusky DB, Scott PM, Trenholm HL, et al. Minimal transmission of zearalenone to milk of dairy cows. J Environ Sci Health B 1990;25(1):87–103.
49. Sundlof SF, Strickland C. Zearalenone and zearanol potential residue problems in livestock. Vet Hum Toxicol 1986;28:242–50.
50. Mirocha CJ, Christensen CM. Oestrogenic mycotoxins synthesis by *Fusarium*. In: Purchase IFH, editor. Mycotoxins. New York: Elsevier; 1974. p. 129–48.
51. Weaver GA, Kurtz HJ, Behrens JC, et al. Effect of zearalenone on the fertility of virgin heifers. Am J Vet Res 1986;47:1395–7.
52. Smith JR, di Menna ME, McGowan LT. Reproductive performance of Coopworth ewes following oral doses of zearalenone before and after mating. J Reprod Fertil 1990;89(1):99–106.
53. Commission of the European Communities. Commission recommendation of 17 August 2006 on the presence of deoxynivalenol, zearalenone, ochratoxin A, T-2 and HT-2 and fumonisins in products intended for animal feeding. Official J of the EU. 2006/576/EC. Available at: https://eur-lex.europa.eu/LexUriServ/LexUriServ.do?uri=OJ:L:2006:229:0007:0009:EN:PDF. Accessed November 18, 2008.
54. Mogensen JP, Frisvad JC, Thrane U, et al. Production of fumonisin B2 and B4 by *Aspergillus niger* on grapes and raisins. J Agric Food Chem 2010;58:954–8.
55. Smith GW, Constable PD. Fumonisin. In: Plumlee KH, editor. Clinical veterinary toxicology. St Louis (MO): Mosby; 2004. p. 250–4.
56. Osweiler GD, Kehrli ME, Stabel JR, et al. Effects of fumonisin-contaminated corn screenings on growth and health of feeder calves. J Anim Sci 1993;71:459–66.
57. Baker DC, Rottinghaus GE. Chronic experimental fumonisin intoxication of calves. J Vet Diagn Invest 1999;11:289–92.
58. Edrington TS, Kamps-Holtzapple CA, Harvey RB, et al. Acute hepatic and renal toxicity in lambs dosed with fumonisin-containing culture material. J Anim Sci 1995;73:508–15.
59. Diaz DE, Hopkins BA, Leonard LM, et al. Effect of fumonisin on lactating dairy cattle. J Dairy Sci 2000;83(abst):1171.
60. Meerdink GL. Citrinin and ochratoxin. In: Plumlee KH, editor. Clinical veterinary toxicology. St Louis (MO): Mosby; 2004. p. 235–9.
61. Ribelin WE, Fukushima K, Still PE. The toxicity of ochratoxin to ruminants. Can J Comp Med 1978;42:172–6.
62. Lloyd WE, Stahr HM. Ochratoxin toxicosis in cattle. In: 22nd Annual Proceedings, American Association Veterinary Laboratory Diagnosticians. San Diego, CA. Visalia, CA: AAVLD 1979. p. 223–8.
63. Fink-Gremmels J. Mycotoxins in forages. In: Diaz DE, editor. The mycotoxin blue book. Nottingham (England): Nottingham University Press; 2005. p. 249–68.
64. Uhlig S, Botha CJ, Vrålstad T, et al. Indole-diterpenes and ergot alkaloids in *Cynodon dactylon* (Bermuda grass) infected with *Claviceps cynodontis* from an outbreak of tremors in cattle. J Agric Food Chem 2009;57:1112–9.

65. Reddy P, Guthride K, Vassiliadis S, et al. Tremorgenic mycotoxins: structure diversity and biological activity. Toxins 2019;11:302–28.

66. Shlosberg A, Zadikov I, Perl S, et al. *Aspergillus clavatus* as the probable cause of a lethal mass neurotoxicosis in sheep. Mycopathologia 1991;114:35–9.

67. Kellerman TS, Newsholme SJ, Coetzer JA, et al. A tremorgenic mycotoxicosis of cattle caused by maize sprouts infested with *Aspergillus clavatus*. Onderstepoort J Vet Res 1984;51:271–4.

68. McKenzie RA, Kelly MA, Shivas RG, et al. *Aspergillus clavatus* tremorgenic neurotoxicosis in cattle fed sprouted grains. Aust Vet J 2004;82:635–8.

69. Van Der Lugt JJ, Kellerman TS, Van Vollenhoven A, et al. Spinal cord degeneration in adult dairy cows associated with the feeding of sorghum beer residues. J S Afr Vet Assoc 1994;65:184–8.

70. Loretti AP, Colodel EM, Driemeier D, et al. Neurological disorder in dairy cattle associated with consumption of beer residues contaminated with *Aspergillus clavatus*. J Vet Diagn Invest 2003;15:123–32.

71. Sabater-Vilar M, Maas RFM, Bosschere HD, et al. Patulin produced by an *Aspergillus clavatus* isolated from feed containing malting residues associated with a lethal neurotoxicosis in cattle. Mycopathologia 2004;158:419–26.

72. O'Brien M, Nielsen KF, O'Kiely P, et al. Mycotoxins and other secondary metabolites produced *in vitro* by *Penicillium paneum* Frisvad and *Penicillium roqueforti* Thom isolated from baled grass silage in Ireland. J Agric Food Chem 2006;54: 9268–76.

73. Sumarah MW, Miller JD, Blackwell BA. Isolation and metabolite production by *Penicillium roqueforti*, *P. paneum* and *P. crustosum* isolated in Canada. Mycopathologia 2005;159:571–7.

74. Gallo A, Giuberta G, Frisvad JC, et al. Review on mycotoxin issues in ruminants: occurrence in forages, effects of mycotoxin ingestion on health status and animal performance and practical strategies to counteract their negative effects. Toxins 2015;7:3057–111.

75. Scudamor K, Livesey C. Occurrence and significance of mycotoxins in forage crops and silage: a review. J Sci Food Agric 1998;77:1–17.

76. Hägglblom P. Isolation of roquefortine C from feed grain. Appl Environ Microbiol 1990;56:2924–6.

77. Tüller G, Armbruster G, Widenmann S, et al. Occurrence of roquefortine in silage – toxicological relevance to sheep. J Anim Physiol Anim Nutr 1998;80:246–9.

78. Muck RE, Nadeau EMG, McAllister TA, et al. Silage review: recent advances and future uses of silage additives. J Dairy Sci 2018;101(5):3890–4000.

79. Ogunade IM, Martinez-Tuppia C, Queiroz OCM, et al. Silage review: mycotoxins in silage: occurrence, effects, prevention, and mitigation. J Dairy Sci 2018; 101(5):4034–59.

80. Colovic R, Puvaca N, Cheli F, et al. Decontamination of mycotoxin-contaminated feedstuffs and compound feed. Toxins 2019;11(11):617–35.

81. Elliott CT, Connolly L, Kolawole O. Potential adverse effects on animal health and performance caused by the addition of mineral adsorbents to feeds to reduce mycotoxin exposure. Mycol Res 2020;36(1):115–26.

82. Dalefield R. Sporidesmin. In: Plumlee KH, editor. Clinical veterinary toxicology. St Louis (MO): Mosby; 2004. p. 264–8.

83. Allen J. Phomopsins. Ergot. In: Plumlee KH, editor. Clinical veterinary toxicology. St Louis (MO): Mosby; 2004. p. 259–62.

84. Kellerman TS, Coetzer JAW, Naudé TW, et al. Neurological disorders without notable pathological lesions. In: Clarke E, editor. Plant poisonings and

mycotoxicoses of livestock in Southern Africa. 2nd edition. Cape Town (SA): Oxford University Press Southern Africa; 2005. p. 63–86.

85. Snyman LD, Kellerman TS, Vleggaar R, et al. Diplonine, a neurotoxin isolated from culture of the fungus *Stenocarpella maydis* (Berk.) Sacc. that induces diplodiosis. J Agric Food Chem 2011;59:9039–44.

86. Odriozola E, Odeón A, Canton G, et al. *Diploidia maydis*: a cause of death of cattle in Argentina. N Z Vet J 2005;53:160–1.

87. Vackavikova M, Malachova A, Veprikova Z, et al. 'Emerging' mycotoxins in cereals processing chains: changes of enniatins during beer and bread making. Food Chem 2013;136:750–7.

88. Panasiuk L, Jedziniak P, Pietruszka K, et al. Frequency and levels of regulated and emerging mycotoxins in silage in Poland. Mycol Res 2019;35:17–25.

89. Khoshal AK, Novak B, Martin PGP, et al. Co-occurrence of DON and emerging mycotoxins in worldwide finished pig feed and their combined toxicity in intestinal cells. Toxins 2019;11(12):727–44.

90. Berthiller F, Schuhmacher R, Adam G, et al. Formation, determination and significance of masked and other conjugated mycotoxins. Anal Bioanal Chem 2009;395:1243–52.

91. Osweiler GD, Trampel DW. Aflatoxicosis in feedlot cattle. J Am Vet Med Assoc 1885;187:636–7.

92. Vesonder RF, Horn BW. Sterigmatocystin in dairy cattle feed contaminated with *Aspergillus versicolor.* Appl Environ Microbiol 1985;49:234–5.

93. Mostrom MS, Raisbeck. Trichothecenes. In: Gupta R, editor. Veterinary toxicology, basic and clinical principles. 1st edition. New York: Academic Press; 2007. p. 951–76.

94. Hintikka EL. Stachybotryotoxicosis in horses. In: Wyllie TD, Morehouse LG, editors. Mycotoxic fungi, mycotoxins, mycotoxicoses. Mycotoxicosis of domestic and laboratory animals, poultry, and aquatic invertebrates and vertebratesvol. 2. New York: Marcel Dekker; 1978. p. 181–5.

95. Tapia MO, Stern MD, Koski RL, et al. Effects of patulin on rumen microbial fermentation in continuous culture fermenters. Anim Feed Sci Technol 2002; 97:239–46.

96. Pal S, Singh N, Ansari KM. Toxicological effect of patulin mycotoxin on the mammalian system: an overview. Toxicol Res (Camb) 2017;6(6):764–71.

97. Naudé TW, Botha CJ, Vorster JH, et al. *Claviceps cyperi*, a new cause of severe ergotism in dairy cattle consuming maize silage and teff hay contaminated with ergotised *Cyperus esculentus* (nut sedge) on the Highveld of South Africa. Onderstepoort J Vet Res 2005;72:23–37.

98. US FDA (Food and Drug Administration). Guidance for industry and FDA: advisory levels for deoxynivalenol (DON) in finished wheat products for human consumption and grains and grain by-products used for animal feed. 2010. Available at: https://www.fda.gov/regulatory-information/search-fda-guidance-documents/guidance-industry-and-fda-advisory-levels-deoxynivalenol-don-finsihed-wheat-products-human. Accessed December 20, 2012.

99. Commission of European Communities (EC). Commission recommendation on the presence of deoxynivalenol, zearalenone, ochratoxin A, T-2 and HT-2 and fumonisins in products intended for animal feeding. 17 August 2006. Official J European Union. 23.8.2006 2006/576/EC. Available at: Eur-lex.europa.eu/LexUriServ.do?uri:OJ:L:2006:229:0007:0009:EN:PDF. Accessed 2010.

100. Canadian Food Inspection Agency (CFIA). Government of Canada. RG (Regulatory guidance) 8: contaminants in Feed. Modified 10.16.2017. p. 30. Available at:

https://www.inspection.gc.ca/animal-health/livestock-feeds/regulatory-guidance/rg-i/eng/1347383943203/1347384015090?chap=0. Accessed February 19, 2020.

101. US FDA. CPG Sec. 683.100 Action levels for aflatoxins in animal feeds. Revised 8/28/94. Available at: http://www.fda.gov/ICECI/ComplianceManuals/CompliancePolicyGuidanceManual/ucm074703.htm. March 30, 2010.

102. US FDA. CPG Sec. 527.400 Whole Milk, Lowfat Milk, Skim Milk - Aflatoxin M1. Updated 11.29.05. Available at: http://www.fda.gov/ICECI/ComplianceManuals/CompliancePolicyGuidanceManual/ucm074482.htm. February 14, 2020.

103. Commission of European Communities (EC). Commission regulation (EC) No. 1881/2006 of 19 December 2006 setting maximum levels for certain contaminants in foodstuffs. 19 December 2006 Official J European Union. Available at: Eur-lex.europa.eu/legal-content/EN/ALL/uri=CELEX%3AE2006R1881. Accessed 2009.

104. FDA US (Food and Drug Administration). Guidance for industry fumonisin levels in human foods and animal feeds. 2001. Available at: http://www.fda.gov/regulatory-information/search-fda/guidance-documents/guidance-industry-fumonisin-levels-human-foods-and-animal-feeds. Accessed October 28, 2009.

105. Alhawatema MD, Gebril S, Cook D, et al. RNAi-mediated down-regulation of a melanin polyketide synthase (*pks*1) gene in the fungus *Slafractonia leguminicola*. World J Microbiol Biotechnol 2017;33:179. Available at: Link.springer.com/content/pdf/10.1007/s11274-017-2346-4.pdf. Accessed February 4, 2020.

Selenosis in Ruminants

Merl F. Raisbeck, DVM, MS, PhD

KEYWORDS

- Selenosis • Selenium • Toxicology • Ruminants

KEY POINTS

- The most common cause of selenium intoxication in livestock is iatrogenic.
- Acute selenosis almost always is the result of over-supplementation or overdosing with parenteral preparations.
- The characteristic features of chronic selenosis in cattle, horses, and swine are bilaterally symmetric alopecia and dystrophic hoof growth.
- Chronic selenosis under range conditions most commonly results from eating high selenium forages.

Selenium (Se) is a metalloid which, in its pure state, may exist as a red amorphous powder, a reddish crystal, a silver-gray crystal, or a brown-black solid. Its potency as both a nutrient and a toxicant, however, is such that, even among Se researchers, few people have ever seen the pure element but rather work with parts per million (ppm) or parts per billion concentrations. To the practicing veterinarian or livestock producer, Se is an abstract number on a feed label or a laboratory report and it is easy to lose sight of the narrow margin between too little and too much.

Although Se originally was discovered during the course of an occupational disease investigation among sulfuric acid workers,[1] the first conclusive identification of naturally occurring Se toxicity in animals came from investigators at the Agricultural Experiment Stations of the University of Wyoming and South Dakota State University.[2-5] These laboratories popularized a model of selenosis in domestic animals, which is still cited in the veterinary literature today. Although some of what was attributed to Se by these early workers seems silly in light of modern knowledge, it must be remembered that at that time, analytical technology was primitive and Se was not known to be essential for health. Thus, there was a tendency on the part of many early investigators to attribute any malady of people or livestock to Se if any amount Se could be identified in tissues or the environment and without considering other possible etiologies.[6,7]

Portions of this work were supported by the Office of Surface Mining Abandoned Coal Mine Lands Reclamation Research Program, the United States Deptartment of Agriculture, and by the Pharmaceutical Manufacturers Association.

Department of Veterinary Sciences, College of Agriculture, University of Wyoming, 2852 Riverside, Laramie, WY 82070, USA

E-mail address: raisbeck@uwyo.edu

Vet Clin Food Anim 36 (2020) 775–789
https://doi.org/10.1016/j.cvfa.2020.08.013
0749-0720/20/© 2020 Elsevier Inc. All rights reserved.

SOURCES

Most of the Se in the geosphere exists in Cretaceous shales and glacial drift, where it forms water-insoluble (and thus biologically unavailable) complexes with iron and sulfur (S). Commercial Se is produced primarily as a byproduct during extraction and refining of other metals, notably copper, nickel, lead, and zinc.[8,9] The element is used extensively in the manufacture of semiconductors (eg, solar cells), nanoparticles, glass, rubber, and various pigments as well as nutritional supplements. It also may become biologically available to livestock and wildlife as the result of human activities, such as strip mining and irrigation (discussed later).

Feed Additives

The most common cause of Se intoxication in livestock is iatrogenic. Because Se is an essential trace element and is relatively cheap, it is commonly added to animal rations at concentrations equivalent to 0.1 ppm to 0.3 ppm of the total diet. Given the relatively narrow range between deficient and toxic dietary concentrations, it is easy for a decimal point mixing error to result in toxic or even lethal exposures. Parenteral solutions used to treat Se deficiency also occasionally cause poisoning, again as the result of either accidental or intentional overdosing.

Natural Sources

Naturally, Se in the geosphere exists as 1 of 5 different oxidation states: Se(VI) (selenate), Se (IV) (selenite), various organic compounds, Se(0) (elemental Se), and Se(-II) (selenide), the latter 2 of which are relatively water-insoluble. Se is mobilized from the insoluble reservoirs in soils, rocks, and so forth by weathering and microbial activity, which oxidize pyritic Se(-II) to water soluble selenite or selenate ions.[9,10] These natural processes are favored under alkaline, oxidizing soil conditions and may be accelerated by human activities, such as surface mining and irrigation. Once converted to a water-soluble form, Se is readily taken up by plants, certain species of which bioconcentrate the element.[8] Se-contaminated runoff water may in turn be concentrated further by evaporation from closed watersheds, such as playas. Although selenosis from water-borne sources is much more common in wild waterfowl, it theoretically may occur in livestock.

Water solubility is the critical determinant in Se bioavailability to plants. All vegetation grown on soils with high water-soluble Se concentrations contain greater than normal Se concentrations. In some regions, soils with very high total Se concentrations produce forages which contain insufficient Se for animal health as the result of environmental factors which render Se unavailable.[11] In most plant species, Se is incorporated into protein as the amino acid analog selenomethionine (Semet).[12,13] Total Se concentrations in such plants seldom exceed 25 ppm to 50 ppm on a dry matter basis, regardless of soil concentration.

In general, plants do not require Se as do mammals and other vertebrates, although there is some evidence that small amounts of Se may facilitate growth in some plant species.[14] In most plant species, excessive soil Se is quite toxic.[15] A few plant species, termed *selenium accumulators*, actually may bioconcentrate Se to hundreds or even thousands of ppm. In these plants, Se is stored as nonphysiologic amino acids and/or eliminated as volatile selenides.[16,17] This adaptation permits them to tolerate soil and tissue concentrations lethal to normal plants. The accumulators are subdivided further into facultative or obligate species depending on whether or not they appear to require Se to survive.[2,18] The former (non-Se requiring) group includes many otherwise useful genera, such as *Atriplex*; the latter (which appear to require

Se) largely are noxious weeds. Although there is some question as whether the so-called obligate accumulators actually require Se (the author raised *Astragalus bisulcatus* in low Se media for 2 years), they are superbly adapted to seleniferous soils and are seldom found on anywhere else.

Although many texts continue to attribute rangeland Se toxicity to obligate accumulators on the basis of the older literature, these plants are so unpalatable that most grazing animals starve before eating any significant amount.[19,20] It also has been suggested that accumulator species mine Se from deeper, less biologically available strata and deposit it in a readily available form in the rooting zone of more desirable forage species.[18] Although this hypothesis theoretically is attractive, there is little evidence to either support or refute it, and the mechanism probably plays only a minor role, if any, in making soil Se available to grazing animals. The principle importance of obligate accumulators under field conditions is as indicators of potentially high soil Se concentrations rather than as sources of Se in themselves.

MODE OF ACTION

Several mechanisms have been postulated to explain the toxic effects of Se on cells and organs. Se chemically is very similar to S and readily substitutes for S in many biochemical reactions, including the disulfide bridges, which provide tertiary structure and thus function to proteins.[21] Substitution of Se for S in keratin was suggested to result in weakened physical protein structure and subsequently failure of keratinized tissues, such as hair and hoof.[22,23] This hypothesis never has been rigorously tested but remains attractive. Ganther[24] demonstrated that the selenite ion reacts with reduced glutathione (GSH) and suggested that the cytotoxic effects of Se are the result of denaturation of critical protein thiols. Wilson and colleagues[25] hypothesized that the Se-induced spinal lesions in swine might involve niacin metabolism, but the single reported experiment testing this hypothesis was inconclusive.

Over the past 50 years, considerable evidence has accumulated that oxidative stress is the pivotal biochemical lesion of selenosis. Spallholz[26] summarized a series of in vitro experiments, which suggested that certain chemical forms (those with unshielded Se atoms, such as selenite or selenocysteine) of Se react with tissue thiols to produce reactive oxygen species. For example, selenite reacts with reduced GSH in vitro to produce superoxide anion and elemental Se.[27] Addition of catalase, super-oxide dismutase, and/or GSH peroxidase to a reaction mixture containing selenite and GSH decreased the generation of free radicals as measured by chemiluminescence.[28] Although selenite is immediately effective in these experimental systems, Semet requires some time and the presence of intact, functioning cells to produce free radicals. This suggests that Semet metabolism to some reactive intermediate is a prerequisite to toxicity.[26]

In animal experiments, Se toxicity is accompanied by numerous indicators of oxidative injury. Ethane (a byproduct of lipid peroxidation) evolution was increased significantly in selenite-treated rats. This effect was not evident in selenate-treated rats.[29] Among rats pretreated with the GSH depletor diethylmaleate and challenged 1 hour later with sodium selenite, 80% to 100% died.[30] Similarly pretreated rats challenged with the same dose of selenite 25 hours later, after GSH levels had recovered, suffered no mortality.[30] In a similar but longer-term experiment, rats treated for several weeks with varying doses of sodium selenite initially exhibited decreased GSH concentrations and increased the ratio of oxidized to reduced GSH (GSSG). GSH concentrations later returned to pretreatment levels as a result of compensatory increases in GSH reductase and glucose-6-phosphate dehydrogenase.[31] Mallard ducks fed toxic concentrations of Se had significantly greater hepatic GSSG and GSSG:GSH ratios.[32] Mallard embryos, incubated with various forms of Se, contained significantly increased thiobarbiturate reactive substances, such as malondialdehyde, compared with controls and supplementation with vitamin E decreased the toxic lesions of Se.[33] Vitamin E–deficient swine were more susceptible to Se toxicity than animals on vitamin adequate diets[34] and supranutritional doses of vitamin E reduced both the mortality[29] and lipid peroxidation[35] in selenite-treated rats.

The link between Se toxicity and oxidative stress is interesting, given that Se commonly is described in the veterinary literature as an "antioxidant" and many veterinarians and nutritionists seem to believe that a diet deficient in any antioxidant can be compensated with extra Se. Given the pathologic similarities between the lesions of vitamin E–Se deficiency and Se toxicity,[6,36] it behooves veterinarians to confirm a diagnosis of deficiency chemically before instituting a Se supplementation program. A classic, if somewhat extreme, example is a flock of sheep in northwestern Wyoming diagnosed as Se deficient on the basis of gross heart lesions and supplemented with selenate. When losses continued, the dose of Se was increased again and the problem worsened. When samples finally were submitted to chemical analysis, it became evident that the animals had been receiving a seleniferous diet from the beginning and that at least a portion of the subsequent deaths actually were due to Se intoxication (Raisbeck, unpublished, 1995).

CLINICAL SIGNS
Acute Selenosis

Acute selenosis almost always is the result of over-supplementation or overdosing with parenteral preparations. Plants that accumulate sufficient Se to be acutely toxic are extremely unpalatable and animals usually starve rather than eat them.[19] Acute selenosis may present as sudden death with few, if any, clinical signs if the dose is large enough. In most cases, however, signs of poisoning begin a few hours to a few days after a toxic dose of Se. Clinical signs, which begin 1 hour to 24 hours post-exposure, generally are referable to the gastrointestinal, cardiovascular, and respiratory systems.[34,37–42]

Initially, intoxicated animals become lethargic and lose interest in eating. Anorexia usually is attributed to the general debility that accompanies poisoning, but conditioned aversion to Se has been demonstrated in otherwise healthy cattle,[43] antelope,[44] and birds.[45] If the toxic dose was given parenterally, the injection site is sore.[34] Poisoned animals often walk with a weak, wobbly gait. Careful clinical observation reveals this ataxia to be the result of generalized weakness and shock rather than any specific neurologic deficit. Although blindness is still mentioned in many textbooks, affected animals are not blind unless there is some complicating factor, such as salt intoxication.[7,46] Severe abdominal pain often is manifested in a stilted gait, teeth grinding, and tucked abdomen, especially if the route of exposure was oral. Excessive sweating is common in horses.[47] The affected animal's breath may have a garlic odor, although this is by no means a consistent finding. Diarrhea may occur, especially in animals that survive for longer periods of time. Vomiting is a common finding in swine and may occur in other species.

Blood pressure is reported to drop even before clinical signs become evident.[40] Heart rate and respiration are elevated, but the pulse is weak and thread, and peripheral circulation is compromised (slow capillary refill and cold extremities). Ventricular arrhythmias have been reported in experimentally poisoned animals. Dyspnea is a prominent finding and poisoned animals may be cyanotic. Auscultation of the thorax reveals moist rales and there often is a serous nasal discharge. Fever, polyuria, and hemolytic anemia have been reported but not always are present. Muscular weakness progresses to prostration and coma. Death is due to circulatory and/or respiratory failure and usually occurs within a day or 2 of exposure.[34,37–42]

Poliomyelomalacia

Flaccid paralysis or tetraplegia may occur in swine 2 days to a month after exposure to toxic amounts of Se.[25,48–50] Although there are scattered reports of neurologic lesions in other species,[51] and epidemiologic evidence of amyotropic lateral sclerosis after long-term Se exposure in people,[52–55] among domestic animals only swine consistently develop neurologic damage as a result of Se toxicity.[6] The onset of signs may be sudden or may occur in individuals that have previously exhibited other signs of acute intoxication (discussed previously). Affected swine exhibit ascending paralysis or tetraplegia but remain alert, have normal vision, and eat if offered food. Very mildly affected swine may recover, but most do not. Clinical signs reflect the underlying bilateral lesions in ventral gray horn of the cervical and lumbar spinal cord for which the condition is named. Poliomyelomalacia often occurs in the portion of a herd, which survives an episode of acute intoxication and usually precedes or coincides with occurrence of classic chronic selenosis, or alkali disease (described later), in the same animals.

Chronic Selenosis

Alkali disease results most frequently from chronic (>30 days) exposure to seleniferous grains or forages, but sometimes it may result from sustained over-feeding of inorganic Se supplements or (anecdotally) by shorter duration exposures.[4] The characteristic features of chronic selenosis in cattle, horses, and swine are bilaterally symmetric alopecia and dystrophic hoof growth (**Fig. 1**). Alopecia typically involves the nape of the neck and tail but, in severe cases, may involve other parts of the body.

The first signs of poisoning are lameness, erythema, and swelling of the coronary bands.[56] These early signs are subtle enough to be easily missed by a herdsman and subside quickly. Earliest signs are followed in a day to as much as 3 weeks by

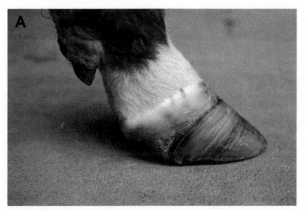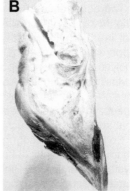

Fig. 1. Forelimb of a steer fed approximately 25 ppm Se as Semet for 120 days. (*A*) Intact hoof prior to necropsy. (*B*) Sagittal section of same hoof through coffin bone and hoof wall. Original hoof wall contained approximately 1 ppm Se; new, underlying hoof, 5 ppm; and the hoof in the area of separation, 15 ppm.

development of a circumferential crack parallel to and just distal to the coronet. Hoof separation and lameness progress apace until the damaged claw is displaced from beneath by new growth and sloughs off. In some cases, the damaged claw is not shed but remains attached, resulting in an extended, upwardly curled toe (slipper toe). Affected animals become so lame they are unable to move to food or water and thus, under range conditions, starve. Sheep are reportedly resistant to the epithelial effects of Se when grazed on toxic pastures,[12] although there are reports of loose wool in experimentally poisoned[57,58] animals. Although there are no definitive experimental comparisons, it is the author's observation that species susceptibility to natural sources of Se is swine (most sensitive) > horses > cattle > sheep (least sensitive).

Se is well-established as a cause of terata and decreased hatchability in egg-laying species,[33,59–61] but is not as well established as a reproductive toxicant in mammals, especially in ruminant livestock. Experimentally, teratogenesis in laboratory mammals requires extremely high (ie, lethal to the dam) dosages and/or artificial measures, such as exposing embryos in vitro.[62,63] Se decreased conception and litter size experimentally in swine,[64] and there are field reports of decreased conception in cattle and sheep[12,65,66] but attempts to produce infertility experimentally have been unsuccessful.[57] Field cases of infertility in cattle herds with clinical alkali disease investigated by the author always have involved other nutritional factors, such as copper deficiency. Whether Se is merely incidental to other factors resulting in decreased conception and infertility or is directly involved as a causative agent has not been conclusively proved, but field data suggest that chronic selenosis potentiates the reproductive effects of, for example, copper deficiency during breeding and early pregnancy (Raisbeck and Waggoner, unpublished, 1994).

Myocardial necrosis has been produced experimentally in cattle, sheep, and swine by both chronic and acute feeding of inorganic Se salts.[42,67–69] Myocardial damage also occurs in calves exposed to selenate in utero.[70] Similar lesions were reported up to 5 weeks after a single parenteral overdose of sodium selenite[41] and death was, in most cases, attributed to heart failure. The lesion is multifocal and does not involve the right ventricle.[6] It is not clear whether natural sources of Se, such as seleniferous grains or forages, cause the same lesion. Early field investigations mentioned a condition referred to as dishrag heart but this has not been reproduced by experimentally feeding naturally either contaminated feedstuffs or L-Semet nor is it mentioned as a finding in modern case reports.

The occurrence of anemia in chronic selenosis in food animals is questionable. Slight (4%–6%) decreases in hematocrit were reported in 1 avian experiment[32] but not in other, virtually identical, studies.[71] Experimentally, rodents develop anemia, apparently as a result of hemolysis, after several weeks on high-Se diets.[3,5,72,73] Hemolytic anemia was reported from 1 spontaneous episode of chronic selenosis in swine[50] but is absent from other field cases and experimental studies in this species.[74–76] Anemia is not a feature of experimental chronic selenosis in cattle and sheep.[43] This may reflect a basic species difference in susceptibility or it may be that some cofactor, such as marginal antioxidant status, is required for hemolysis.

Se has been recognized as immunotoxic in waterfowl and rodents for many years.[77–79] Recently, it has been demonstrated that Se also suppresses the immune system in ruminants. High dietary Se from inorganic Se salts, L-Semet, or contaminated hay suppressed primary antibody response in yearling calves and antelope[44,80] Feeding Se, 12 ppm, as sodium selenite suppressed the leukocyte mitogenic response in adult beef cows.[70] Immunotoxicity seems to require the presence of elevated Se concentrations in the immediate leukocyte environment during antigen processing because it does not occur when cells are manipulated in vitro.[81]

Measurable immune suppression occurs at dietary concentrations less than half that required for other effects.[80] The practical implications of these findings remain to be determined under field conditions but these results suggest that animals chronically exposed to high dietary Se are at increased risk of infectious disease. It also calls into question the common practice of simultaneously administering vaccines and parenteral Se supplements.

Other spontaneous conditions that have been attributed to chronic selenosis in food animals include neurologic disease (so-called blind staggers [BSs]) and hepatopathy. There are few detailed studies of liver morphology and function in chronic selenosis. Early accounts, which attribute severe hepatic damage to Se, generally are unreliable,[6,82] and more recent investigators have discovered only minimal morphologic changes in cattle,[56,83,84] pigs,[4] and sheep.[42,68] There are, however, reports of serum chemistry changes indicative of liver disease in horses[83] and multifocal hepatic necrosis in cattle that died acutely of selenosis.[41,85] Veterinarians should remain alert to the possibility that the liver may be involved in selenosis.

BSs purportedly result from ingestion of Se accumulators and present as blindness, circling, head pressing, dysphagia, and paralysis.[86] There only are 2 original reports of BSs[87,88] and no well-documented reports of BSs resulting from experimentally feeding seleniferous plants or purified Se compounds. There is compelling evidence that BSs actually were a potpourri of infectious, nutritional, and toxic diseases unrelated to Se.[7]

PATHOLOGY

Acute Se intoxication produces myocardial necrosis in cattle, sheep, pigs, and possibly horses. This may be evident grossly as pale streaks and hemorrhagic areas in the myocardium and accumulation of edema in the lungs. In one of the more morphologically detailed chronic feeding experiments with selenate, intoxicated ewes often had acute myocardial necrosis with postnecrotic fibrosis.[89] Similarly, in a heifer fed selenite and that subsequently died of heart failure, there was a mixture of acute (necrosis) and resolved (fibrosis) lesions (Raisbeck and O'Toole, unpublished, 1995). Lesions were similar to vitamin E–Se deficiency in that they did not involve the right ventricle.

Porcine poliomyelomalacia is the only form of Se intoxication reported in domestic mammals that consistently involves the nervous system.[6] In affected swine, there is bilaterally symmetric necrosis of the cervical and lumbar intumescences of the ventral gray columns of the spinal cord.[25,48,50] This lesion is similar to that produced by the niacin antagonist 6-aminonicotinamide.[82] In some pigs, lesions were reported also to involve portions of the brainstem.[90]

Given the S-rich nature of keratin and the chemical similarity of S to Se, it is not surprising that keratinocytes, especially those that produce hard keratin, are a Se target common to most, if not all animal species. The earliest lesions consist of abnormal maturation of keratinocytes in the stratum spinosum and mild cases may progress no further.[6] More advanced lesions involved ballooning degeneration and necrosis of these same cells. Alopecia results from atrophy of primary hair follicles; secondary follicles are not affected. Most atrophic follicles are collapsed and lack a hair shaft. The inner root sheath is atrophic or absent and the outer sheath contains dyskeratotic keratinocytes. In the hoof, affected cells on the coronary papillae and the primary laminae of the stratum internum produce dyskeratotic debris, which accumulates in the horn tubules and distort the normal architecture of the hoof wall.[56,84] These changes are concentrated in a small area parallel to the coronary band by virtue of the fact that tubular keratin formation is a continuous process, with cellular damage occurring simultaneously in all papillae when Se concentrations peak. Hooves are designed to divert proximally directed cracks to a lateral direction.[91] Dilatation of horn tubules, combined with Se-induced defects in the intertubular keratin, exaggerate this tendency, resulting in focused circumferential cracks in the proximal part of the hoof wall.

DIAGNOSIS

A diagnosis of Se intoxication rests on the traditional triad of clinical signs, biochemical and pathologic lesions, and chemical analysis. Sudden death, or sudden onset of lassitude, inappetence, pulmonary edema, cardiac arrhythmia, and shock, especially after a change in feed, should make an astute diagnostician include acute selenosis in the list of differential diagnoses. Progressive posterior ataxia in swine, especially if coupled with a previous episode of gastrointestinal and cardiovascular signs, should do likewise. Loss of mane and tail in horses[92] or cattle, coupled with characteristic transverse hoof cracks several weeks or months after introduction to potentially seleniferous feedstuffs, suggests chronic selenosis.

Tissue Se concentrations are less reliably predictive of tissue and organ damage than with many other toxicants. Specific concentrations in any particular case may vary with the tissue sampled, the chemical form of Se involved (Semet > inorganic forms of Se), the type of analysis used, and the presence of other elements, such as mercury, which bind Se in unavailable forms.[93–95] In general, inorganic Se is cleared more rapidly than Se from natural sources, such as forages and grains. Natural Se (specifically Semet) accumulates to greater concentrations in most tissues with chronic feeding than Se from inorganic sources yet appears less biologically available for either beneficial or toxic functions.[96] In seabirds, Se has been shown to form biologically inert complexes in tissues with other elements (notably mercury), which are chemically indistinguishable from biologically available forms.[93] This observation has since been extended to terrestrial ecosystems.[97] Chemical analysis of Se in tissues is somewhat tricky and, although the situation is improving, normal or toxic ranges from 1 laboratory may not translate well to results from another laboratory or to numbers from the older literature.

Blood GSH peroxidase activity, which normally increases with Se exposure, may briefly dip into the deficient range in some horses and cattle near the onset of clinical chronic selenosis (Raisbeck and Hammar, unpublished, 1990). Because the usual reason for depression of this enzyme is Se deficiency, depressed enzyme activity together with higher than normal blood concentrations is a strong indicator of Se intoxication. Unfortunately, this phenomenon is not consistent so its absence cannot be used to rule out selenosis.

The samples traditionally recommended for Se analysis include blood, serum, urine, liver, kidney, hoof, and hair. Each has advantages and disadvantages. Urine and serum Se concentrations increase quickly after a toxic dose but are fairly ephemeral and may return to normal range by the time an animal shows overt signs of chronic selenosis (Raisbeck, unpublished, 1993-1997). Whole blood and liver concentrations are less prone to short-term fluctuations and remain elevated longer after a toxic dose. In general, blood and liver Se concentrations greater than 1 ppm (wet weight basis) should raise the possibility of selenosis in domestic livestock, especially after exposure to inorganic forms of Se, such as feed supplements.[20] These specific concentrations are not, in themselves, sufficient for a diagnosis. Under some conditions, blood and liver concentrations may reach more than 5 ppm in apparently healthy cattle, which grow to maturity without apparent ill effects.[43] The latter is true especially if the source of Se was contaminated forage. Some investigators have suggested the ratio of liver to kidney Se concentrations as a definitive diagnostic test. In normal animals, kidney Se concentration is greater than liver; this ratio is reversed in Se-intoxicated animals. This reversal, however, seems more an indicator of high Se intake than a diagnostic test per se because such ratios have also been observed in healthy animals grazing seleniferous pastures.

Theoretically, Se, once deposited in keratinized structures, such as hoof and hair, is metabolically inert and thus a more reliable long-term indicator of Se intake than liver or blood. Hair Se concentrations usually are less than 1 ppm in cattle or horses on normal Se diets. Concentrations greater than 5 ppm are indicative of excessive Se exposure. Some caution in interpretation is warranted, however, because hair and hoof concentrations may be influenced by seasonal or nutritional influences on growth, shedding, or exogenous contamination It is not unusual to see 10-fold or greater variation in Se concentration along a hair shaft or between different parts of a hoof. Used judiciously, this variation in hair Se concentration can be used to approximate the temporal pattern of Se exposure; segments closer to the skin represent more recent exposure.[98,99] It is important to select hair shafts that were actively growing during the presumed period of exposure. In cattle, the best sample is the tail switch and in horses, the mane, and tail.

Treatment

There is no proven specific therapy for acute Se intoxication. Symptomatic and supportive therapy may be useful in some cases, but the prognosis for any animal afflicted with acute selenosis is poor. Experimentally, massive doses of vitamin E ameliorate many of the cytotoxic effects of Se in laboratory rodents,[35] if given before or soon after intoxication. This strategy has not been tested in domestic livestock species, but, based on rodent and avian studies, would require 10 times to 20 times a normal therapeutic dose. Bromosulfophthalein (BSP) enhanced biliary excretion and decreased urinary excretion of ^{75}Se-selenite in rats.[100] This process involves scavenging nucleophilic Se metabolites prior to their methylation and excretion. Because these same reactive Se species are believed to be ultimately be responsible for the cytotoxic effects of Se, scavenging them before they react with cellular components may be protective. BSP treatment did decrease embryo lethality in Se-treated duck embryos (Raisbeck and Orsted, unpublished, 1996). These experiments were designed, however, to test biochemical hypotheses and may not be directly applicable to clinical therapy.

Uncomplicated chronic selenosis has been treated successfully with low-Se, high-protein, high-quality diets, and supportive measures in horses.[20] The nursing care required is extensive, however, and often not justified in food animals. Frequent therapeutic hoof trimming should be used to minimize abnormal posture and resultant secondary joint and skeletal problems. Measures to reduce pain, such as heart-bar shoes and soft, sandy footing, enable affected animals to maintain normal food and water intake and thus condition. Nonsteroidal anti-inflammatory agents and analgesics likewise serve to keep affected animals eating and nourished.

Prevention

Prevention consists of avoiding exposure to excessive dietary or parenteral Se. Total dietary Se concentrations, as low as 5 ppm (dry matter), may, under some circumstances, be toxic. Dietary imbalances, such as low protein or vitamin E, increase susceptibility to Se toxicity. A diet deficient in Se, itself, predisposes animals to selenosis. Se , like many essential trace elements, has a narrow safety margin and iatrogenic poisoning easily may result from relatively simple miscalculations in dose. Thus, an extra degree of caution is in order when working with Se-containing dietary supplements or drugs.

In areas with seleniferous forages, it may be impossible to completely avoid excess dietary Se, yet many ranchers in seleniferous areas have developed empirical strategies to minimize economic losses. Se concentrations in edible forage grasses peak between heading and maturity.[65] Although the precise timing of this peak may be different in other regions and with different forage mixtures,[101] it is consistent for any given locale. Utilizing known seleniferous pastures before or after this critical period lessens the exposure to Se. Seleniferous vegetation in any given pasture often is concentrated in hot spots, where plant concentrations may be 2 times to 10 times greater than the rest of the pasture. Identifying these areas by forage sampling and fencing them out may lower total dietary intake below toxic thresholds. Because chronic selenosis usually requires several weeks of exposure to a toxic pasture, some ranchers intensively graze such pastures with for a relatively short period and then retreat to lower-Se areas.

Experimentally, feeding arsenic compounds, such as arsanilic acid, has lessened the severity of selenosis, especially in monogastric animals, such as swine.[66,102] This approach has not, however, proven beneficial under field conditions with natural cases of selenosis. Feeding linseed oil meal protects rats and chickens against some of the effects of chronic selenosis,[94,103] but again the practice has not lived up to its promise under field conditions.

There is anecdotal evidence of genetically mediated resistance or sensitivity to Se in cattle and possibly other species. Closed herds on seleniferous ranges will go for years with few selenosis cases and then suddenly experience a rash of alkali disease after introduction of new bulls. Although the phenomenon is not well proved experimentally, common sense dictates caution when introducing new bloodlines to impacted herds.

Chronic selenosis is exacerbated under field conditions by other nutritional disorders endemic to arid grasslands, such as copper deficiency. Correction of these underlying problems often dramatically decreases the severity of Se-related syndromes. Before focusing on efforts to control selenosis, veterinarians should consider the full spectrum of nutritional and toxic possibilities.

SUMMARY

Despite more than 8 decades of research, some aspects of the natural history of selenosis remain confused in modern texts. The primary targets of acute Se toxicity in food animal species are the cardiovascular, gastrointestinal, and possibly hematopoietic systems. Swine may develop neurologic lesions; however, the signs and pathology of poliomyelomalacia are quite distinct from those described as BSs by early workers. The most characteristic signs of chronic selenosis are hair and hoof loss; however, other, less specific damage to the immune system and reproduction may be economically more important. Given the numerous interactions of chronic Se with other dietary factors, it is important to examine the whole environment when dealing with a potential selenosis case.

REFERENCES

1. Sharma S, Singh R. Selenium in soil, plant and animal systems. CRC Crit Rev Environ Contr 1983;13:23–50.

2. Beath OA, Draize JH, Eppson HF, et al. Certain poisonous plants of Wyoming activated by selenium and their association with respect to the soil. J Am Pharm Assoc 1934;23:94–7.
3. Franke KW. A new toxicant occurring naturally in certain samples of plant food-stuffs. I. Results obtained in preliminary feeding trials. J Nutr 1934;8:596–608.
4. Franke KW. A new toxicant occurring naturally in certain samples of plant food-stuffs. II. The occurrence of the toxicant in the protein fraction. J Nutr 1934;8:609–13.
5. Franke KW, Potter VR. A new toxicant occurring naturally in certain samples of plant foodstuffs. III. Hemoglobin in rats fed toxic wheat. J Nutr 1934;8:615–24.
6. O'Toole D, Raisbeck MF. Magic numbers, elusive lesions: comparative pathology and toxicology of selenosis in waterfowl and mammalian species. In: Frankenberger WT, Engberg RA, editors. Environmental chemistry of selenium. New York: Marcel Dekker; 1998. p. 355–95.
7. O'Toole D, Raisbeck MF, Case JC, et al. Selenium-induced "Blind Staggers" and related myths. A commentary on the extent of historical livestock losses attributed to selenosis on western rangelands. Vet Pathol 1996;33:104–16.
8. Bodnar A, Konieczka P, Namiesnik. The properties, functions, and use of selenium compounds in living organisms. J Environ Sci Health C Environ Carcinog Ecotoxicol Rev 2012;30:225–52.
9. Ullah H, Liu G, Yousaf B, et al. A comprehensive review on environmental transformation of selenium: recent advances and research perspectives. Environ Geochem Health 2019;41:1003–35.
10. Presser TS, Sylvester MA, Low WH. Bioaccumulation of selenium from natural geologic sources in western states and its potential consequences. Environ Manage 1994;18:423–36.
11. Gissel-Nielsen G. Effects of selenium supplementation of field crops. In: Frankenberger WT, Engberg RA, editors. Environmental chemistry of selenium. New York: Marcel Dekker; 1998. p. 99–112.
12. Olson OE. Selenium in plants as a cause of livestock poisoning. In: Keeler RF, Van Kampen KR, James LF, editors. Effects of poisonous plants on livestock. New York: Academic Press; 1978. p. 121–35.
13. Olson OE, Novacek EJ, Whitehead EI, et al. Investigations on selenium in wheat. Phytochemistry 1970;9:1181–8.
14. Ulhassan Z, Gill RA, Ali S, et al. Dual behavior of selenium: insights into physio-biochemical, anatomical and molecular analyses of four *Brassica napus* cultivars. Chemosphere 2019;225:329–41.
15. Kolbert Z, Lehota N, Molnar A. "The roots" of selenium toxicity: a new concept. Plant Signal Behav 2016;11:e1241935.
16. Neuhierl B, Bock A. On the mechanism of selenium tolerance in selenium-accumulating plants. Eur J Biochem 1996;239:235–8.
17. Wang Y, Bock A, Neuhierl B. Acquisition of selenium tolerance by a selenium non-accumulating Astragalus species via selection. Biofactors 1999;9:3–10.
18. Rosenfeld I, Beath OA. Selenium. New York: Geobotany, Biochemistry, Toxicity and Nutrition, Academic Press; 1964.
19. Beath OA: Chemical examination of Astragalus bisulcatus. University of Wyoming Agricultural Experiment Station 31st Annual Report. 1920. p. 127.
20. Raisbeck MF, Dahl ER, Sanchez DA, et al. Naturally occurring selenosis in Wyoming. J Vet Diagn Invest 1993;5:84–7.
21. Burk RF. Molecular biology of selenium with implications for its metabolism. FASEB J 1991;5:2274–9.

22. Dudley HC. Toxicology of selenium: 1. A study of the distribution of selenium in acute and chronic cases of selenium poisoning. Am J Hyg 1937;23:169–80.

23. Moxon AL. Alkali disease or selenium poisoning. South Dakota State College of Agricultural and Mechanical Arts, Agricultural Experiment Station Bulletin 1937; 311:1–91.

24. Ganther HE. Selenotrisulfides. Formation by reaction by thiols with selenous acid. Biochemistry 1968;7:2898–905.

25. Wilson TM, Cramer PG, Owen RL, et al. Porcine focal symmetrical poliomyelomalacia: test for interaction between dietary selenium and niacin. Can J Vet Res 1989;53:454–61.

26. Spallholz JE. On the nature of selenium toxicity and carcinostatic activity. Free Radic Biol Med 1994;17:45–64.

27. Seko Y, Saito Y, Kitahara J, et al. Active oxygen generation by the reaction of selenite with reduced glutathione *in vitro*. In: Wendel A, editor. Selenium in biology and medicine. Berlin: Springer Verlag; 1989. p. 70–3.

28. Yan L, Spallholz JE. Generation of reactive oxygen species from the reaction of selenium compounds with thiols and mammary tumors. Biochem Pharmacol 1993;45:429–37.

29. Dougherty JJ, Hoekstra WG. Stimulation of lipid peroxidation in vivo by injected selenite and lack of stimulation by selenate. Biochim Biophys Acta 1982;169: 209–15.

30. Nonavinakere VK, Potmis RA, Rasekh HR, et al. Selenium lethality: role of glutathione and metallothionein. Toxicol Lett 1993;66:273–9.

31. LeBoeuf RA, Zentner KL, Hoekstra WG. Effect of dietary selenium concentration and duration of selenium feeding on hepatic glutathione concentrations in rats. Proc Soc Exp Biol Med 1985;180:348–52.

32. Hoffman DJ, Heinz GH, Lecaptain LJ, et al. Toxicity and oxidative stress of different forms of organic selenium and dietary protein in mallard ducklings. Arch Environ Contam Toxicol 1996;31:120–7.

33. Orsted KM. Investigations in mechanisms of selenium induced teratogenesis: oxidative stress, MS Pathobiology Thesis. Laramie (WY): University of Wyoming; 1998. p. 101.

34. Van Vleet JF, Meyer KB, Olander HJ. Acute selenium toxicosis induced in baby pigs by parenteral administration of selenium-vitamin E preparations. J Am Vet Med Assoc 1974;165:543–7.

35. Csallany AS, Su L-C, Menken BZ. Effect of selenite, vitamin E and N,N'-diphenyl-p-phenylenediamine on liver organic solvent-soluble libofuscin pigments in mice. J Nutr 1984;114:1582–7.

36. Herigstad RR, Whitehair CK, Olson OE. Inorganic and organic selenium toxicosis in young swine: comparison of pathologic changes with those in swine with vitamin E-selenium deficiency. J Am Vet Med Assoc 1973;34:1227–38.

37. Ahmed KE, Adam SE, Idrill OF, et al. Experimental selenium poisoning in nubian goats. Vet Hum Toxicol 1990;32:249–51.

38. Blodgett DJ, Bevill RF. Acute selenium toxicosis in sheep. Vet Hum Toxicol 1987; 29:233–6.

39. MacDonald DW, Christian RG, Strausz KI, et al. Acute selenium toxicity in neonatal calves. Can Vet J 1981;22:279–81.

40. Moxon AL, Rhian M. Selenium poisoning. Physiol Rev 1943;23:305–37.

41. Shortridge EH, O'Hara PH, Marshall PM. Acute selenium poisoning in cattle. N Z Vet J 1971;19:47–51.

42. Smyth JBA, Wang JH, Barlow RM, et al. Experimental acute selenium intoxication in lambs. J Comp Pathol 1990;102:197–209.
43. Raisbeck MF, O'Toole D, Belden EL, et al. Chronic selenosis in ruminants. In: Garland T, Barr AC, editors. Toxic plants and other toxicants. Wallingham (United Kingdom): CAB International; 1998. p. 389–96.
44. Raisbeck MF, O'Toole D, Schamber RA, et al. Toxicologic effects of a high-selenium hay diet in captive adult and yearling pronghorn antelope (Antilocapra americana). J Wildl Dis 1996;32:9–16.
45. O'Toole D, Raisbeck MF. Experimentally induced selenosis of adult mallard ducks: clinical signs, lesions and toxicology. Vet Pathol 1997;34:330–40.
46. Casteel SW, Osweiler GD, Cook WO, et al. Selenium toxicosis in swine. J Am Vet Med Assoc 1985;186:1084–5.
47. Crinion RAP, O'Connor JP. Selenium intoxication in horses. Irish Vet J 1978; 32:81–6.
48. Wilson TM, Drake TR. Porcine focal symmetrical poliomyelomalacia. Can J Comp Med 1982;46:218–20.
49. Wilson TM, Scholz R, Drake T. Porcine focal symmetrical poliomyelomalacia and selenium toxicity: description of a field outbreak and preliminary observations on experimental reproduction. Proc Am Assn Vet Lab Diagn 1982;25:135–42.
50. Wilson TM, Scholz RW, Drake TR. Selenium toxicity and porcine focal symmetrical encephalomalacia: description of a field outbreak and experimental reproduction. Can J Comp Med 1983;47:412–21.
51. Maag DD, Glenn MW. Toxicity of selenium: farm animals. In: Muth OH, editor. Selenium in biomedicine. Westport (CN): AVI; 1967. p. 127–40.
52. Vinceti M, Botteci I, Fan A, et al. Are environmental exposures to selenium, heavy metals, and pesticides risk factors for amyotrophic lateral sclerosis? Rev Environ Health 2012;27(1):19–41.
53. Vinceti M, Crespi CM, Malagoli C, et al. Friend or Foe? The current epidemiologic evidence on selenium and human cancer risk. J Environ Sci Health C Environ Carcinog Ecotoxicol Rev 2013;31:305–41.
54. Vinceti M, Mandrioli J, Borella P, et al. Selenium neurotoxicity in humans: bridging laboratory and epidemiologic studies. Toxicol Lett 2014;230:295–303.
55. Wahlstrom RC, Kamstra LD, Olson OE. The effect of arsanilic acid and 3-nitrophenylarsonic acid on selenium poisoning in the pig. J Anim Sci 1955;14:105–9.
56. O'Toole D, Raisbeck MF. Pathology of experimentally induced chronic selenosis ("alklai disease") in yearling cattle. J Vet Diagn Invest 1995;7:364–73.
57. Panter KE, James LF, Mayland HF. Reproductive response of ewes fed alfalfa pellets containing sodium selenate or Astragalus bisulcatus as a selenium source. Vet Hum Toxicol 1995;37:30–2.
58. Tucker JO. (1960): Preliminary Report of selenium toxicity in sheep. Proceedings American College of Veterinary Toxicologists, Denver, Colorado, August 14, 1960. p. 41–5.
59. Franke KW, Tully WC. A new toxicant occurring naturally in certain samples of plant foodstuffs. Poult Sci 1936;15:316–8.
60. Heinz GH, Hoffman D, Krynitsky AJ, et al. Reproduction in mallards fed selenium. J Toxicol Environ Health 1987;6:423–33.
61. Shi M, Zhang C, Xia IF, et al. Maternal dietary exposure to selenium nanoparticle led to malformation in offspring. Ecotoxicol Environ Saf 2018;156:34–40.
62. Usami M, Tabata H, Ohno Y. Effects of glutathione depletion on selenite- and selenate-induced embryotoxicity in cultured rat embryos. Teratog Carcinog Mutagen 1999;19:257–66.

63. Willhite CC. Selenium teratogenesis. Ann N Y Acad Sci 1993;678:169–71.
64. Wahlstrom RC, Olson OE. The effect of selenium on reproduction in swine. J Anim Sci 1959;18:141–5.
65. Dinkel CA, Minyard JA, Ray DE. Effects of season of breeding on reproductive and weaning performance of beef cattle grazing seleniferous range. J Anim Sci 1963;22:1043–5.
66. Dinkel CA, Minyard JA, Whitehead EI, et al. Agricultural research at the reed ranch substation. South Dakota Agricultural Experiment Station Circular 1957; 135:1–35.
67. Gardiner MR. Chronic selenium toxicity studies in sheep. Aust Vet J 1966;42: 442–8.
68. Glenn MW, Jensen R, Griner LA. Sodium selenate toxicosis: the effects of extended oral administration of sodium selenate on mortality, clinical signs, fertility and early embryonic development in sheep. Am J Vet Res 1964;25: 1479–99.
69. Morrow DA. Acute selenite toxicity in lambs. J Am Vet Med Assoc 1968;152: 1625–9.
70. Yaeger MJ, Neiger RD, Holler L, et al. The effect of subclinial selenium toxicosis on pregnant beef cattle. J Vet Diagn Invest 1998;10:268–73.
71. Green DE, Albers PH. Diagnostic criteria for selenium toxicosis in aquatic birds: histologic lesions. J Wildl Dis 1997;33:385–404.
72. Das PM, Sadan JR, Gupta RK, et al. Experimental selenium toxicity in guinea pigs: haematological studies. Ann Nutr Metab 1989;33:347–53.
73. Halverson AW, Ding-Tsay KC, Treibwasser KC, et al. Development of hemolytic anemia in rats fed selenite. Toxicol Appl Pharmacol 1970;17:151–9.
74. Baker DC, James LF, Hartley WJ, et al. Toxicosis in pigs fed selenium-accumulating Astragalus plant species or sodium selenate. Am J Vet Res 1989;50:1396–9.
75. Goehring TB, Palmer IS, Olson OE, et al. Toxic effects of selenium on growing swine fed corn-soybean meal diets. J Anim Sci 1984;59:733–7.
76. Harrison LH, Colvin BM, Stuart BP, et al. Paralysis in swine due to focal symmetrical poliomalacia: possible selenium toxicosis. Vet Pathol 1983;20:265–73.
77. Fairbrother A, Fowles J. Subchronic effects of sodium selenite and selenomethionine on several immune functions in mallards. Arch Environ Contam Toxicol 1990;19:836–44.
78. Koller LD, Exon JH, Talcott PT, et al. Immune responses in rats supplemented with selenium. Clin Exp Immunol 1986;63:570–6.
79. Wang Y, Li J, He J. The adverse effects of Se toxicity on inflammatory and immune responses in chicken spleens. Biol Trace Elem Res 2018;185:170–6.
80. Raisbeck MF, Schamber RA, Belden EL. Immunotoxic effects of selenium in mammals. In: Garland T, Barr C, editors. Toxic plants and other natural toxicants. Wallingford (United Kingdom): CAB International; 1997. p. 260–6.
81. Schamber RA. Selenium immunotoxicity, MS Thesis. Laramie (WY): University of Wyoming; 1994. p. 268.
82. O'Sullivan BM, Blakemore WF. Acute nicotinamide deficiency in the pig induced by 6-aminonicotinamide. Vet Pathol 1980;103:748–56.
83. Knott SG, McCray CWR. Two Naturally occurring outbreaks of selenosis in Queensland. Aust Vet J 1959;35:161–5.
84. Raisbeck MF, O'Toole D. Morphologic studies of selenosis in herbivores. In: Garland T, Barr AC, editors. Toxic plants and other natural toxicants. Wallingford (United Kingdom): CAB International; 1998. p. 380–8.

85. Twomey T, Crinion RAP, Glazier DB. Selenium toxicity in cattle in Comeath. Irish Vet J 1977;31:41–6.
86. Beath OA. The story of selenium in Wyoming. In: Laramie WY, editor. Rosefeld (IL): University of Wyoming, Agricultural Experiment Station; 1982. p. 1–23.
87. Draize JH, Beath OA. Observations on the pathology of blind staggers and alkali disease. J Am Vet Med Assoc 1935;39:753–63.
88. Rosenfeld I, Beath OA. Pathology of selenium poisoning. In: Laramie WY, editor. Wyoming agricultural experiment station bulletin. University of Wyoming; 1946. p. 1–27.
89. Glenn MW, Jensen R, Griner LA. Sodium selenate toxicosis: pathology and pathogensis of sodium selenate toxicosis in sheep. Am J Vet Res 1964;25: 1486–94.
90. Panter KE, Hartley WJ, James LF, et al. Comparative toxicity of selenium from seleno-DL-methionine, sodium selenate, and Astragalus bisulcatus in pigs. Fundam Appl Toxicol 1996;32:217–23.
91. Bertram JE, Gosline JM. Fracture toughness design in horse hoof keratin. J Exp Biol 1986;125:29–47.
92. Witte ST, Will LA, Olsen CR, et al. Chronic selenosis in horses fed locally produced alfalfa hay. J Am Vet Med Assoc 1993;202:406–9.
93. Goode AA, Wolterbeek HT. Have high selenium concentrations in wading birds their origins in mercury? Sci Total Environ 1994;144:247.
94. Jensen LS, Werho DB, Leyden DE. Selenosis, hepatic selenium accumulation, and plasma glutathione peroxidase activity in chicks as affected by a factor in linseed meal. J Nutr 1977;107:391–6.
95. Nuttal KL. Evaluating selenium poisoning. Ann Clin Lab Sci 2006;36:409–20.
96. Waschulewski IH, Sunde RA. Effect of dietary methionine on tissue selenium and glutathione peroxidase activity in rats given selenomethionine. Br J Nutr 1988; 60:57–68.
97. Qiu G, Abeysinghe KS, Xiao-Dong Y, et al. Effects of selenium on bioaccumulation in a Terrestrial food chain from an abandoned mercury mining region. Bull Environ Contam Toxicol 2019;102:329–34.
98. Davis TZ, Stegelmeier BL, Hall JO. Analysis of horse hair as a means of evaluationg selenium toxicosis and long-term exposures. J Agric Food Chem 2014;62: 7393–7.
99. Davidson-York D, Galey FD, Blanchard P, et al. Selenium elimination in pigs after an outbreak of selenium toxicosis. J Vet Diagn Invest 1999;11:352–7.
100. Gregus Z, Perjesi P, Gyurasics A. Enhancement of selenium excretion bile by sulfobromophthalein: elucidation of the mechanism. Biochem Pharmacol 1998;56:1391–402.
101. Raisbeck MF, O'Toole D, Sanchez DA, et al. Re-evaluation of selenium toxicity in grazing mammals. In: Schuman G, Vance G, editors. Decades later: a time for reassessment. Princeton (WV): American Society for Surface Mining and Reclamation; 1995. p. 372–83.
102. Minyard JA, Dinkel CA, Olson OE. Effect of arsanilic acid in counteracting selenium poisoning in beef cattle. J Anim Sci 1960;19:260–4.
103. Palmer IS, Olson OE, Halverson AW, et al. Isolation of factors in linseed oil meal protective against chronic selenosis in rats. J Nutr 1980;110:145–50.

Moving?

Make sure your subscription moves with you!

To notify us of your new address, find your **Clinics Account Number** (located on your mailing label above your name), and contact customer service at:

Email: journalscustomerservice-usa@elsevier.com

800-654-2452 (subscribers in the U.S. & Canada)
314-447-8871 (subscribers outside of the U.S. & Canada)

Fax number: 314-447-8029

Elsevier Health Sciences Division
Subscription Customer Service
3251 Riverport Lane
Maryland Heights, MO 63043

*To ensure uninterrupted delivery of your subscription, please notify us at least 4 weeks in advance of move.

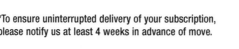